Atlas of
*A*NESTHESIA

Volume VIII
Cardiothoracic Anesthesia

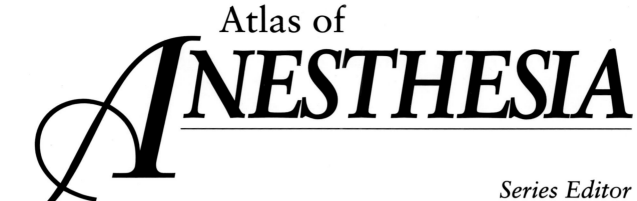

Atlas of
ANESTHESIA

Series Editor
Ronald D. Miller, MD

Professor and Chairman of Anesthesia
Professor of Cellular and Molecular Pharmacology
University of California, San Francisco, School of Medicine
San Francisco, California

Volume VIII
Cardiothoracic Anesthesia

Volume Editor
J.G. Reves, MD

Professor and Chairman
Department of Anesthesiology
Duke University Medical Center
Durham, North Carolina

With 20 contributors

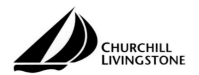

CHURCHILL
LIVINGSTONE

Developed by Current Medicine, Inc., Philadelphia

Current Medicine, Inc.
400 Market Street
Suite 700
Philadelphia, PA 19106

Director of Product Development: Lori J. Bainbridge
Senior Developmental Editor: Marian A. Bellus
Assistant Editor: Deborah Singer
Art Director: Paul Fennessy
Design and Layout: Christine Keller-Quirk
Illustration Director: Ann Saydlowski
Illustrators: Marie Dean, Wieslawa Langenfeld, Larry Ward, Debra Wertz
Cover Design: Christine Keller-Quirk
Cover Illustration: Wieslawa Langenfeld
Production: Lori Holland, Amy Giuffi
Typesetting: Ryan Walsh
Indexing: Alexandra Nickerson

Cardiothoracic anesthesia/volume editor, J. G. Reves.
        p. cm. –(Atlas of anesthesia: v. 8)
    Includes bibliographical references and index.
    ISBN 0-443-07974-9
    1. Anesthesia in cardiology–Atlases. I. Reves, J. G. II. Series.
RD87.3.H43 C37 1998
617.9′67412–dc21

                    98-35854
                    CIP

ISBN 0-443-07974-9

Although every effort has been made to ensure that drug doses and other information are presented accurately in this publication, the ultimate responsibility rests with the prescribing physician. Neither the publishers nor the author can be held responsible for errors or for any consequences arising from the use of the information contained therein. Any product mentioned in this publication should be used in accordance with the prescribing information prepared by the manufacturers. No claims or endorsements are made for any drug or compound at present under clinical investigation.

Printed in Hong Kong by Paramount Printing Group Limited.
10 9 8 7 6 5 4 3 2 1

SERIES PREFACE

This multi-volume series *Atlas of Anesthesia* organizes the largest and most comprehensive collection of teaching visuals in the field of anesthesiology. The publisher, volume editors, and I have invited the most prominent members of the anesthesiology community to provide the most up-to-date information in a format that offers not only the finest images available but also unique schematic presentations of how and why we feel pain. Combined with the slide atlas and CD-ROM, *Atlas of Anesthesia* provides teaching materials of the finest quality in easily accessible formats and allows anesthesiology to become a visual specialty in a way that has never been attempted previously. The topics of the volumes include Critical Care, Scientific Principles, Preoperative Preparation and Intraoperative Monitoring, Principles of Anesthetic Techniques and Anesthetic Emergencies, Subspecialty Care, Pain Management, Pediatric Anesthesia, and Cardiothoracic Anesthesia.

The specialty of anesthesia originally was restricted to operating room anesthesia with some involvement in preoperative evaluation. Furthermore, in the past patients with severe medical conditions were considered too high risk to be anesthetized (*eg,* those who had suffered a myocardial infarction within the previous 3 to 6 months or those with severe obstructive pulmonary disease). In the past 25 years, it has become possible for patients with extensive medical disease (*eg,* acute myocardial infarction, failure of one or more organs, immunosuppression) to be successfully anesthetized for major invasive surgery.

With far more challenging situations, the specialty has responded by the development of new drugs, monitoring techniques, and subspecialties. The new drugs act on receptors that were not even known a few years ago, necessitating extensive knowledge of receptors (*eg,* opioid) of various functions and selection of drugs for specific effects. Improvements in monitoring include the development of the pulmonary artery catheter, transesophageal echocardiography, evoked potentials, pulse oximetry, and multiple gas analysis. New techniques such as hemodilution, infusion and warming devices, and fiberoptic endotracheal intubation have also been introduced. Cardiac, neurologic, pediatric, transplant, ambulatory, and obstetric subspecialties have expanded to encompass the entire perioperative period, including extensive preoperative evaluation and therapy, critical care medicine, and pain management, in both acute and chronic settings.

In response to the impressive expansion of the specialty, many educational devices (including books and journals) have been developed. The educational transmission of the combined cognitive and technical aspects of anesthesia can be markedly facilitated by illustrations, including images, graphs, decision-making trees, and algorithms.

In bringing this series to publication, credit is due to the volume editors and to the many contributors who have shared their expertise and their time. Credit is also due to Abe Krieger, President of Current Medicine, who conceived the atlas; to Marian Bellus, Senior Developmental Editor; and to Jackie Dunn, who coordinated work on this project in my office.

Ronald D. Miller, MD

FOREWORD

I am writing the foreword to this volume from the perspective of a cardiologist who, for the past 15 years, has had a front-row seat watching the development of cardiothoracic anesthesia at Duke University Medical Center under the tutelage of Dr. J. G. Reves. The extremely complex nature of modern cardiothoracic anesthesia is clearly illustrated by the titles of the chapters in this book, which range in scope from cardiovascular physiology and pharmacology and the preoperative evaluation of patients to a series of descriptions of techniques dealing with anesthesia and intraoperative care for specific cardiac and pulmonary diseases, ending with a description of the postoperative intensive care of patients. The modern cardiothoracic anesthesiologist is obviously much more than a single-purpose physician. The dramatic decrease in both morbidity and mortality in surgical patients that has occurred in the past decade is due in no small part to the expanded role of these specialists. Extensive basic and clinical research has provided a foundation for a number of new evaluative and treatment modalities. This excellent volume provides a clear, concise overview of the multiple roles played by the cardiothoracic anesthesiologist in caring for patients with complex cardiac and pulmonary diseases.

Joseph C. Greenfield, Jr., MD
James B. Duke Professor of Medicine
Duke University Medical Center
Duham, North Carolina

Cardiothoracic anesthesia during the past 30 years has become a major anesthesiology subspecialty. This is evident in a number of ways: Textbooks have been written on the subject; the Society of Cardiovascular and Thoracic Anesthesia sponsors a major annual meeting; countless scientific papers have been authored by practitioners and investigators in the field; and hundreds of anesthesia fellows have spent a year or more in educational programs designed to produce cardiothoracic anesthesiologists. Additionally, cardiac surgery has grown in volume, and with the increase in the elderly population, there are certain to be more cardiothoracic operations. All of these facts argue for redoubled education in cardiothoracic anesthesiology.

This volume of *Atlas of Anesthesia* is an attempt to satisfy the need for education in the specialized anesthesia area of cardiothoracic anesthesia. The format appeals to the reader since it condenses much of our knowledge to pictorial and highly organized tabular presentations. This conveys to the reader a very clear, although not exhaustive, treatment of what we all recognize are complex clinical and basic science issues. The contributors have done their work well and have organized their knowledge into this highly efficient form of communication. I congratulate each contributor on this achievement.

The growth and maturity of cardiothoracic anesthesia into a major medical subspecialty is the product of the need for specialists and the willingness of clinicians and investigators to confine their practice and inquiry to this area. Anesthesiologists who practice in this area have been recognized by their cardiology and surgical peers as authorities who have helped advance cardiac surgery in the recent past. I was struck in 1979 by the comments of the Emory University surgeon, Charles Hatcher, MD, in the foreword to Dr. Joel Kaplan's first textbook, *Cardiac Anesthesia*, in which Hatcher wrote: " A major factor, if not *the* major factor, in the current remarkably low operative mortality for open heart surgery has been the emergence of the cardiac anesthesiologist." And in 1986, the pioneering cardiac surgeon, John Kirklin, MD, wrote in his classic textbook *Cardiac Surgery*: "Continuous communication and coordination between anesthesiologist and surgeon is vitally important....For the anesthesiologist to reach his or her potential and for the patient to receive the best care, the anesthesiologist should be a specialist in cardiovascular anesthesia and supportive treatment." These comments from our surgical colleagues reflect on the stature that the cardiothoracic anesthesiologist, as a specialist, achieved early in the development of modern cardiac surgery. The words signal a challenge to live up to the confidence that others have placed in us. Gratefully, we can report that cardiothoracic anesthesiologists now make many clinical contributions in this field, and also are working with our other medical specialty colleagues to make cardiac surgery safer for our patients. Much of the progress in organ protection and the more expeditious care of patients has been led by anesthesiologists. These advances are incorporated in this atlas, and we look for further progress in the future.

J.G. **Reves**, MD

CONTRIBUTORS

John T. Apostolakis, MD
Assistant Staff Anesthesiologist
Department of Cardiothoracic Anesthesia
Cleveland Clinic Foundation
Cleveland, Ohio

Richard L. Applegate II, MD
Associate Professor
Department of Anesthesiology
Loma Linda University School of Medicine;
Director of Clinical Anesthesiology Service
Loma Linda University Medical Center
Loma Linda, California

George J. Crystal, PhD
Associate Professor
Departments of Anesthesiology, Physiology, and Biophysics
University of Illinois College of Medicine;
Director of Research Laboratory
Department of Anesthesiology
Illinois Masonic Medical Center
Chicago, Illinois

B. Hugh Dorman, MD, PhD
Professor and Director, Cardiothoracic Anesthesiology
Department of Anesthesiology
Medical University of South Carolina
Charleston, South Carolina

Lee A. Fleisher, MD
Associate Professor of Anesthesiology
 Joint Appointments in Medicine, Health Policy, and
  Management
The Johns Hopkins Medical Institutions;
Attending Anesthesiologist
The Johns Hopkins Hospital
Baltimore, Maryland

Katherine P. Grichnik, MD
Assistant Professor
Department of Anesthesia
Division of Cardiothoracic Anesthesia
Duke University Medical Center
Durham, North Carolina

Andrew K. Hilton, MB, FANZCA
Assistant Professor
Departments of Anesthesia and Surgery
Duke University School of Medicine;
Attending Anesthesiologist
Duke University Medical Center;
Co-director Surgical Intensive Care Unit
Durham Veteran Affairs Medical Center
Durham, North Carolina

Jacqueline M. Leung, MD, MPH
Associate Professor
Department of Anesthesia
University of California, San Francisco, School of
  Medicine;
Attending Anesthesiologist
University of California, San Francisco–Mount Zion
  Medical Center
San Francisco, California

Mark F. Newman, MD
Associate Professor
Department of Anesthesiology
Duke University School of Medicine;
Chief, Division of Cardiothoracic Anesthesia
Duke University Medical Center
Durham, North Carolina

Christopher J. O'Connor, MD
Assistant Professor
Department of Anesthesiology
Rush Medical College;
Director, Cardiothoracic Anesthesia
Rush–Presbyterian–St. Luke's Medical Center
Chicago, Illinois

J. G. Reves, MD
Professor and Chairman
Department of Anesthesiology
Duke University Medical Center;
Durham, North Carolina

Joseph L. Romson, MD, PhD
Assistant Clinical Professor
Department of Anesthesia
University of California, San Francisco, School of Medicine;
Staff Anesthesiologist
Department of Cardiovascular Anesthesia
Kaiser-Permanente Medical Center
San Francisco, California

Roger L. Royster, MD

Professor and Vice Chairman
Department of Anesthesiology
Wake Forest University School of Medicine
Winston-Salem, North Carolina

Robert M. Savage, MD, FACC

Staff Anesthesiologist
Department of Cardiothoracic Anesthesia and Cardiology
Cleveland Clinic Foundation
Cleveland, Ohio

Randall M. Schell, MD

Associate Professor of Anesthesiology
Director of Medical Student Education in Anesthesiology
Loma Linda University Medical Center
Loma Linda, California

Thomas F. Slaughter, MD

Assistant Professor
Department of Anesthesiology
Duke University School of Medicine;
Attending Physician
Durham Veterans' Affairs Medical Center
Durham, North Carolina

Mark Stafford Smith, MD, CM, FRCPC

Assistant Professor
Department of Anesthesiology
Duke University School of Medicine;
Cardiothoracic Anesthesiologist
Duke University Medical Center
Durham, North Carolina

Kenneth J. Tuman, MD

Professor
Department of Anesthesiology
Rush Medical College;
Vice Chairman
Department of Anesthesiology
Rush-Presbyterian-St. Luke's Medical Center
Chicago, Illinois

Christopher C. Young, MD

Assistant Professor
Departments of Anesthesiology and Surgery
Duke University School of Medicine;
Chief, Division of Critical Care Medicine
Duke University Medical Center
Durham, North Carolina

David A. Zvara, MD

Assistant Professor
Department of Anesthesiology
Wake Forest University School of Medicine
Winston-Salem, North Carolina

CONTENTS

Cardiovascular Physiology

George J. Crystal

An understanding of basic concepts of cardiovascular physiology is essential for effective and safe patient management in the perioperative period. This information provides a theoretic rationale for the use of drugs and physiologic interventions, *eg*, mechanical ventilation and cardiopulmonary bypass, to maintain and control the patient's vital functions. Furthermore, it offers a foundation for appreciating the theory and limitations of current methods of blood conservation, including controlled hypotension and acute normovolemic hemodilution. Finally, it provides insight into steps that can be taken clinically to avoid various pathophysiologic conditions, such as tissue edema and myocardial ischemia.

This chapter presents a review of the fundamental mechanisms controlling function of the heart and the various types of blood vessel, *ie*, the large arteries, arterioles, capillaries, and veins. Other subjects covered include 1) the carriage of oxygen in the blood and its delivery to the body tissues; 2) the role of capillary recruitment in the maintenance of tissue oxygenation; 3) the concept of critical oxygen delivery; and 4) the response of the cardiovascular system to acute normovolemic hemodilution. In light of the critical role of the heart in maintaining adequate blood flow and oxygen delivery to the body tissues, particular focus is given to this organ. The factors regulating coronary blood flow and myocardial oxygen consumption are addressed, and how imbalances among these variables may produce myocardial ischemia. The role of endothelium-derived nitric oxide in coronary vascular control is given special attention. Mechanisms underlying coronary steal are described. Normal values for hemodynamic and oxygen transport variables are presented to encourage quantitative thinking.

Because of space limitations, the chapter is not comprehensive. It is confined to cardiovascular mechanisms in the adult; differences at the extremes of youth and old age are not considered. Furthermore, several important subjects are not at all covered, including the functions of the pericardium and the electrical properties of the heart. Information concerning these and other related subjects can be obtained from the references listed at the end of the chapter.

CARDIAC PHYSIOLOGY

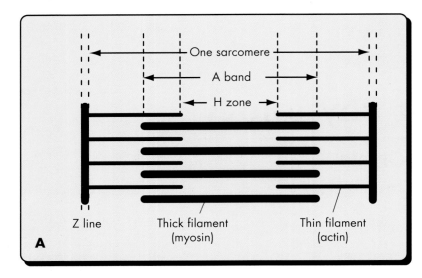

A

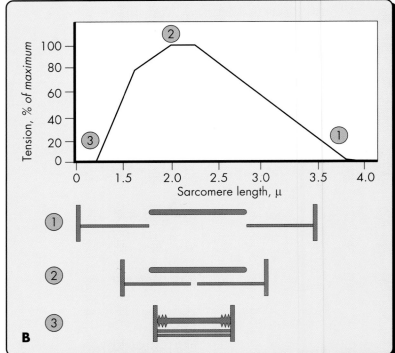

B

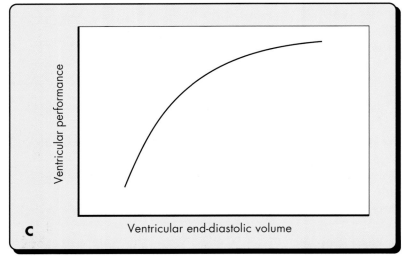

C

Figure 1-1. Molecular basis of Starling's law. **A,** The sarcomere is the basic functional unit of the myocardium. The ultrastructural arrangement of the thick (myosin) and thin (actin) myofilaments within the sarcomere and their interaction can explain much of the mechanical behavior of cardiac muscle. The Z lines mark the ends of the individual sarcomere. Within the confines of the sarcomere are alternating light and dark bands, giving the myocardium its striated appearance. At the center of the sarcomere is a broad dark area of constant width, termed the A band. The H zone is created in the center of the A band by withdrawal of the active filaments. Cardiac muscle contraction is initiated by an increase in intracellular calcium, which results in the formation of cross-bridges between the adjacent actin and myosin filaments. This process tends to draw the thin myofilaments and the Z lines toward the center of the sarcomere. **B,** The total developed tension is a direct function of the number of cross-bridges pulling in parallel, and thus on the amount of overlap between the thin and thick filaments prior to activation. The length–active tension relationship intrinsic to cardiac muscle is the basis for Starling's law of the heart, which states that the strength of contraction of the intact heart is proportional to the initial length of the cardiac muscle fiber, *ie,* the end-diastolic volume (preload). **C,** This can be demonstrated using the cardiac function curve, which is a plot of ventricular performance, *eg,* stroke volume, as a function of end-diastolic volume. In vivo, the cardiac muscle fibers are stretched by venous inflow. Normally, the volume in the ventricle before contraction, *ie,* the preload, sets the sarcomere to a suboptimal length; the active tension that can be developed from that length is only about 20% of maximum. Thus, increases in end-diastolic volume owing to enhanced venous return cause an improvement in ventricular performance. The factors affecting end-diastolic volume are 1) total blood volume, 2) atrial contribution to ventricular filling, 3) pumping action of skeletal muscle, 4) venous tone, 5) body position, 6) intrathoracic pressure, 7) intrapericardial pressure, and 8) ventricular compliance. (*Parts A and B adapted from* Braunwald and coworkers [1].)

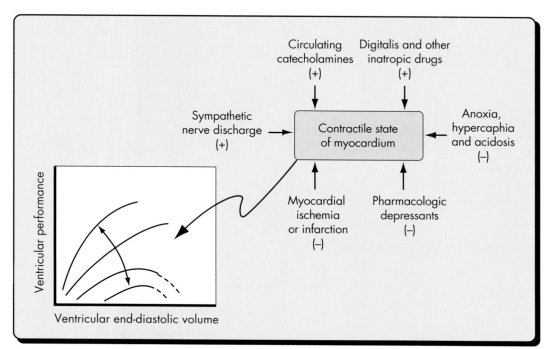

Figure 1-2. Family of cardiac function curves demonstrating the effect of contractility on cardiac performance. Changes in contractility may augment cardiac performance (positive inotropic effect), or depress it (negative inotropic effect). The effects of inotropic factors on cardiac performance can be demonstrated using a family of cardiac function curves. Movement of an entire curve upward or downward signifies a positive or negative inotropic effect, respectively. Examples of positive inotropic factors are circulating catecholamines, and the cardiac sympathetic nerves, whereas examples of negative inotropic factors are acidosis and anesthetics. (*Adapted from* Braunwald and coworkers [1]; with permission.)

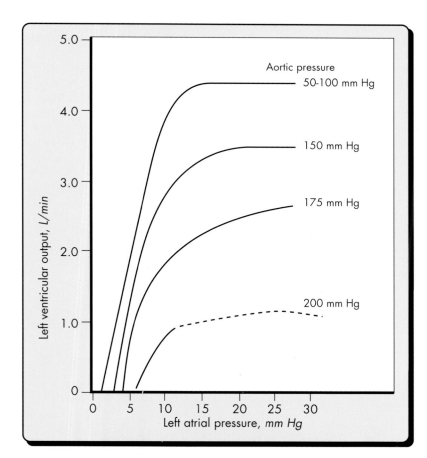

Figure 1-3. The inverse relationship between afterload and cardiac performance. Afterload is an important determinant of ventricular function. Afterload may be defined as the tension, force, or stress in the ventricular wall during ventricular ejection. In accordance with the law of Laplace, afterload is directly related to intraventricular pressure and size and inversely related to wall thickness. Because of changing size and pressure, afterload varies continuously during ventricular ejection. Thus, it is difficult to quantify with precision. Aortic pressure for the left ventricle and pulmonary artery pressure for the right ventricle will usually provide a reasonable estimate of afterload in vivo. In isolated heart preparations in which preload, inotropic state, and beating rate are held constant, increases in afterload cause reductions in left ventricular output, *ie*, stroke volume (shown in figure). In the intact circulation, this impairment of cardiac performance may be avoided when the level of contractility is high, or when venous return and preload increase sufficiently. The conditions of hypovolemia and cardiac depression increase the vulnerability to reduced stroke volume in the face of increased afterload. Afterload-reducing vasodilating drugs, *eg*, nitroprusside, have been used to augment cardiac performance in acute cardiac failure. (*Adapted from* Sagawa [2]; with permission.)

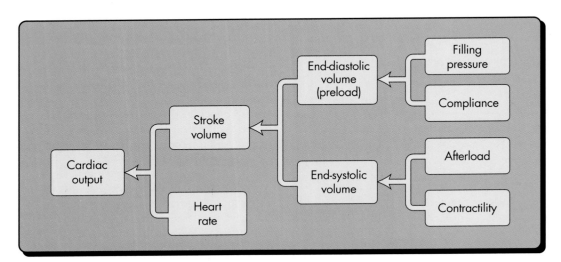

Figure 1-4. The major determinants of cardiac output. Cardiac output is the product of stroke volume and heart rate. Stroke volume is increased by increases in end-diastolic volume (Starling's law) and in myocardial contractility, whereas it is decreased by increases in afterload, *ie*, wall tension.

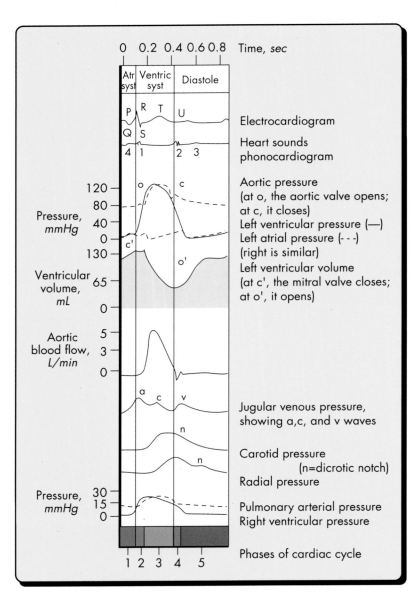

Figure 1-5. Events of the cardiac cycle. The phases of the cardiac cycle are identified at the bottom as follows: 1) atrial systole, 2) iso-volumetric ventricular contraction, 3) ventricular ejection, 4) isovolumetric relaxation, and 5) ventricular filling. At o, the heart valve opens, and at c, it closes. Salient points: 1) Atrial systole begins after the P wave of the electrocardiogram; ventricular systole begins near the end of the R wave and ends just after the T wave. 2) When ventricular pressure exceeds aortic pressure, the aortic valve opens, and ventricular ejection begins. 3) The amount of blood ejected by the ventricle (the stroke volume) is about 65% of the end-diastolic volume. This is termed the ejection fraction. 4) About 80% of ventricular filling is passive, *ie*, it occurs before atrial systole. 5) Events on the right side of the circulation are similar to those on the left side, but they are somewhat asynchronous. Right atrial systole precedes left atrial systole, and contraction of the right ventricle begins after that of the left ventricle. However, since pulmonary arterial pressure is less than aortic pressure, right ventricular ejection precedes left ventricular ejection. Atr syst—atrial systole; ventric syst—ventricular systole. (*Adapted from* Ganong [3]; with permission.)

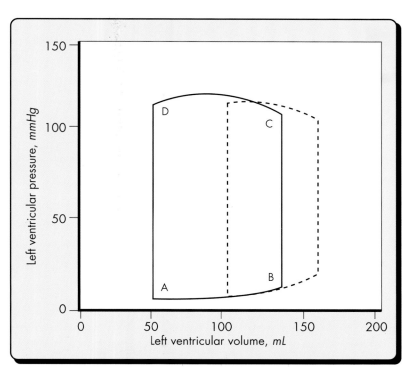

Figure 1-6. The relationship between ventricular pressure and volume during a cardiac cycle. The data presented are for the left ventricle. A similar plot (with a reduced pressure range) could be generated for the right ventricle. For the normal left ventricle (*solid line*), diastolic filling starts at *A*, and ends at *B*, when the mitral valve closes. The increase in ventricular pressure during this period of filling reflects the compliance of the ventricular wall. During iso-volumetric contraction (*B* to *C*), pressure increases steeply while volume remains constant. At *C*, ventricular pressure rises to a level in excess of aortic pressure, the aortic valve opens, and blood is ejected. Ventricular ejection (systole) continues until the ventricular pressure falls below aortic pressure and the aortic valve closes (*D*). The volume of blood ejected by the ventricle per beat (the stroke volume) is approximately 65% of the end-diastolic volume (ejection fraction). The period of isovolumetric relaxation follows (*D* to *A*), which is characterized by a sharp decrease in pressure and no change in volume. The mitral valve opens at *A*, thus completing one cardiac cycle. Effects of variations in loading conditions, and contractile state can be demonstrated using the pressure-volume relationship. In the figure, the *dashed line* shows the effect of heart failure, *ie*, decreased contractility, on the pressure-volume relationship. The area within the pressure-volume loop represents the mechanical work of the heart.

HEMODYNAMICS AND SYSTEMIC VASCULAR CONTROL

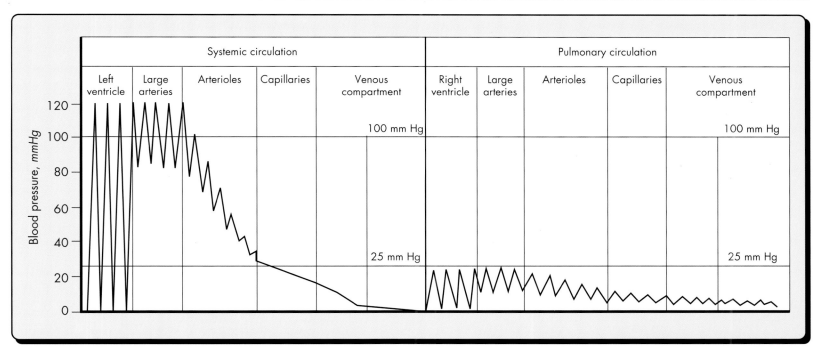

Figure 1-7. Pressure changes as blood passes through the series-coupled vascular elements in the systemic and pulmonary circulations. The heart is composed of two parallel pumps, each composed of an atrium and a ventricle. The right side of the heart supplies the pulmonary circulation, where exchange of oxygen and carbon dioxide occurs in the lung alveoli, while the left side of the heart supplies the systemic circulation, which carries oxygenated blood to the body tissues. Salient features of the figure are 1) The developed pressure of the right ventricle is approximately one sixth that of the left ventricle. This results in a smaller workload for the right ventricle, which is in keeping with its much thinner wall. 2) Although pressure in the ventricles falls nearly to zero during diastole, pressure is maintained in the large arteries. This is possible because the large arteries are very distensible. A portion of the energy released by cardiac contraction during systole is stored in the vessels. During diastole, the elastic recoil of the vessels converts this potential energy into forward blood flow, which ensures that capillary flow is continuous throughout the cardiac cycle. 3) The most severe drop in pressure occurs in the arterioles; hence, they are often termed the resistance vessels. The diameter of the arteriole is regulated by the contractile activity of the smooth muscle contained in its wall. Variations in arteriolar diameter are an important determinant of capillary blood flow and hydrostatic pressure (*Adapted from Folkow and Neil (4); with permission.*)

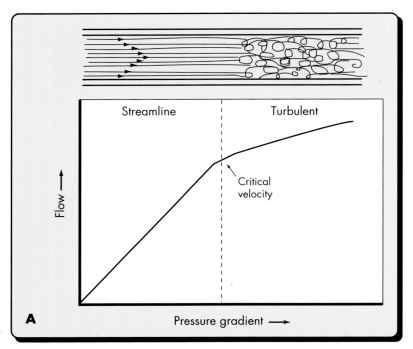

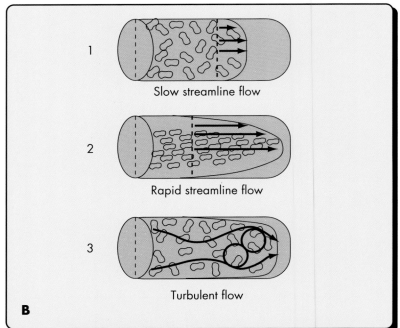

Figure 1-8. Determinants of blood flow according to Poiseuille's law. Effect of turbulent flow on this relationship. Poiseuille's law defines the influence of various factors on the flow of fluid through a tube: $F = [\Pi\,(P_i - P_o)r^4]/8\eta l$, where F is flow, $\Pi/8$ is a constant of proportionality, P_i is the pressure in, and P_o is the pressure out, r^4 is the fourth power of the radius of the tube, η is the viscosity of fluid, and l is the tube length. Rearranging Poiseuille's law, it can be shown that resistance to flow is directly dependent on tube length and viscosity, and inversely dependent on the fourth power of the radius of the tube. In the circulation, it is vessel radius that is the major determinant of resistance to blood flow. Because this factor is raised to the fourth power, small changes in radius cause marked changes in resistance. **A,** relationship between the pressure gradient (ΔP) and flow. At a given resistance, a plot of ΔP versus F yields a straight line. The resistance is reflected by the slope of the line, *ie*, the

greater the slope, the less the resistance. Pouiseuille's law applies to streamline, laminar flow. B, However, blood flow in vessels can be pulsatile, and in large vessels at high flow rates, may not be laminar. This is termed turbulent flow. The tendency for turbulence is given by the Reynolds number (Re): $Re = VD\gamma/\eta$, where V is linear velocity, D is diameter, γ is density, and η is viscosity. Re is dimensionless because it is the ratio of inertial and cohesive forces. The former tend to disrupt the stream, whereas the latter tend to maintain it. It is difficult to induce turbulence during steady flow in an unbranched tube of constant diameter if Re is below 2000. The critical Re in vivo, however, is much less because pulsation and vessel geometry distort the stream. Turbulence causes non-linearity in the ΔP versus F relationship (*panel A*). (Panel A *adapted from* Feigl [5] and panel B *from* Keele and Neil [6]; with permission.)

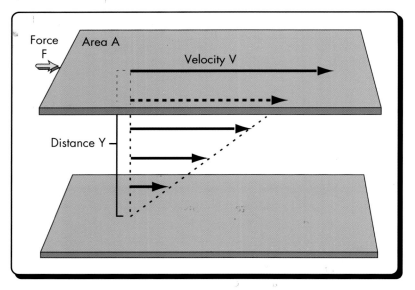

Figure 1-9. Viscosity. Viscosity is a primary determinant of blood flow resistance. An understanding of the term viscosity can be gained from the model shown in the figure. A homogeneous fluid is confined between two closed-spaced, parallel plates (analogous to playing cards). Assume the area of each plate is A, the distance between the plates is Y, and the bottom plate is stationary. If a tangential force (a shear stress) is applied to the upper plate, this plate will move with velocity V in the direction of the applied force and a velocity gradient (or shear rate) is developed in the fluid. Viscosity is defined as the factor of proportionality relating shear stress and shear rate for the fluid, *ie*, viscosity = shear stress/shear rate. Newton assumed that viscosity was a constant property of a particular fluid and independent of shear rate. Fluids that demonstrate this behavior are termed newtonian. Because blood consists of erythrocytes suspended in plasma, it does not behave like a newtonian fluid; the viscosity of blood increases sharply with reductions in shear rate. The non-newtonian behavior is localized in vivo on the venous side of the circulation because of its lower shear rates, but this behavior can be attenuated or abolished by hemodilution. The tendency for increased hematocrit to raise blood viscosity is attenuated when blood flows through tubes of capillary diameter. This is because the erythrocytes are normally very deformable, and thus they can squeeze through the capillary lumen in single file. Blood viscosity varies inversely with temperature. (*Adapted from* Fahmy [7]; with permission.)

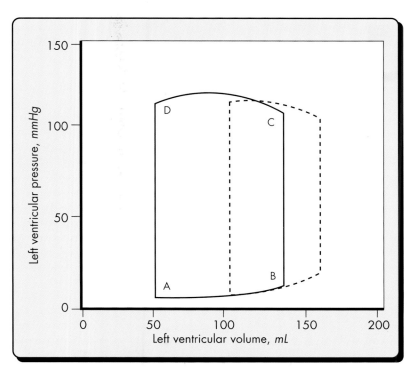

Figure 1-6. The relationship between ventricular pressure and volume during a cardiac cycle. The data presented are for the left ventricle. A similar plot (with a reduced pressure range) could be generated for the right ventricle. For the normal left ventricle (*solid line*), diastolic filling starts at *A*, and ends at *B*, when the mitral valve closes. The increase in ventricular pressure during this period of filling reflects the compliance of the ventricular wall. During iso-volumetric contraction (*B* to *C*), pressure increases steeply while volume remains constant. At *C*, ventricular pressure rises to a level in excess of aortic pressure, the aortic valve opens, and blood is ejected. Ventricular ejection (systole) continues until the ventricular pressure falls below aortic pressure and the aortic valve closes (*D*). The volume of blood ejected by the ventricle per beat (the stroke volume) is approximately 65% of the end-diastolic volume (ejection fraction). The period of isovolumetric relaxation follows (*D* to *A*), which is characterized by a sharp decrease in pressure and no change in volume. The mitral valve opens at *A*, thus completing one cardiac cycle. Effects of variations in loading conditions, and contractile state can be demonstrated using the pressure-volume relationship. In the figure, the *dashed line* shows the effect of heart failure, *ie*, decreased contractility, on the pressure-volume relationship. The area within the pressure-volume loop represents the mechanical work of the heart.

HEMODYNAMICS AND SYSTEMIC VASCULAR CONTROL

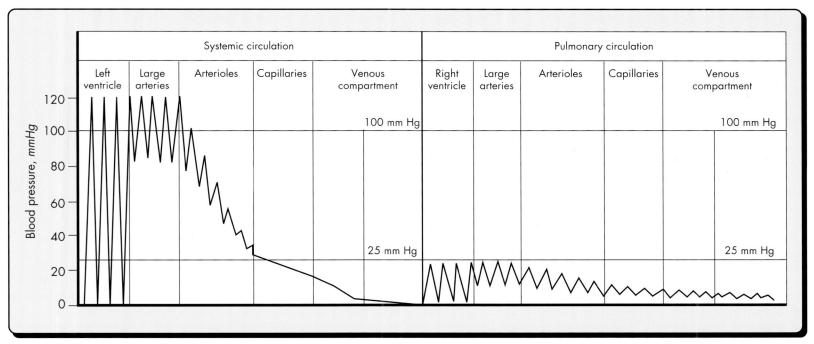

Figure 1-7. Pressure changes as blood passes through the series-coupled vascular elements in the systemic and pulmonary circulations. The heart is composed of two parallel pumps, each composed of an atrium and a ventricle. The right side of the heart supplies the pulmonary circulation, where exchange of oxygen and carbon dioxide occurs in the lung alveoli, while the left side of the heart supplies the systemic circulation, which carries oxygenated blood to the body tissues. Salient features of the figure are 1) The developed pressure of the right ventricle is approximately one sixth that of the left ventricle. This results in a smaller workload for the right ventricle, which is in keeping with its much thinner wall. 2) Although pressure in the ventricles falls nearly to zero during diastole, pressure is maintained in the large arteries. This is possible because the large arteries are very distensible. A portion of the energy released by cardiac contraction during systole is stored in the vessels. During diastole, the elastic recoil of the vessels converts this potential energy into forward blood flow, which ensures that capillary flow is continuous throughout the cardiac cycle. 3) The most severe drop in pressure occurs in the arterioles; hence, they are often termed the resistance vessels. The diameter of the arteriole is regulated by the contractile activity of the smooth muscle contained in its wall. Variations in arteriolar diameter are an important determinant of capillary blood flow and hydrostatic pressure (*Adapted from* Folkow and Neil (4); with permission.)

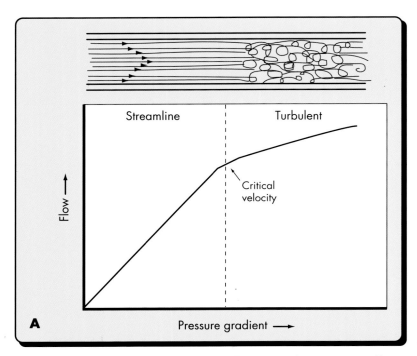

A

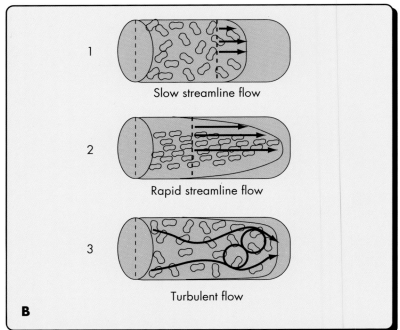

B

Figure 1-8. Determinants of blood flow according to Poiseuille's law. Effect of turbulent flow on this relationship. Poiseuille's law defines the influence of various factors on the flow of fluid through a tube: $F = [\Pi \, (Pi-Po)r^4]/8\eta l$, where F is flow, $\Pi/8$ is a constant of proportionality, Pi is the pressure in, and Po is the pressure out, r^4 is the fourth power of the radius of the tube, η is the viscosity of fluid, and l is the tube length. Rearranging Poiseuille's law, it can be shown that resistance to flow is directly dependent on tube length and viscosity, and inversely dependent on the fourth power of the radius of the tube. In the circulation, it is vessel radius that is the major determinant of resistance to blood flow. Because this factor is raised to the fourth power, small changes in radius cause marked changes in resistance. A, relationship between the pressure gradient (ΔP) and flow. At a given resistance, a plot of ΔP versus F yields a straight line. The resistance is reflected by the slope of the line, *ie*, the greater the slope, the less the resistance. Poiuseuille's law applies to streamline, laminar flow. B, However, blood flow in vessels can be pulsatile, and in large vessels at high flow rates, may not be laminar. This is termed turbulent flow. The tendency for turbulence is given by the Reynolds number (Re): $Re = VD\gamma/\eta$, where V is linear velocity, D is diameter, γ is density, and η is viscosity. Re is dimensionless because it is the ratio of inertial and cohesive forces. The former tend to disrupt the stream, whereas the latter tend to maintain it. It is difficult to induce turbulence during steady flow in an unbranched tube of constant diameter if Re is below 2000. The critical Re in vivo, however, is much less because pulsation and vessel geometry distort the stream. Turbulence causes non-linearity in the ΔP versus F relationship (*panel A*). (Panel A *adapted from* Feigl [5] and panel B *from* Keele and Neil [6]; with permission.)

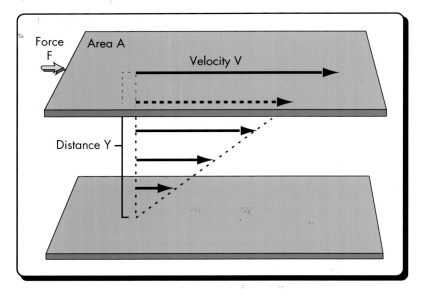

Figure 1-9. Viscosity. Viscosity is a primary determinant of blood flow resistance. An understanding of the term viscosity can be gained from the model shown in the figure. A homogeneous fluid is confined between two closed-spaced, parallel plates (analogous to playing cards). Assume the area of each plate is A, the distance between the plates is Y, and the bottom plate is stationary. If a tangential force (a shear stress) is applied to the upper plate, this plate will move with velocity V in the direction of the applied force and a velocity gradient (or shear rate) is developed in the fluid. Viscosity is defined as the factor of proportionality relating shear stress and shear rate for the fluid, *ie*, viscosity = shear stress/shear rate. Newton assumed that viscosity was a constant property of a particular fluid and independent of shear rate. Fluids that demonstrate this behavior are termed newtonian. Because blood consists of erythrocytes suspended in plasma, it does not behave like a newtonian fluid; the viscosity of blood increases sharply with reductions in shear rate. The non-newtonian behavior is localized in vivo on the venous side of the circulation because of its lower shear rates, but this behavior can be attenuated or abolished by hemodilution. The tendency for increased hematocrit to raise blood viscosity is attenuated when blood flows through tubes of capillary diameter. This is because the erythrocytes are normally very deformable, and thus they can squeeze through the capillary lumen in single file. Blood viscosity varies inversely with temperature. (*Adapted from* Fahmy [7]; with permission.)

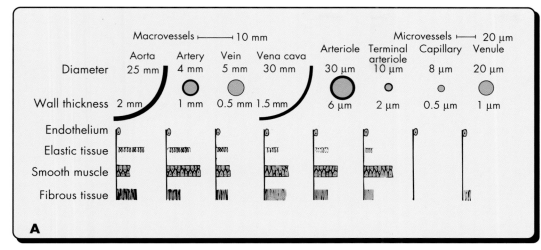

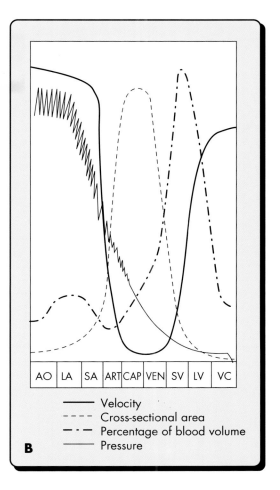

Figure 1-10. Characteristics of blood vessels. **A,** Dimensions and structural attributes of the various vessel types. **B,** Pressure, velocity, cross-sectional area, and capacity of blood vessels. The salient points in this figure are: 1) The large conduit arteries are predominantly elastic structures that convert the intermittent cardiac output into continuous flow. Because the cross-sectional area is small, the flow velocity in the arteries is high. The resistance to flow in the arteries is small, and thus the pressure drop is also small. 2) The arterioles and the terminal arterioles are the major sites of resistance (and of pressure drop) in the vascular bed. Adjustments in tone of smooth muscle in the arterioles are the primary mechanism for local regulation of blood flow. 3) The capillaries have a very large aggregate cross-sectional area (which decreases flow velocity), and a thin wall, which is keeping with their function as a site of blood-tissue exchange. 4) The veins and venules are the primary sites for blood storage. AO—aorta; ART—arterioles; CAP—capillaries; LA—large arteries; LV—large veins; SA—small arteries; SV—small veins; VC—venae cavae; VEN—venules. (*Adapted from* Berne and Levy [8]; with permission.)

Legend for B:
— Velocity
--- Cross-sectional area
-·-·- Percentage of blood volume
— Pressure

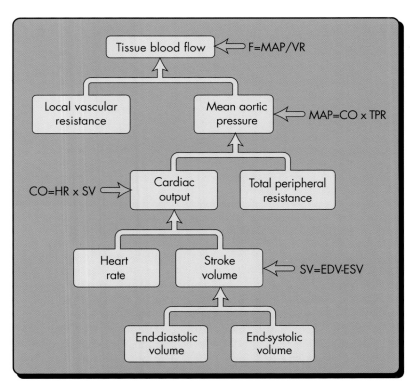

Figure 1-11. Flow diagram demonstrating the factors and the interrelationships determining tissue blood flow. The fundamental function of the circulation is to provide sufficient blood to the body tissues to sustain their metabolic demands. Tissue blood flow (F) is essentially dependent on the ratio between mean aortic pressure (MAP), and local vascular resistance (VR). MAP is determined by function within the heart and the peripheral vasculature, and their interaction. These relationships are shown in the figure. The main determinant of VR is radius of the local arterioles, which is under the control of metabolic, neural, and humoral influences. CO—cardiac output; EDV—end-diastolic volume; ESV—end-systolic volume; HR—heart rate; SV—stroke volume; TPR—total peripheral resistance. (*Adapted from* Rothe [9]; with permission.)

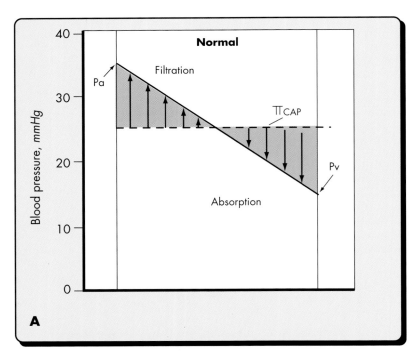

A

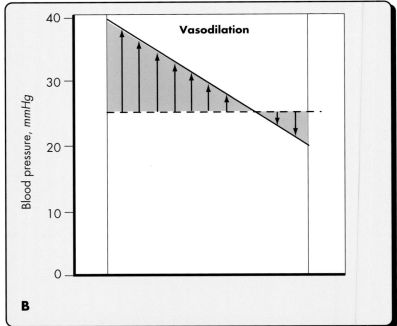

B

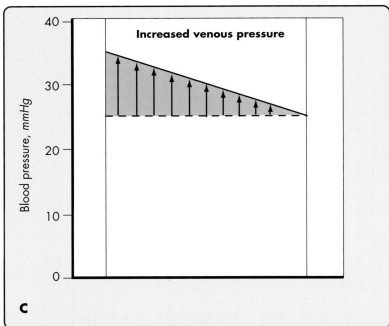

C

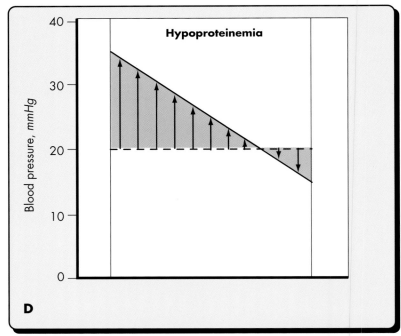

D

Figure 1-12. Factors influencing the balance between capillary filtration and absorption: mechanisms of edema. Because the capillary wall is highly permeable to water and to almost all the solutes of the plasma with the exception of the plasma proteins, it acts like a porous filter through which protein-free plasma moves by bulk flow under the influence of a hydrostatic pressure gradient. Transcapillary filtration is defined by the equation: Fluid filtration= C_F [(P_{cap}-P_{IF}) - (Π_{cap}-Π_{IF})], where C_F is capillary filtration coefficient; P_{cap} is capillary hydrostatic pressure; P_{IF} is interstitial fluid hydrostatic pressure; Π_{IF} is interstitial fluid oncotic pressure; and Π_{cap} is capillary oncotic pressure. P_{cap} and Π_{IF} are forces of filtration. P_{cap} is determined by arterial pressure, venous pressure, and the ratio of postcapillary to precapillary resistance. An increase in any of these factors will increase P_{cap}. P_{cap} is approximately 35 mm Hg at the arterial end of the capillaries and approximately 15 mm Hg at the venous end. Π_{IF} is due to plasma proteins that have passed through the capillary wall and is normally very low compared with P_{cap}. Thus, P_{cap} is normally the major force of filtration. P_{IF} and Π_{cap} are forces favoring absorp-

tion. P_{IF} is determined by the volume of fluid and the distensability of the interstitial space, and is normally nearly equal to zero. Π_{cap} is due to to the plasma proteins (most predominantly albumin), and has a value of approximately 25 mm Hg. Π_{cap} is normally the major force for absorption. *The direction and magnitude of capillary bulk flow is essentially a function of the ratio of P_{cap} to Π_{cap}.* Filtered fluid that reaches the extravascular spaces is returned to the circulatory system via the lymphatic network. Under normal conditions (**A**), filtration dominates at the arterial end of the capillary, and absorption at the venous end because of the gradient of hydrostatic pressure; there is a small net filtration, which is compensated for by lymph flow. Edema is a condition of excess accumulation of fluid in the interstitial space. It occurs when net filtration exceeds drainage via the lymphatics. This can be caused by 1) increased capillary pressure, 2) decreased plasma protein concentration, 3) accumulation of osmotically active substances in the interstitial space, 4) increased capillary permeability, or 5) inadequate lymph flow. **B to D**, Conditions resulting in edema. (*Adapted from* Rothe [9]; with permission.)

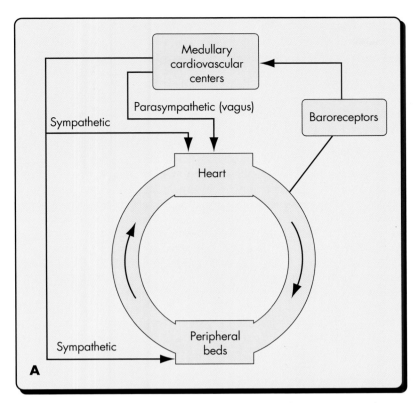

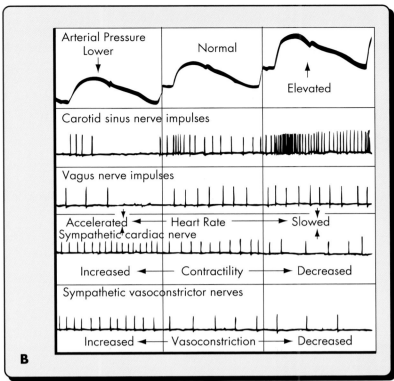

Figure 1-13. Baroreceptor control of the circulation. Arterial blood pressure is maintained within narrow limits by a negative feedback system. **A,** The major components of this system are 1) an afferent limb composed of the baroreceptors in the carotid and aortic arch and their respective sensory nerves, the glossopharyngeal and vagus nerves; 2) the cardiovascular centers in the medulla that receive and integrate the sensory information; and 3) an efferent limb composed of the sympathetic nerves to the heart and blood vessels and the parasympathetic (vagus) nerve to the heart. The baroreceptors are stimulated by stretch of the vessel wall, which results from an increase in transluminal pressure. Impulses originating in the baroreceptors tonically inhibit discharge of the sympa-

thetic nerves to the heart and blood vessels, and tonically facilitate discharge of the vagus nerve to the heart. **B,** A rise in arterial pressure reduces baroreceptor afferent activity resulting in further inhibition of the sympathetic nerves and facilitation of the vagus nerves. This produces vasodilation, venodilation, and reductions in stroke volume, heart rate, and cardiac output, which tend to normalize arterial pressure. A decrease in arterial pressure has opposite effects. The cardiovascular centers in the medulla are also under the influence of neural mechanisms arising in the arterial chemoreceptors, hypothalamus, and cerebral cortex, and of local changes in P_{CO_2} and P_{O_2}. (Panel A *adapted from* Rothe and Friedman [10] and panel B *adapted from* Rushmer [11]; with permission.)

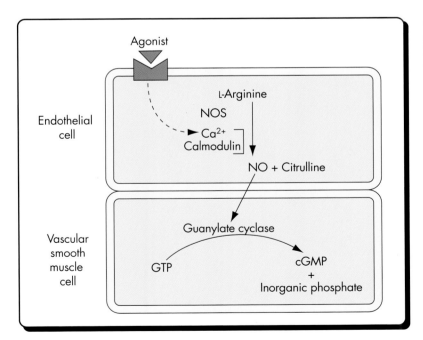

Figure 1-14. Nitric oxide (NO): its source, release, and functions in the cardiovascular system. NO is a ubiquitous inter- and intracellular signaling molecule with important roles in many physiologic processes [12]. NO is produced in cardiac endocardial cells and vas-

cular endothelial cells from the amino acid L-arginine in a reaction requiring the constitutive enzyme nitric oxide synthase (NOS). NOS activity is stimulated by increases in intracellular calcium concentration, which occur in response to the interaction of a chemical agent in the blood, *eg*, bradykinin or acetylcholine, with its specific membrane receptor or by increases in shear stress. Endothelium-derived nitric oxide (EDNO) diffuses into the underlying vascular smooth muscle where it stimulates production of cyclic guanosine monophosphate (cGMP), thus causing vascular relaxation. Inhibitors of NOS have been shown to produce hypertension in animals, implying that basally released NO maintains a tonic vasodilator tone in the systemic resistance vessels. EDNO is a potent inhibitor of platelet aggregation and adhesion to the endothelial surface. Furthermore, aggregating platelets release serotonin and adenosine diphosphate, which in turn act on the endothelium to cause massive release of NO causing vasodilation and a flushing out of the developing thrombus. EDNO has been suggested as a physiologic modulator of myocardial contractility and oxygen consumption, although these roles are controversial [13,14]. EDNO release is inhibited in a number of pathologic conditions, including atherosclerosis, diabetes mellitus, and hypercholesterolemia [12,15]. Vascular endothelial dysfunction may promote coronary vasospasm [12]. The vasodilating effects of sodium nitroprusside and nitroglycerin have been explained by their ability to provide exogenous NO [12]. Inhaled NO has been used as a treatment for pulmonary hypertension. GTP—guanosine triphosphate.

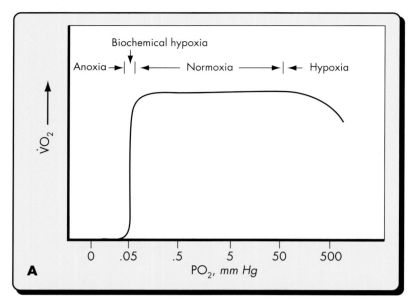

Figure 1-15. The oxygen delivery system. The cardiovascular and respiratory systems act in concert in transporting oxygen from the environment to tissue mitochondria. **A,** The objective of the oxygen delivery system in vivo is to ensure that PO_2 in the vicinity of all mitochondria is maintained above 0.1 mm Hg, which is the level required for unimpaired oxygen consumption ($\dot{V}O_2$). The only function of a PO_2 above 0.1 mm Hg is to provide sufficient driving force for diffusion of oxygen to mitochondria remote from capillaries. **B,** The integrated oxygen transport system can be viewed as a series of steps, each with a PO_2 cost. The three primary determinants of oxygen transport are oxygen saturation, hemoglobin concentration, and cardiac output. A decrease in any of these three factors will reduce oxygen transport unless compensated for by an increase in the others. If all three components decrease simultaneously, reductions as little as 30% of each component may prove intolerable unless rapidly corrected. If the reduction in oxygen transport is severe, it can produce tissue hypoxia, *ie,* cause a fall in tissue PO_2 that is sufficient to limit mitochondrial $\dot{V}O_2$ and to stimulate lactate production. (Panel A *adapted from* Honig [16] and panel B *adapted from* Nunn [17]; with permission.)

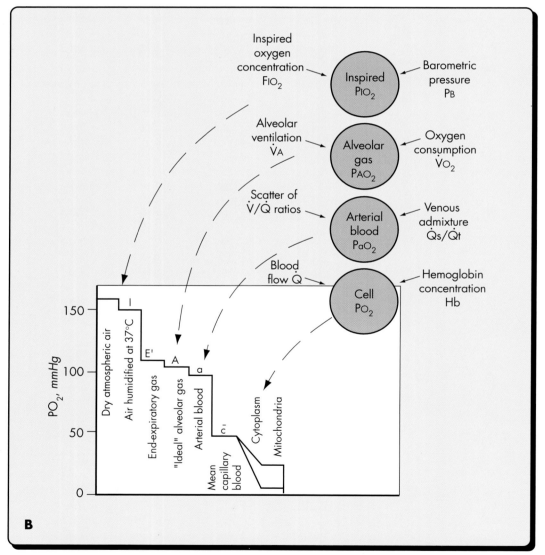

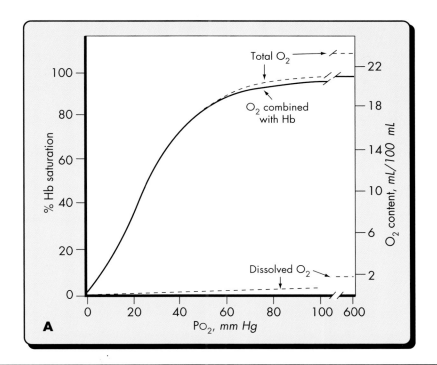

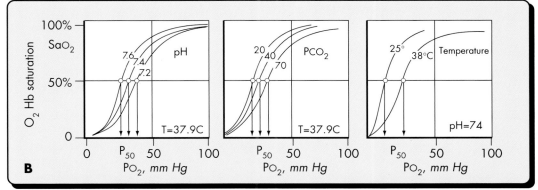

Figure 1-16. Oxygen carriage in the blood: oxyhemoglobin dissociation curve. **A,** Arterial oxygen content (CaO_2) is composed of oxygen bound to hemoglobin (Hb) and dissolved in plasma. Bound oxygen (vol%) is a direct function of Hb concentration (g/100 mL), oxyhemoglobin saturation (SaO_2), and the oxygen-carrying capacity for Hb (mL/g) (O_2 bound = (Hb × SaO_2 × 1.39). Oxyhemoglobin saturation is dependent on PO_2 and the oxyhemoglobin dissociation curve. The sigmoid shape of the curve reflects the fact that the four binding sites on a given hemoglobin molecule interact with each other. The result is a curve that is steep up to a PO_2 of 60 mm Hg and then becomes more shallow thereafter, approaching 100% saturation asymptotically. At a PO_2 of 100 mm Hg to which human arterial blood is equilibrated, 97% of the binding sites have bound oxygen. The shape of the oxyhemoglobin dissociation curve has important physiologic implications. The flatness of the curve above a PO_2 of 80 mm Hg ensures a relatively constant oxyhemoglobin saturation for arterial blood despite wide variations in alveolar oxygen pressure. The steep portion of the curve between 20 and 60 mm Hg permits unloading of oxygen from hemoglobin at relatively high PO_2 values, which permits the delivery of large amounts of oxygen into the tissue by diffusion. **B,** The oxygen binding properties of hemoglobin are influenced by a number of factors, including pH, PCO_2, and temperature. These factors cause shifts of the oxyhemoglobin dissociation curve to the right or left without changing the slope of the curve.

Rightward shifts of the curve facilitate unloading of oxygen at the tissue. To quantify the extent of a shift in the oxyhemoglobin dissociation curve, the so-called P_{50} is used, *ie,* the PO_2 required for 50% saturation. The P_{50} of normal adult hemoglobin at 37°C and normal pH and PCO_2 is 26 to 27 mm Hg. The compound 2, 3-diphosphoglycerate (2,3-DPG) is an intermediate in anaerobic glycolysis (the biochemical pathway by which red blood cells produce adenosine triphosphate), which binds to hemoglobin. Increases in intraerythrocytic 2,3-DPG concentration reduce the affinity of hemoglobin for oxygen, *ie,* they shift the oxyhemoglobin dissociation curve to the right, whereas decreases have opposite effects. Several factors have been found to influence red cell 2,3-DPG concentrations. After storage in a blood bank for only 1 week, 2,3-DPG concentrations are one third normal, resulting in a shift to the left of the oxyhemoglobin dissociation curve. On the other hand, conditions associated with chronic hypoxia, *eg,* living at high altitude or chronic anemia, stimulate production of 2,3-DPG, which causes a rightward shift of the oxyhemoglobin dissociation curve. Dissolved oxygen (vol.%) is linearly related to PO_2 [O_2 dissolved = 0.003 vol%/mm × PO_2 (mm Hg)]. Dissolved oxygen normally accounts for only 1.5% of total oxygen but this contribution increases when the bound component is reduced during hemodilution. (Panel A *adapted from* West [18] and panel B *adapted from* Weibel [19]; with permission.)

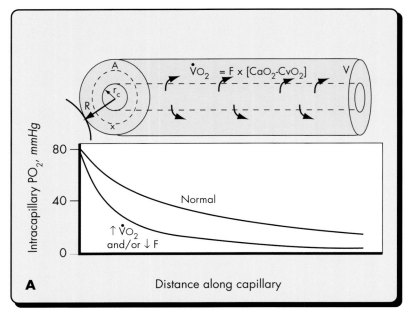

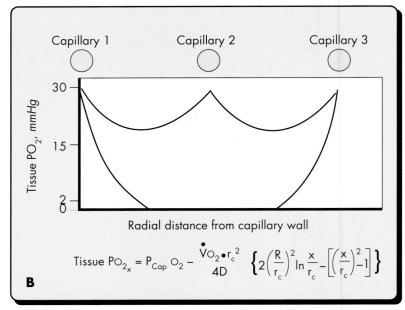

$$\text{Tissue PO}_{2_x} = \text{P}_{\text{Cap}}\text{O}_2 - \frac{\dot{\text{V}}\text{O}_2 \cdot r_c^2}{4D} \left\{ 2\left(\frac{R}{r_c}\right)^2 \ln\frac{x}{r_c} - \left[\left(\frac{x}{r_c}\right)^2 - 1\right] \right\}$$

Figure 1-17. Diffusion of oxygen to tissues; capillary-to-cell oxygen delivery. The final step in the delivery of oxygen to tissue mitochondria is diffusion from the capillary blood. According to the law of diffusion, this process is determined by the capillary-to-cell PO₂ gradient and the diffusion parameters, capillary surface area and blood-cell diffusion distance. In 1919, Krogh formulated the capillary recruitment model to describe the processes underlying oxygen transport in tissue [20]. The basic model was later expanded and refined [16,21]. The model consists of a single capillary and the surrounding cylinder of tissue that it supplies. Two interrelated oxygen gradients are involved: a longitudinal gradient within the capillary (**A**), and a radial oxygen gradient extending into the tissue (**B**). Most oxygen in capillary blood is bound to hemoglobin and cannot leave the capillary. This bound oxygen is in equilibrium with the small amount of oxygen dissolved in the plasma. The consumption of oxygen by the tissue (V̇O₂) creates a transcapillary gradient for oxygen. Diffusion of oxygen into the surrounding tissue shifts the equilibrium between bound and dissolved oxygen, so that more oxygen is released from hemoglobin. By this mechanism, oxygen dissociation from hemoglobin is controlled by tissue oxygen consumption. The longitudinal oxygen gradient within the capillary is created by the extraction of oxygen by tissue as blood passes from the arterial to venous ends of the capillary. In accordance with the Fick equation, the arteriovenous oxygen difference (CaO₂-CvO₂) is equivalent to the ratio of oxygen consumption to blood flow (F). An increase in oxygen consumption, a decrease in blood flow, or both, will steepen the longitudinal oxygen gradient. Proportional changes in oxygen consumption and blood flow are required to maintain the longitudinal oxygen gradient constant. A corresponding value for capillary PO₂ (P_cap O₂) can be estimated from the value for capillary oxygen content taking into account hemoglobin concentration and the oxyhemoglobin dissociation curve. The shape of the longitudinal gradient in PO₂ within the capillary is approximately exponential because of the influence of the oxyhemoglobin dissociation curve. The P_cap O₂ is the driving force for diffusion of oxygen into the tissue. Because P_cap O₂ is minimum at the venous end of the capillary, the mitochondria in this region are most vulnerable to oxygen deficits. The radial drop in PO₂ to any point "x" within the tissue cylinder is described from the equation shown in *panel B*, where R is the radius of the tissue cylinder, r_c is the radius of the capillary, and D is the oxygen diffusion coefficient. This equation can be simplified to provide a value for mean tissue PO₂ in the tissue cylinder: mean PtO₂=P_cap O₂-A(V̇O₂×R²/4D), where P̄_cap O₂ is blood oxygen tension at a midway point in the capillary and A is a constant related to the relationship between capillary radius and tissue cylinder radius. R is determined by the number of capillaries perfused with red blood cells per volume of tissue and is controlled by the precapillary sphincters. The favorable influence of capillary recruitment on tissue PO₂ is evident in *panel B*. If only capillaries 1 and 3 are open, diffusion distance is so large that PO₂ falls to zero toward the center of the tissue cylinder. The low tissue PO₂ causes relaxation of the precapillary sphincter controlling capillary 2. Perfusion of capillary 2 decreases diffusion distance, and increases tissue PO₂ to an adequate level throughout the tissue. (*Adapted from* Honig [16]; with permission.)

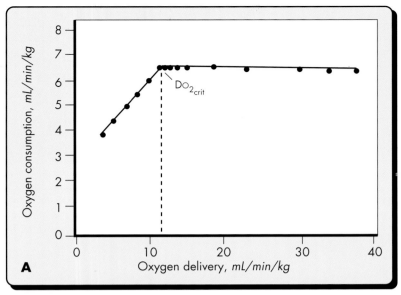

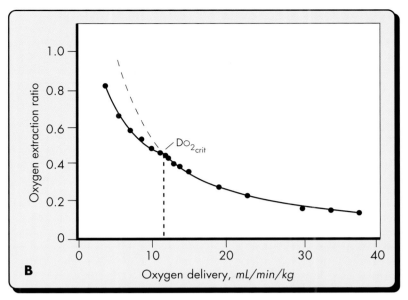

Figure 1-18. Critical oxygen delivery. The Fick equation can be used to calculate oxygen consumption of the whole body (V_{O_2}): $V_{O_2} = CO \times (Ca_{O_2} - Cv_{O_2})$ (Equation 1), where CO is cardiac output, and Ca_{O_2} and Cv_{O_2} are arterial and mixed venous oxygen content, respectively. Cardiac output is usually measured by thermodilution using a Swan-Ganz catheter situated in the pulmonary artery. Samples of blood are collected from an artery and from the pulmonary artery (mixed venous sample) and analyzed for oxygen content. Whole-body oxygen delivery can also be calculated: $D_{O_2} = CO \times Ca_{O_2}$ (Equation 2). The oxygen extraction ratio (E_{O_2} in %) is defined by the equation: $E_{O_2} = Ca_{O_2} - Cv_{O_2})/ Ca_{O_2}$ (Equation 3). Combining equations 1 and 2 and rearranging terms, it can be demonstrated that ER is also equal to the ratio of V_{O_2} and D_{O_2}. Measurements of ER, as well as Pv_{O_2}, are frequently used clinically to assess overall adequacy of D_{O_2} (and CO) in critically ill patients. At rest, D_{O_2} greatly exceeds V_{O_2} and thus E_{O_2} is relatively modest (approximately 23% to 25%), resulting in a substantial reserve for oxygen extraction [22]. **A,** At normal or high levels of oxygen delivery, V_{O_2} is constant and independent of D_{O_2}. As D_{O_2} is gradually reduced, an increased E_{O_2} maintains V_{O_2}. Eventually a critical point is reached where oxygen extraction cannot increase adequately, and V_{O_2} begins to fall. Below this threshold, the so-called critical D_{O_2} (or $D_{O_{2crit}}$), the level of V_{O_2} is limited by the supply of oxygen. In anesthetized dogs, the critical D_{O_2} was found to be approximately 10 mL/min/kg [22]. The normal biphasic D_{O_2}–V_{O_2} relationship has been demonstrated in patients without respiratory failure undergoing coronary artery bypass surgery [23], whereas a direct linear relationship between D_{O_2} and V_{O_2} has been demonstrated in patients with acute adult respiratory distress syndrome [24], implying a pathologic impairment of oxygen tissue extraction in these patients. (*Adapted from* Schumacker and Cain [22]; with permission.)

INTERORGAN VARIATION IN BASELINE OXYGEN EXTRACTION

	Blood flow, mL/min/100 g	Oxygen consumption, mL/min/100 g	(a–v) O_2 difference, vol%	Oxygen extraction, %
Left ventricle	80	8	14	70
Brain	55	3	6	30
Liver	85 }	2	6	30
GI tract	40 }			
Kidneys	400	5	1.3	6.5
Muscles	3	0.15	5	25
Skin	10	0.2	2.5	12.5
Rest of body	3	0.15	4.4	22

Figure 1-19. Interorgan variation in baseline values for blood flow, oxygen consumption, and oxygen extraction in average humans. The individual body tissues vary widely with respect to the relationship between blood flow (oxygen delivery) and oxygen consumption, and thus in their baseline oxygen extraction. For example, in the left ventricle baseline oxygen extraction is 70% to 75%, whereas in the kidney it is 5% to 10%. The high baseline oxygen extraction in the left ventricle renders it extremely dependent on blood flow to maintain adequate oxygen transport. GI—gastrointestinal. (*Adapted from* Folkow and Neil [4]; with permission.)

CHARACTERISTIC VALUES FOR HEMODYNAMIC AND WHOLE-BODY O₂ TRANSPORT VARIABLES FOR THE NORMAL RESTING ADULT

Hemodynamic variables

Systemic arterial blood pressure (systolic/diastolic) = 120/80 mm Hg
Pulmonary arterial blood pressure (systolic/diastolic) = 21/9 mm Hg
Left ventricular end-diastolic pressure = < 12 mm Hg
Right ventricular end-diastolic pressure = < 6 mm Hg
Cardiac output = 5 L/min
Ejection fraction = 0.6–0.8

O₂ transport variables

Arterial P_{O_2} = 100 mm Hg
Arterial hemoglobin saturation = 97%
Mixed venous P_{O_2} = 40 mm Hg
Mixed venous hemoglobin saturation = 75%
Hemoglobin = 15 g/100 mL
Arterial O₂ content = 20.5 vol%
O₂ delivery = 1025 mL/min
Mixed venous O₂ content = 15.8 vol%
Arteriovenous O₂ difference = 4.7 vol%
O₂ consumption = 235 mL/min
O₂ extraction ratio = 23%

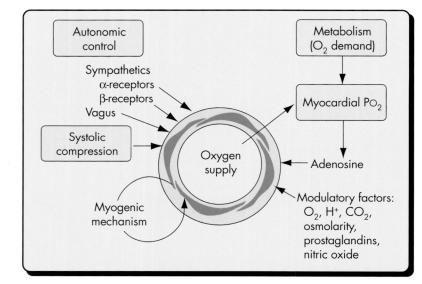

Figure 1-21. Coronary blood flow regulation: factors influencing coronary vascular resistance. Coronary vascular resistance is determined by the throttling effect caused by extravascular compressive forces during systole and by active changes in the tone of arteriolar smooth muscle. The mechanical impediment to coronary blood flow is most prominent in the subendocardial layers of the left ventricular wall. This factor results in blood flow in the left coronary circulation being higher during diastole, rather than during systole, as is the case in other vascular beds, including the right ventricular wall. The pressure gradient for blood flow in the left ventricular wall is approximated by the difference between aortic diastolic pressure and left ventricular end-diastolic pressure. Local metabolic control mechanisms predominate in the active control of coronary vasomotor tone. These mechanisms provide a close coupling between coronary blood flow and myocardial oxygen demand, which serves to maintain myocardial P_{O_2} (and coronary venous P_{O_2}) nearly constant. Adenosine, a breakdown product of adenosine triphosphate, is a potent endogenous vasodilator that is thought to play a central role in metabolic regulation of coronary perfusion. Other metabolites may also contribute, including carbon dioxide, oxygen, hydrogen ions, and nitric oxide (released from the vascular endothelium). Autoregulation refers to the intrinsic capability of the coronary circulation to maintain a relatively constant coronary blood flow over a wide range of perfusion pressures. This may be due to metabolic or myogenic mechanisms. A myogenic response refers to the intrinsic tendency of vascular smooth muscle to contract in response to increased distending pressure and to relax in response to decreased distending pressure. A higher tissue pressure results in a reduced autoregulatory capability in the subendocardium compared with the subepicardium. This contributes to the greater vulnerability of that region to infarction during coronary insufficiency. The coronary arterioles are endowed with α (constrictor) and β₂ (dilating) adrenergic receptors, and with muscarinic-cholinergic (dilating) receptors, and they are supplied by sympathetic and parasympathetic (vagus) nerves. These autonomic pathways normally play a secondary role in coronary vascular regulation. (*Adapted from* Rubio and Berne [25]; with permission.)

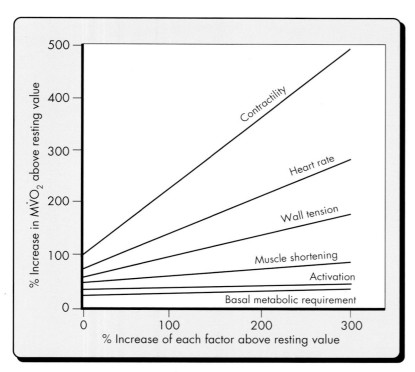

exclusively on aerobic metabolism to meet its energy demands. Although the left ventricle constitutes less than 0.5% of the weight of the body, in humans it accounts for approximately 7% of the body's basal oxygen consumption [1]. The utilization of substrates by the heart depends on their availability as well as on the heart's nutritional status and hormonal influences. Although various substances, including fatty acids, glucose, lactate, pyruvate, acetate, ketone bodies, and amino acids can serve as energy sources, under physiologic conditions fatty acids and glucose are preferred [1]. The most important determinants of myocardial oxygen consumption are contractility, heart rate, and wall tension. Other points worthy of mention are [1]: 1) Wall tension is directly proportional to the pressure and radius of the heart and inversely proportional to the wall thickness (law of Laplace). The area beneath the left ventricular pressure pulse per minute, *ie*, the time-tension index, bears a direct relationship to myocardial oxygen consumption. 2) When external work (pressure × stroke volume) is considered, pressure work has a much greater oxygen cost than does flow work. Muscle shortening per se has only a small influence on myocardial oxygen consumption. 3) Basal metabolism reflects adenosine triphosphate–requiring processes not directly related to contraction, such as activity of cell membrane Na-K ATPase for maintaining the ionic environment, and other cellular processes, such as protein synthesis. 4) The oxygen cost of activation comprises two components: electrical activation, and release and uptake of calcium by the sarcoplasmic reticulum. $M\dot{V}O_2$—myocardial oxygen consumption. (*Adapted from* Marcus [26]; with permission.)

Figure 1-22. Determinants of myocardial oxygen consumption. The heart is a continuously active organ that normally depends almost

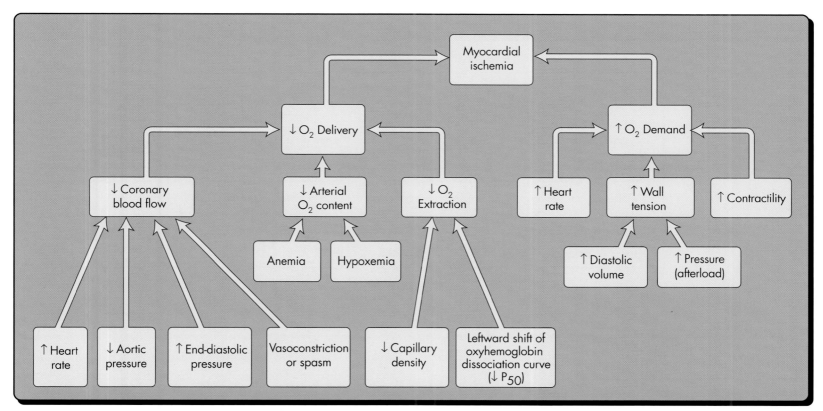

Figure 1-23. Conditions having detrimental influence on myocardial oxygen balance: mechanisms of myocardial ischemia. In normal hearts, myocardial oxygen supply (coronary blood flow) is matched to the prevailing myocardial oxygen demand via adjustments in vascular tone by local metabolic mechanisms. When the vasodilator reserve of the coronary bed is limited by a proximal stenosis, the myocardium becomes more vulnerable to ischemia, *ie*, oxygen demand exceeds oxygen supply. The factors tending to promote this condition are presented in the figure. Several points to be made are 1) An increase in heart rate decreases myocardial oxygen delivery by decreasing coronary blood flow (via a shortening of the diastolic period), while it also increases

myocardial oxygen demand. 2) An increase in preload reduces myocardial oxygen delivery (by reducing the pressure gradient for coronary blood flow), while it also increases myocardial oxygen demand (via an increase in wall tension). 3) A decrease in aortic pressure decreases myocardial oxygen delivery by decreasing coronary blood flow, but it decreases myocardial oxygen demand via a decrease in wall tension. Thus, its net effect depends on the balance between these factors. Under conditions of restricted coronary vasodilator reserve, the most favorable hemodynamic situation is characterized by a low heart rate and preload, a normal aortic pressure, and a normal to moderate inotropic state [27]. P_{50}—PO_2 required for 50% saturation.

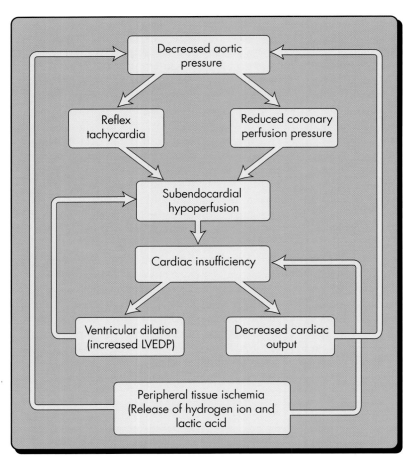

Figure 1-24. Myocardial blood flow and oxygen delivery during acute normovolemic hemodilution (ANH). The heart, particularly the left ventricular wall, is the principal organ at risk during ANH [28]. This is because of several factors, including 1) an augmented contractile demand; 2) a low baseline coronary venous P_{O_2} resulting in a small reserve for oxygen extraction; and 3) the tendency for subendocardial ischemia, when tachycardia or aortic hypotension occurs in the presence of a dilated vasculature. Moderate ANH (hematocrit about 20% to 25%) is accompanied by transmurally uniform increases in myocardial blood flow that are sufficient to maintain myocardial oxygen consumption and myocardial oxygen delivery, and to avoid lactate production. The increases in myocardial blood flow are due to a reduction in coronary vascular resistance because of the combined effects of reduced blood viscosity and dilation of coronary resistance vessels by local metabolites. The minimum safe hematocrit has been determined to be approximately 10%. Below this level, aortic pressure decreases because the increase in cardiac output does not compensate for the fall in systematic vascular resistance. This initiates a vicious cycle (shown in figure), which, if not interrupted by blood transfusion, may lead to irreversible cardiac failure and circulatory collapse. LVEDP—left ventricular end-diastolic pressure.

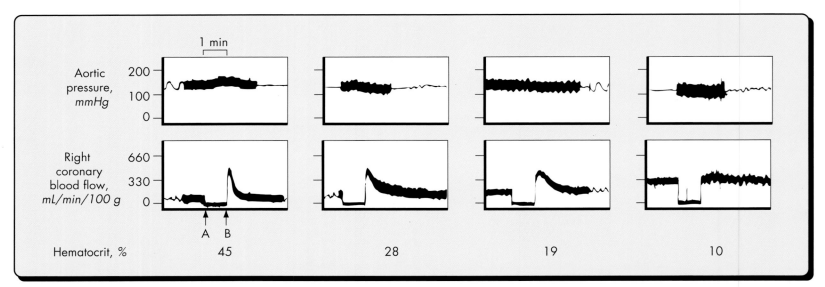

Figure 1-25. Coronary reserve assessed by analysis of the reactive hyperemic response in the right coronary circulation of a dog: diminution during hemodilution. The transient increase in blood flow above the control rate that follows an interval of arterial occlusion (from *A* to *B*) is termed reactive hyperemia [26]. The temporal characteristics of the reactive hyperemia have been explained by metabolites produced in ischemic tissue to first dilate the resistance vessels, and then to be washed out during reperfusion. A coronary occlusion of 60 seconds is usually required to maximally dilate the coronary circulation, and thus to assess the coronary reserve. Longer occlusions only increase the duration of the reactive hyperemic response. Coronary reserve in the normal right and left ventricular walls is appreciable (400% to 500%), but it is reduced in a variety of conditions, including left ventricular hypertrophy, coronary obstruction, and hemodilution (shown in the figure) [29]. A diminished coronary reserve renders the myocardium more vulnerable to ischemia secondary to increases in cardiac work or reductions in perfusion pressure. (*Adapted from* Crystal and coworkers [29]; with permission.)

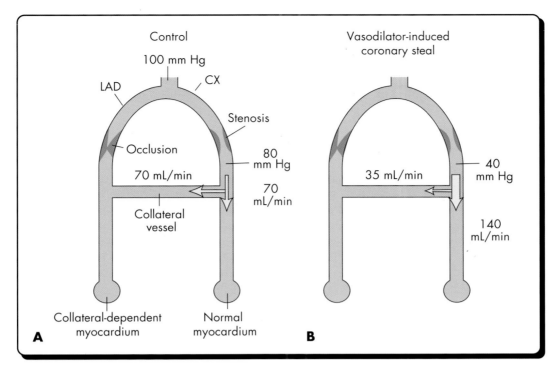

Figure 1-26. Determinants of coronary steal. Coronary steal refers to the phenomenon in which small-vessel dilation and an increase in flow to an area of already well-perfused myocardium leads to a decrease in flow to another area of myocardium with borderline perfusion and limited coronary reserve. Coronary steal can occur between two arteries connected by collateral vessels, *ie*, intercoronary steal, or from subendocardium to subepicardium distal to a coronary stenosis, *ie*, transmural steal. **A** and **B** demonstrate the hemodynamic basis of intercoronary steal. In this hypothetical situation, 1) the left anterior descending (LAD) coronary artery is completely occluded, and the myocardium in its perfusion territory is receiving flow via collateral vessels originating at the circumflex (CX) artery, and 2) the CX has a significant stenosis. Under control conditions, the resistance vessels in the LAD bed are maximally dilated; thus, blood flow in this region is pressure-dependent. Coronary steal occurs when a coronary vasodilating drug (or a physiologic factor such as hypercapnia) reduces vascular resistance in the distal CX bed, which increases the rate of blood flow through the CX artery. This steepens the pressure drop within this artery, resulting in a reduced pressure at the source of the collateral vessels, and a decrease in collateral flow to the pressure-dependent LAD bed. Transmural steal occurs because the subepicardium has a greater capacity for autoregulation than does the subendocardium. This is probably the result of the higher tissue pressures in the subendocardium. Coronary steal can precipitate myocardial ischemia if the decrease in flow is not accompanied by a proportional decrease in myocardial oxygen demand.

REFERENCES

1. Braunwald E, Ross Jr J, Sonnenblick EH: *Mechanisms of Contraction of the Normal and Failing Heart.* Boston: Little, Brown; 1976:72–81, 269–282.

2. Sagawa K: Analysis of the ventricular pumping capacity as function of input and output pressure loads. In *Physical Bases of Circulatory Transport: Regulation and Exchange.* Edited by Reeve EB, Guyton AC. Philadelphia: WB Saunders; 1967:141–149.

3. Ganong WF. *Review of Medical Physiology.* Norwalk, CT: Appleton & Lange; 1987:467–470.

4. Folkow B, Neil E: *Circulation.* New York: Oxford University Press; 1971:12.

5. Feigl, EO: Physics of the Cardiovascular System. In *Physiology and Biophysics II: Circulation, Respiration, and Fluid Balance.* Edited by Ruch TC, Patton HD. Philadelphia: WB Saunders; 1974:10–22.

6. Keele CA, Neil E: *Samson Wright's Applied Physiology.* London: Oxford University Press; 1971:60–62, 73–75.

7. Fahmy NR: Techniques for deliberate hypotension: haemodilution and hypotension. In *Hypotensive Anaesthesia.* Edited by Enderby GEH. Edinburgh: Churchill-Livingstone; 1985:164–183.

8. Berne RM, Levy MN: *Principles of Physiology.* St. Louis: CV Mosby; 1990:194–195.

9. Rothe CF: Cardiodynamics. In *Physiology.* Edited by Selkurt EE. Boston: Little, Brown; 1971:321–344.

10. Rothe CF, Friedman JJ: Control of the cardiovascular system. In *Physiology.* Edited by Selkurt EE. Boston: Little, Brown; 1971:371–393.

11. Rushmer RF: *Cardiovascular Dynamics.* Philadelphia: WB Saunders; 1970:165.

12. Moncada S, Palmer RMJ, Higgs EA: Nitric oxide: physiology, pathophysiology, and pharmacology. *Pharmacol Rev* 1991, 43:109–141.

13. Crystal GJ, Gurevicius J: Nitric oxide does not modulate myocardial contractility acutely in in situ canine hearts. *Am J Physiol* 1996, 270:H1568–H1576.

14. Kelly RA, Balligand J-L, Smith TW: Nitric oxide and cardiac function. *Circ Res* 1996, 79:363–380.

15. de Belder AJ, Radomski MW, Martini JF, Moncada S: Nitric oxide and the pathogenesis of heart muscle disease. *Eur J Clin Invest* 1995, 25:1–8.

16. Honig CR. *Modern Cardiovascular Physiology.* Boston: Little, Brown; 1981:181–187.

17. Nunn JF: *Nunn's Applied Respiratory Physiology.* Oxford: Butterworth Heinemann; 1993:255–268.

18. West JB. *Respiratory Physiology: The Essentials.* Baltimore: Williams & Wilkins; 1990:69–73.

19. Weibel ER. *The Pathway for Oxygen.* Cambridge: Harvard University Press; 1984:149.

20. Krogh A: The number and distribution of capillaries in muscles with calculations of the oxygen pressure head necessary for supplying the tissue. *J Physiol (Lond)* 1919, 52:409–415.

21. Kety SS: Determinants of tissue oxygen tension. *Fed Proc* 1957, 16:666–670.

22. Schumacker PT, Cain SM: The concept of critical oxygen delivery. *Intensive Care Med* 1987, 13:223–229.

23. Shibutani K, Komatsu T, Kubal K, et al.: Critical level of oxygen delivery in anesthetized man. *Crit Care Med* 1983, 11:640–643.

24. Danek SJ, Lynch JP, Weg JG, Dantzker DR: The dependence of oxygen uptake on oxygen delivery in the adult respiratory distress syndrome. *Am Rev Respir Dis* 1980, 122:387–395.

25. Rubio R, Berne RM: Regulation of Coronary blood flow. *Progr Cardiovasc Dis* 1975, 18:105–122.

26. Marcus ML: *The Coronary Circulation in Health and Disease.* New York: McGraw-Hill; 1983:70.

27. Hug CC Jr, Shanewise JS: Anesthesia for adult cardiac surgery. In *Anesthesia.* Edited by Miller RD. New York: Churchill-Livingstone; 1994, 1757–1809.

28. Crystal GJ, Salem MR: Acute normovolemic hemodilution. In *Blood Conservation in the Surgical Patient.* Edited by Salem MR. Baltimore: Williams & Wilkins; 1996, 168–188.

29. Crystal GJ, Kim S-J, Salem MR: Right and left ventricular O_2 uptake during hemodilution and β-adrenergic stimulation. *Am J Physiol* 1993, 265:H1769–H1777.

2

Cardiovascular Pharmacology

David A. Zvara and Roger L. Royster

There are many facets to the study of cardiovascular pharmacology. The pharmacologic treatment of heart failure, myocardial ischemia and myocardial infarction, and hypertension with drugs such as inotropes, vasodilators, and diuretics are major subject areas for whole disciplines of study. For example, the principles of anti-ischemic drug therapy rest on the physiology of myocardial oxygen supply and demand. The heart functions at a high metabolic rate and oxygen extraction is nearly complete regardless of heart rate. Therefore, myocardial oxygen delivery is of paramount importance. Oxygen delivery is dependent on the oxygen content of the blood and coronary blood flow. Any disruption in either of these two areas leads to profound regional or global myocardial ischemia. Oxygen demand depends largely on heart rate, contractility, and wall tension, which is a function of afterload and preload. Pharmacologic intervention in ischemic patients is targeted at improvements in oxygen supply or demand.

This chapter focuses on three major drug categories that are effective in treating myocardial ischemia: nitrates, β-blockers, and calcium channel blockers. These three groups of drugs work through very different mechanisms, yet the net result is improvement in ischemic syndromes. Nitrates and calcium channel blockers work primarily through coronary artery vasodilation as well as improvements in myocardial performance. β-Blockers, in contrast, reduce the inotropic state of the heart, as well as the heart rate. Nitrates and β-blockers are indicated for the acute treatment of ischemic syndromes and in some cases, myocardial infarction. Calcium channel blockers are effective for long-term control of myocardial ischemic syndromes, but are less commonly employed for acute myocardial ischemia.

Another major area of study is pharmacologic support of the failing heart. There are many causes of myocardial failure and a specific drug therapy cannot successfully treat every patient. Therefore, as with myocardial ischemic syndromes, the underlying cause of myocardial failure must be determined. For example, it is not uncommon to care for patients with chronic congestive heart failure. Similarly, one may be confronted with profound left ventricular dysfunction after coronary artery bypass grafting in a patient with previously good ventricular function. In each of these cases, cardiovascular pharmacologic support is required, yet these patients are remarkably different in the pathophysiology involved. This chapter evaluates the effects of digoxin, vasodilators, β-adrenergic agonists, phosphodiesterase inhibitors, and other drugs used to support the acute or chronically failing heart.

This chapter thus contains a broad overview of the two major areas of cardiovascular drug support: pharmacologic treatment of myocardial ischemia and pharmacologic support of the failing heart. Commonly used agents by a perioperative physician either in the operating room or the intensive care unit are discussed.

CARDIOVASCULAR PHARMACOLOGY AND MYOCARDIAL ISCHEMIA

MYOCARDIAL ISCHEMIA: FACTORS GOVERNING O_2 SUPPLY AND DEMAND

O_2 supply	O_2 Demand
Heart rate*	Heart rate*
O_2 Content	Contractility
Hemoglobin, O_2 saturation %, Pa_{O_2}	Wall tension
Coronary blood flow	Afterload (impedance)
CPP = DBP - LVEDP*	Preload (LVEDP)*
CVR	

* Variable effects, both supply and demand.

Figure 2-1. Myocardial ischemia: factors governing oxygen supply and demand. Myocardial ischemia results from an imbalance between myocardial oxygen supply and myocardial oxygen demand. Oxygen supply is a product of oxygen content of the blood and coronary blood flow. Myocardial oxygen demand increases with increasing heart rate, the contractile state of the heart, and ventricular wall tension [1]. Changes in heart rate and left ventricular end-diastolic pressure affect both oxygen supply and demand. An increasing heart rate increases the metabolic demand of the heart, yet at the same time reduces oxygen supply secondary to a shortened diastolic interval. Increasing left ventricular end-diastolic pressure (LVEDP) decreases endomyocardial coronary perfusion pressure thereby inhibiting oxygen supply. CCP—coronary perfusion pressure; CVR—coronary vascular resistance; DBP—diastolic blood pressure (*Modified from* Royster [2].)

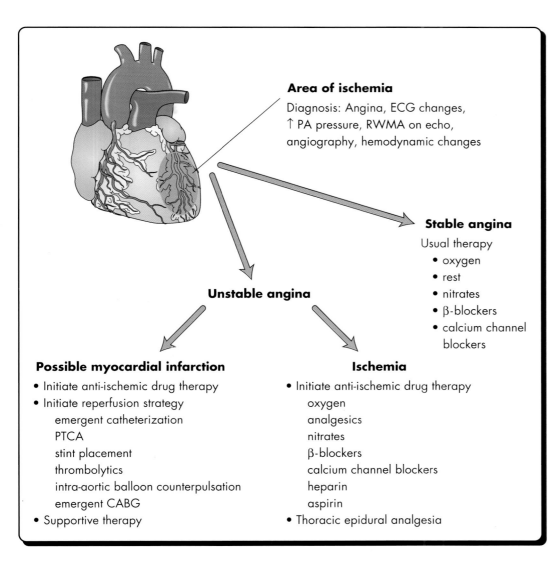

Area of ischemia

Diagnosis: Angina, ECG changes,
↑ PA pressure, RWMA on echo,
angiography, hemodynamic changes

Stable angina

Usual therapy
- oxygen
- rest
- nitrates
- β-blockers
- calcium channel
  blockers

Unstable angina

Possible myocardial infarction

- Initiate anti-ischemic drug therapy
- Initiate reperfusion strategy
  emergent catheterization
  PTCA
  stint placement
  thrombolytics
  intra-aortic balloon counterpulsation
  emergent CABG
- Supportive therapy

Ischemia

- Initiate anti-ischemic drug therapy
  oxygen
  analgesics
  nitrates
  β-blockers
  calcium channel blockers
  heparin
  aspirin
- Thoracic epidural analgesia

Figure 2-2. Therapy for acute myocardial ischemia. In an awake patient, ischemia is often heralded by the symptoms of angina. In the anesthetized patient, however, ischemia is manifest by changes in the electrocardiogram (ECG), increasing pulmonary artery (PA) pressures, regional wall motion abnormalities (RWMA), or other changes in hemodynamics. In cases of stable angina usual therapy includes supplemental oxygen, rest, and continuation of usual anti-ischemic medications such as nitrates, β-blockers, and calcium channel blockers. Unstable angina, however, requires more aggressive intervention. Possible myocardial infarction must be evaluated rapidly [3]. Early intervention may include angiography, percutaneous transluminal coronary angioplasty (PTCA), intra-aortic balloon counterpulsation, or emergent coronary artery bypass grafting (CABG). Treatment of unstable angina without infarction requires prompt pharmacologic intervention. Thoracic epidural anesthesia may provide relief in some patients with unremittent angina [4].

PHYSIOLOGIC EFFECTS OF INTRAVENOUS NITROGLYCERIN	
Decreased myocardial O_2 demand	**Enhanced myocardial O_2 supply**
Decreased preload, wall stress	Dilation of coronary arteries: epicardial vessels, eccentric stenosis, and collaterals
Decreased afterload, impedance	Decreased LVEDP enhances subendocardial flow
Decreased cardiac output decreases arterial pressure	Inhibition of coronary spasm or reduction of coronary vasomotor tone
	Decreased platelet aggregation

Figure 2-3. Physiologic effects of intravenous nitroglycerin. Nitroglycerin effectively works on both sides of the myocardial oxygen supply-demand equation. Nitroglycerin decreases myocardial oxygen demand by decreasing preload, thereby decreasing wall stress. Arterial vasodilation reduces afterload and ventricular impedance. There may be an associated decrease in cardiac output with lowering of arterial pressure. Myocardial oxygen supply is enhanced via coronary artery dilation. Left ventricular end-diastolic pressure (LVEDP) is decreased. Nitroglycerin decreases platelet aggregation in vitro [5]. It is unknown if this observed effect reduces the risk of thrombotic complications in patients with recurrent ischemia. (*Modified from* Thadani [6].)

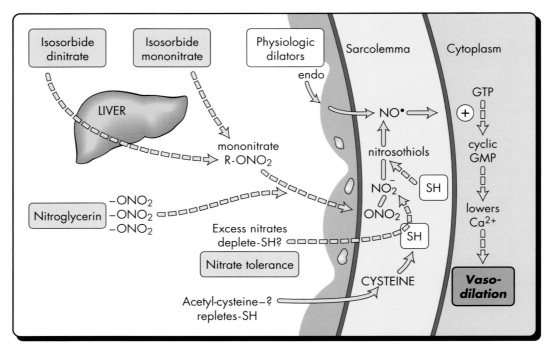

Figure 2-4. Nitrates for treatment of myocardial ischemia. Mechanisms of the effects of nitrates in the generation of nitric oxide (NO) and the stimulation of guanylate cyclase and cyclic guanosine monophosphate (cyclic GMP), which mediates vasodilation. Sulfhydryl (SH) groups are required for the formation of NO and the stimulation of guanylate cyclase. Isosorbide dinitrate is metabolized by the liver, whereas this route of metabolism is bypassed by the mononitrates. endo—endothelium; GTP—guanosine triphosphate; (*From* Opie [7].)

ORGANIC NITRATES AVAILABLE FOR CLINICAL USE

Nonproprietary Names and Trade Names	Chemical Structure	Preparations, Usual Doses, and Routes of Administration
Amyl nitrate (isoamyl nitrite)	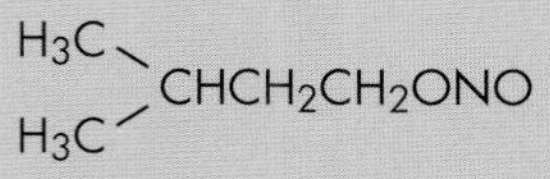 H_3C $CHCH_2CH_2ONO$ H_3C	Inh: 0.18 or 0.3 mL
Nitroglycerin (glyceryl trinitrate)	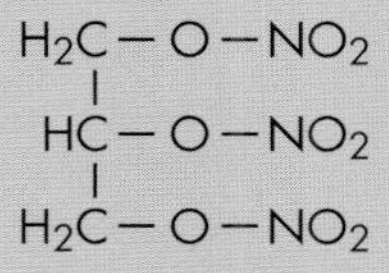 $H_2C-O-NO_2$ $HC-O-NO_2$ $H_2C-O-NO_2$	T: 0.15–0.6 mg as needed S: 0.4 mg per spray as needed C: 2.5–9 mg two to four times daily B: 1 mg every 3–5 h O: 1.25–5 cm (1/2 to 2 in), topically to skin every 4–8 h D: 1 disc (2.5–15 mg) every 24 h IV: 5 µg/min; increments of 5 µ/min
Isosorbide dinirtrate	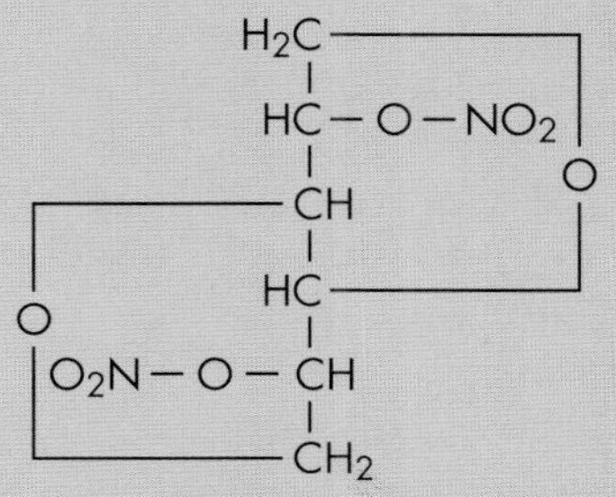 (structure)	T: 2.5–10 mg every 2–3 h T(C): 5–10 mg every 2–3 h T(O): 10–40 mg every 6 h C: 40–80 mg every 8–12 h
Isosorbide-5-mononitrate	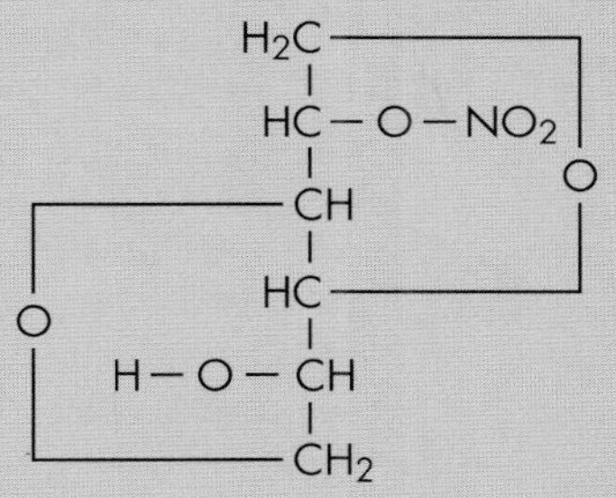 (structure)	T: 10–40 mg twice daily C: 60 mg daily
Erythrityl tetranitrate	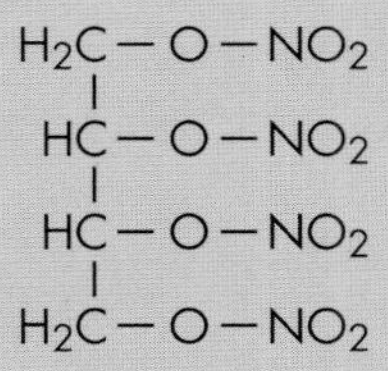 $H_2C-O-NO_2$ $HC-O-NO_2$ $HC-O-NO_2$ $H_2C-O-NO_2$	T: 5–10 mg as needed T(O): 10 mg three times daily

Figure 2-5. Organic nitrates available for clinical use. B—buccal (transmucosal tablet); C—sustained-release capsule or tablet; D—transdermal disc; Inh—inhalant; IV—intravenous injection; O—ointment; S—lingual spray; T—tablet for sublingual use; T(C)—chewable tablet; T(O)—oral tablet or capsule. (*From* Robertson and Robertson [8]; with permission.)

RECOMMENDATIONS FOR INTRAOPERATIVE NITROGLYCERIN

Class I*	High-risk patients previously on nitroglycerin who have active signs of myocardial ischemia without hypotension.
Class II†	As a prophylactic agent for high-risk patients to prevent myocardial ischemia and cardiac morbidity, particularly in those who have required nitrate therapy to control angina. The recommendation for prophylactic use of nitroglycerin must take into account the anesthetic plan and patient hemodynamics and must recognize that vasodilation and hypovolemia can readily occur during anesthesia and surgery.
Class III‡	Patients with signs of hypovolemia or hypotension.

* Conditions for which there is evidence for and/or general agreement that a procedure be performed or a treatment is of benefit.
† Conditions for which these is a divergence of evidence and/or opinion about the treatment.
‡ Conditions for which there is evidence and/or general agreement that the procedure is not necessary.

Figure 2-6. Recommendations for intraoperative nitroglycerin. Nitroglycerin is clearly indicated for the perioperative treatment of patients with active ischemia without hypotension. Nitroglycerin used as a prophylactic agent to prevent ischemia is less clear. Current literature both supports and refutes a beneficial effect of nitroglycerin in both cardiac and noncardiac surgical patients [9–12]. The American College of Cardiology and the American Heart Association have collaborated to provide guidelines for perioperative nitroglycerin administration, shown in the table. (*From* Eagle and coworkers [13]; with permission.)

β-ADRENERGIC BLOCKADE

EFFECTS OF β-ADRENERGIC BLOCKERS ON MYOCARDIAL ISCHEMIA

Reductions in myocardial oxygen consumption
Improvements in coronary blood flow
   Prolonged diastolic perfusion period
   Improved collateral flow
   Increased flow to ischemic areas
Overall improvement in supply/demand ratio
Stabilization of cellular membranes
Improved oxygen dissociation from hemoglobin
Inhibition of platelet aggregation
Reduced mortality after myocardial infarction

Figure 2-7. Effect of β-adrenergic blockers on myocardial ischemia. β-Adrenergic blockers reduce oxygen consumption by reducing heart rate, blood pressure, and myocardial contractility. Heart rate reduction also increases diastolic coronary blood flow thereby improving oxygen supply. Other important effects of β-blockade include activity as an antihypertensive agent, and its effects on cardiac rhythm and automaticity. The pulmonary system and the metabolic regulation of carbohydrates and lipids are affected. Platelet aggregation is inhibited with β-blockade [14]. (*From* Royster and Zvara [15]; with permission.)

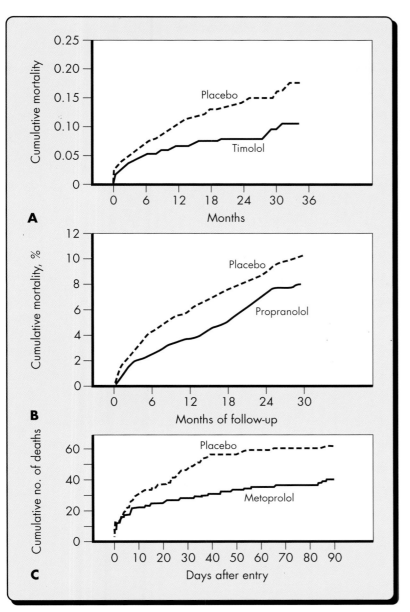

A

B

C

Figure 2-8. Blockade and postmyocardial infarction morbidity. A–C, Mortality following timolol, propranolol, and metoprolol, respecively. Patients with an evolving myocardial infarction should receive early intravenous β-adrenergic blocker therapy, followed by oral therapy, provided there are no contraindications to these medications [3]. β-Blocker therapy may immediately improve an ischemic condition by improving oxygen supply-demand ratios and result in a reduction in infarct size and rate of reinfarction in patients receiving thrombolytic therapy. Long-term β-blockade after infarction is associated with improved survival. Relative contraindications to β-blocker therapy include heart rate less than 60 beats/min, systolic blood pressure less than 100 mm Hg, moderate or severe left ventricular failure, signs of peripheral hypoperfusion, PR interval greater than 0.24 secs, second- or third-degree atrioventricular block, severe chronic obstructive pulmonary disease, history of asthma, severe peripheral vascular disease, or insulin-dependent diabetes mellitus. (*Modified from* Turi and Braunwald [16]; with permission.)

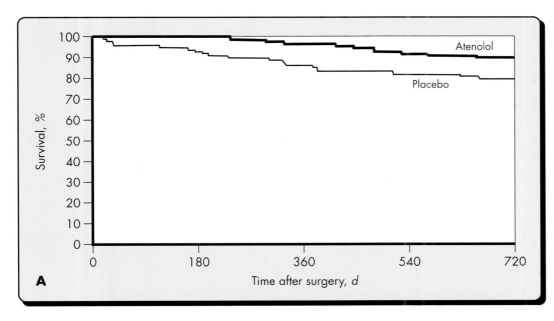

A

Figure 2-9. β-Blockade and mortality and cardiovascular morbidity after noncardiac surgery. Perioperative ischemia and nonfatal myocardial infarction increase the risk of serious cardiovascular outcomes in the 2 years after surgery [17–19]. Elevations in heart rate during the days after surgery may be associated with an increased number of ischemic events [20]. A perioperative course of β-blockade reduces heart rate and is associated with improved patient outcome up to 2 years after surgery. A, In a randomized, placebo controlled trial, perioperative atenolol administration reduced 2-year mortality and cardiovascular morbidity.

A, Overall survival in the 2 years after surgery among 192 patients in the two groups. The rate of survival at 6 months was 100% in the atenolol group and 92% in the placebo group (*P*<0.001); at 1 year the rates were 97% and 86% (*P* = 0.005); and at 2 years, survival rates were 90% and 79%, respectively (*P* = 0.019).

(*Continued on next page*)

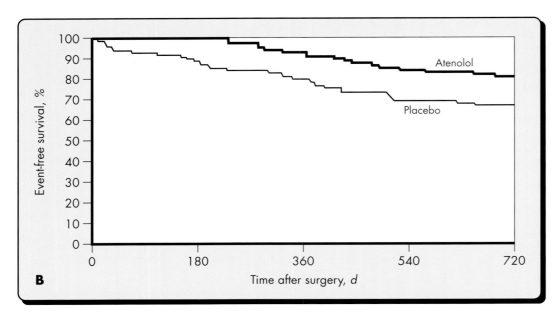

Figure 2-9. (*Continued*) B, Event-free survival in the 2 years after noncardiac surgery among 192 patients in the atenolol and placebo groups who survived to hospital discharge. The outcome measure combined the following events: myocardial infarction, unstable angina, the need for coronary artery bypass surgery, and congestive heart failure. The rate of event-free survival at 6 months (180 days) was 100% in the atenolol group and 88% in the placebo group (*P*<0.001); at 1 year (360 days), the rates were 92% and 78%, respectively (*P* = 0.003); and at 2 years (720 days), the rates were 83% and 68%, respectively (*P* = 0.008). (*From* Mangano and coworkers [21]; with permission.)

β-ADRENERGIC BLOCKERS: PHARMACOLOGIC PROFILE

Drug Name	ISA	Lipid solubility	Metabolism	Serum half-life, *h*	Intravenous + preparation (U.S.A.)	Dosage
Nonselective						
Propranolol	-	++	Hepatic	3–6	+	IV: 0.5–1 mg titrated Oral: 10–80 mg qid
Timolol	-	+	Hepatic, renal	4–6	-	Oral: 10–20 mg bid
Nadolol	-	-	Renal	16–24	-	Oral: 40–240 mg qd
Pindolol	+	+	Hepatic, renal	3–4	-	Oral: 5–60 mg bid
Labetalol	-	+	Hepatic	4–6	+	IV: 0.25–2 mg/kg Oral: 100–300 mg bid
Cardioselective						
Esmolol	-	-	Erythrocyte	9 min	+	IV: 0.5–1 mg/kg loading 50–300 µg/kg/min infusion
Metoprolol	-	+	Hepatic	3–4	+	IV:1–2 mg titrated Oral: 25–50 mg qid
Atenolol	-	-	Renal	6–9	-	Oral: 50–200 mg qd
Acebutolol	+	-	Hepatic, renal	8–12	-	Oral: 200–400 mg qd

Figure 2-10. β-Adrenergic blockers: pharmacologic profile. Several β-blockers (acebutolol, carteolol, celiprolol, penbutolol, and pindolol) have agonist as well as antagonist properties and are characterized as having intrinsic sympathomimetic activity (ISA). Propranolol is the most lipid-soluble β-blocker and generally has the most central nervous system side effects. First-pass liver metabolism is very high with propranolol, approximately 90%. Because of the high hepatic extraction of propranolol, factors that affect hepatic blood flow markedly affect propranolol plasma levels. In contrast, esmolol, a cardioselective β-blocker, undergoes a rapid hydrolysis by erythrocyte esterases resulting in a half-life of 9 minutes. Esmolol produces significant reductions in blood pressure, heart rate, and cardiac index after a loading dose of 500 µg/kg and an infusion of 300 µg/kg/min in patient with coronary artery disease; however, the effects are completely reversed within 30 minutes after discontinuation of the infusion [22]. Labetalol provides selective α_1-receptor blockade and nonselective β_1- and β_2-blockade. The potency of β-adrenergic blockade is 5- to 10-fold greater than α_1-adrenergic blockade. In contrast to other β-blockers, labetalol can be considered a peripheral vasodilator that does not cause reflex tachycardia. Metoprolol is an intravenous (IV) β_1-selective agent often used for heart rate control perioperatively. Sudden withdrawal of β-adrenergic blockade may be associated with an imbalance of the sympathetic nervous system resulting in enhanced adrenergic activity. Such a condition may result in tachycardia, hypertension, arrhythmias, myocardial ischemia, and infarction. This period of hypersensitivity may occur from 2 to 6 days after withdrawal of β-blockade.

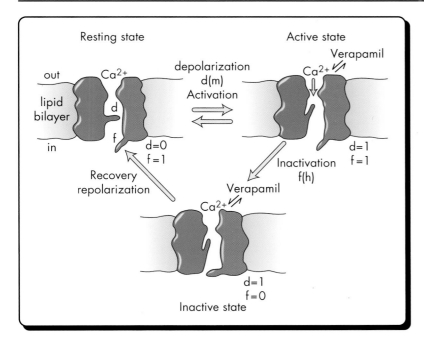

Figure 2-11. Physiology of the calcium channel. In the resting state the d(m) gate (activation gate) is closed and the f(h) gate (inactivation gate) is open (d = 0, f = 1). Depolarization to the threshold activates the slow channel to the active state, the d gate opening rapidly and the f gate still being open (d = 1; f = 1). The activated channel spontaneously inactivates to the inactive state due to closure of the f gate (d = 1; f = 0). The recovery process after repolarization returns the channel from the inactive state back to the resting state, and the channel is again available for reactivation. Also depicted is the possible binding of verapamil to the outer mouth of the slow channel in the active state channel or slowing the recovery process for converting from the inactive state back to the resting state. (*Modified from* Sperelakis [23,24]; with permission.)

CARDIOVASCULAR EFFECTS OF CALCIUM ANTAGONISTS

Effects	Diltiazem	Verapamil	Dihydropyridines	Bepridil
Coronary vasodilation	↑	↑	↑	↑
Systemic vasodilation	↑	↑	↑↑	↑
Myocardial contraction	↓	↓↓	0 or ↓	0 or ↓
Myocardial oxygen demand	↓	↓	↓	↓
Heart rate	↓↓	↓	0 or ↑	↓
Atrioventricular nodal conduction	↓	↓↓	0	0 or ↓

↑—increase; ↓—decrease; 0—no effect.

Figure 2-12. Cardiovascular effects of calcium antagonists. Calcium channels exist in cardiac muscles, smooth muscles, and probably many other cellular membranes. These channels are also present in cellular organelle membranes such as the sarcoplasmic reticulum and mitochondria. Calcium functions as a generator of the cardiac action potential and an intracellular second messenger to regulate intracellular events. Calcium channel blockers interact with the L-type calcium channel and include drugs from four different classes: 1) the 1,4-dihydropyridine derivatives represented by nifedipine, nimodipine, nicardipine, isradipine, amlodipine, and felodipine; 2) the phenylalkyl amines represented by verapamil; 3) the benzothiazepines represented by diltiazem; and 4) a diarylaminopropylamine ether, bepridil. Bepridil is a newer calcium channel blocker with antianginal, antihypertensive, and type 1 arrhythmic properties. Bepridil has a marked effect on myocardial conduction and is contraindicated in patients with a history of serious ventricular arrhythmias, sick sinus syndrome, second- or third-degree atrioventricular block, and patients with congenital prolonged QT interval. (*From* Weiner [25].)

THERAPEUTIC APPLICATIONS OF CALCIUM CHANNEL BLOCKERS

Established clinical indications

Ischemic myocardial syndromes
Prinzmetal's angina
Unstable angina
Chronic stable angina
Cardiac arrhythmias
Hypertension and hypertensive emergencies
Hypertrophic cardiomyopathies

Potential indications

Cardioprotection
Pulmonary hypertension and afterload reduction
Migraine and cluster headaches
Cerebral insufficiency and vasospasm
Raynaud's phenomenon
Disorders of gastrointestinal motility
Exercise-induced bronchospasm
Prevention of atherosclerosis

Figure 2-13. Therapeutic applications of calcium channel blockers. Calcium channel blockers reduce myocardial oxygen demand by decreasing contractility, heart rate, and arterial blood pressure. Myocardial oxygen supply may be improved by dilation of coronary and collateral vessels. All calcium channel blockers are effective at reversing coronary spasm, reducing ischemic episodes, and reducing nitroglycerin consumption in patients with variant, or Prinzmetal's, angina. Caution must be extended when dihydropyridines are used during initial therapy for myocardial ischemia. The dihydropyridines may cause reflex tachycardia and may exacerbate anginal symptoms. Significant adverse effects associated with calcium channel blockers include adverse or exaggerated hemodynamic effects related to the arterial vasodilation, as well as negative inotropy, chronotropy, and dromotropy. Hypotension, heart failure, bradycardia, asystole, and atrioventricular nodal block have all been reported with calcium channel blocker use. (*From* Singh and coworkers [26].)

A. PHARMACOKINETICS OF CALCIUM ANTAGONISTS USED COMMONLY FOR ANGINA PECTORIS*

Parameter	Diltiazem	Nicardipine	Nifedipine	Nifedipine GITS
Usual adult dose	IV: 0.25 mg/kg bolus then 0.15 mg/kg/h Oral: 30–90 mg tid or qid	IV: 10–15 mg/h for 30 min then 3–5 mg/h Oral: 20–30 mg tid	SL: 10–30 mg tid or qid Oral: 10–30 mg tid or qid	Oral: 30–60 mg daily
Extent of absorption (%)	80–90	100	90	> 90
Extent of bioavailability (% of dose)	40–70	30	65–75	45–75
Onset of action	Oral: <15 min	< 20 min	SL: < 3 min Oral: < 20 min	≈ 6 h
Peak effect	Oral: 30 min	1 h	Oral: 1–2 h	After 6 h
Therapeutic serum levels (ng/mL)	50–200	30–50	25–100	25–100
Elimination half–life (h)	3.5–6.0	2.0–4.0	2.0–5.0	2.0–5.0
Elimination	60% metabolized by liver; remainder excreted by kidneys	High first-pass hepatic metabolism	High first-pass hepatic metabolism	High first-pass hepatic metabolism
Heart rate	↓	↑	↑↑	↑
Peripheral vascular resistance	↓	↓	↓↓	↓↓
FDA-approved indications				
Hypertension	Yes	Yes	Yes	Yes
Angina	Yes	Yes	Yes	Yes
Coronary spasm	Yes	No	Yes	Yes

Figure 2-14. Pharmacokinetics of calcium antagonists commonly used for angina pectoris (**A** and **B**). FDA—Food and Drug Administration; GITS—gastrointestinal therapeutic system; IV—intravenous; SL—sublingual. (*From* Gersh and coworkers [27]; with permission.)

(*Continued on next page*)

B. PHARMACOKINETICS OF CALCIUM ANTAGONISTS USED COMMONLY FOR ANGINA PECTORIS*

	Verapamil	Amlodipine	Felodipine	Isradipine	Bepridil
Usual adult dose	IV: 0.075 to 0.015 mg/kg Oral: 80–120 mg tid or qid	2.5–10 mg qd	5–20 mg qd	2.5–5.0 mg bid	200–400 mg qd
Extent of absorption (%)	90	> 90	> 90	> 90	> 90
Extent of bioavailability (% of dose)	20–35	60–65	20	15–24	> 80
Onset of action	IV: 2 min Oral: 2 h	1–2 h	2 h	20 min	2–3 h
Peak effect	IV: 3–5 min Oral: 3–4 h	6–12 h	2–5 h	1.5 h	8 h
Therapeutic serum levels (ng/mL)	80–300	5–20	1–5	2–10	500–2000
Elimination half–life (h)	3.0–7.0[†]	30–50	9	8	26–64
Elimination	85% eliminated by first-pass hepatic metabolism	Hepatic	High first-pass hepatic metabolism	High first-pass hepatic metabolism	Hepatic
Heart rate	↓	0	↑	0	↓
Peripheral vascular resistance	↓	↓↓↓	↓↓↓	↓↓↓	↓
FDA-approved indications					
Hypertension	Yes	Yes	Yes	Yes	Yes
Angina	Yes	Yes	No	No	Yes
Coronary spasm	Yes	Yes	No	No	No

* All agents approved by FDA for treatment of angina pectoris.
† 4.5–12 h with multiple dosing.

Figure 2-14. (*Continued*)

GENERAL PRINCIPLES OF PERIOPERATIVE CARDIAC FAILURE

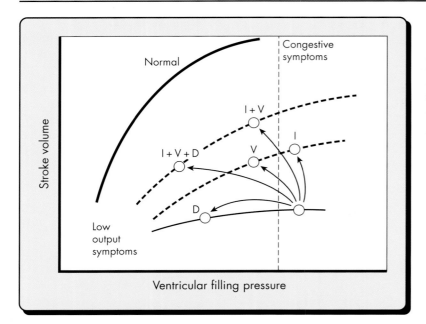

Figure 2-15. Response to pharmacologic intervention in heart failure. The relationships between diastolic filling pressure (or preload) and cardiac output (ventricular performance) are illustrated for a normal heart (*uppermost tracing*) and for a patient with heart failure (*lowermost tracing*). When a patient starts in a low-output syndrome with congestive symptoms, inotropic agents, vasodilators, and diuretics can be used to move the patient to a more desirable physiologic state. D—diuretic; I—inotropic agent; V—vasodilation. (*From* Kelly and Smith [28]; with permission.)

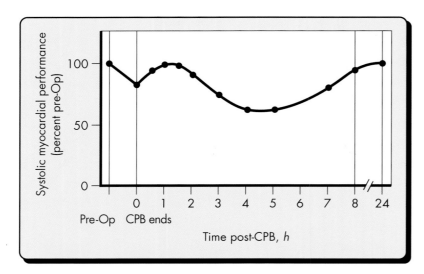

Figure 2-16. Myocardial performance after cardiopulmonary bypass (CPB). Myocardial performance after cardiopulmonary bypass is a dynamic phenomenon. The heart is recovering from a period of ischemic diastolic arrest, hypothermia, surgical trauma, and potential reperfusion injury. Cardiac index, mean arterial pressure, right ventricular ejection fraction, and left ventricular ejection fraction initially decrease soon after separation from CPB reaching a nadir at approximately 5 hours later. With the exception of mean arterial pressure, these values subsequently rise over the next several hours [29]. This plot illustrates the changing requirements for post-CPB cardiovascular support.

FACTORS THAT PREDICT THE USE OF INOTROPIC DRUG SUPPORT AFTER CPB	
Variable	*P* value
Low ejection fraction	0.002
Long duration of bypass	0.004
Older age	0.005
Longer duration of aortic cross-clamping	0.009
Cardiac enlargement	0.021
Female sex	0.027

Figure 2-17. Factors that predict the use of inotropic drug support after cardiopulmonary bypass (CPB). Inotropic support is common after CPB. In a recent study, various preoperative and intraoperative factors associated with the use of inotropes were analyzed by logistic regression. The overall incidence of inotropic support in patients with ejection fraction less than 0.55 was approximately 60% to 70% [30].

CARDIAC GLYCOSIDES: DIGOXIN

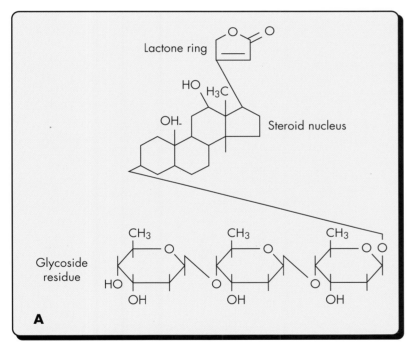

A

Figure 2-18. Digoxin. Digoxin is one of the most widely prescribed cardiac glycosides [31]. The actions of digitalis glycosides on the heart can be separated into two major areas: 1) a positive inotrope action in the failing heart, and 2) a profound effect on the myocardial conduction system. **A,** The chemical structure of digoxin demonstrates a steroid nucleus containing an unsaturated lactone at the C17 position and one or more glycosidic residues at C3.

(Continued on next page)

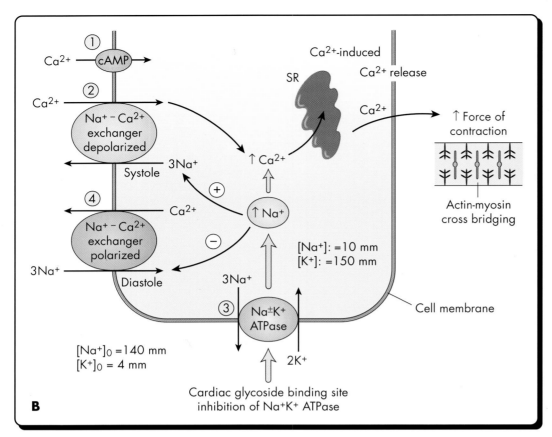

Figure 2-18. (*Continued*) B, Mechanism of action. During depolarization, both sodium and calcium rapidly enter the myocardial cell. Calcium enters by cyclic adenosine monophosphate (cAMP)-dependent L-type channels (*1* and by reversal of cation transport in the sodium-calcium exchanger (*2*). Restoration of the resting cell ionic balance requires active transport of these ions against electrical gradients (*3* and *4*). The energy for this process is controlled to some degree by adenosine triphosphatase (ATP-ase). Cardiac glycosides inhibit the sodium potassium ATP-ase (*3*). Calcium balance is maintained by the sodium-calcium exchanger (*4*). However, when there is a high concentration of intracellular sodium, there is an inhibition of the sodium-intracellular calcium exchanger during the resting state, resulting in an increase of intracellular calcium. The intracellular calcium exchangeable pool increases, and the calcium is available for uptake into the sarcoplasmic reticulum (SR), and myocardial contractility increases.

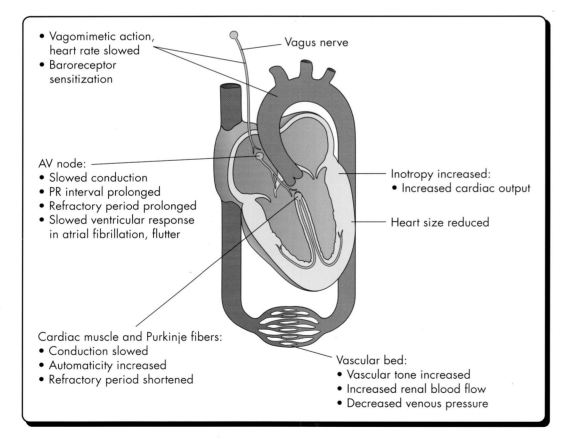

Figure 2-19. Physiologic action of digitalis glycosides. Digitalis glycosides have an effect on myocardial performance that is dose related up to serum digoxin levels of 1.5 ng/mL. There is both a direct action on cardiac muscle and the specialized conduction system, and indirect actions on the cardiovascular system as mediated by the autonomic nervous system. There are three primary actions: 1) an increase in the force and velocity of myocardial systolic contraction; 2) a negative chronotropic effect; and 3) a decreased conduction velocity through the atrioventricular (AV) node. These actions lead to the two main therapeutic uses of digitalis glycosides: the treatment of chronic congestive heart failure and the treatment of ventricular rate in atrial fibrillation. (*Modified from* Netter [32].)

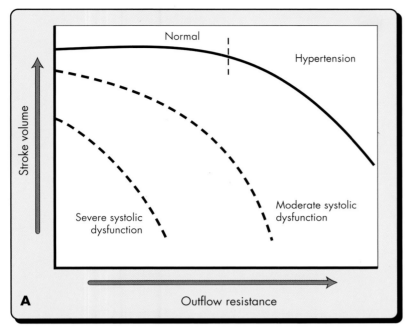

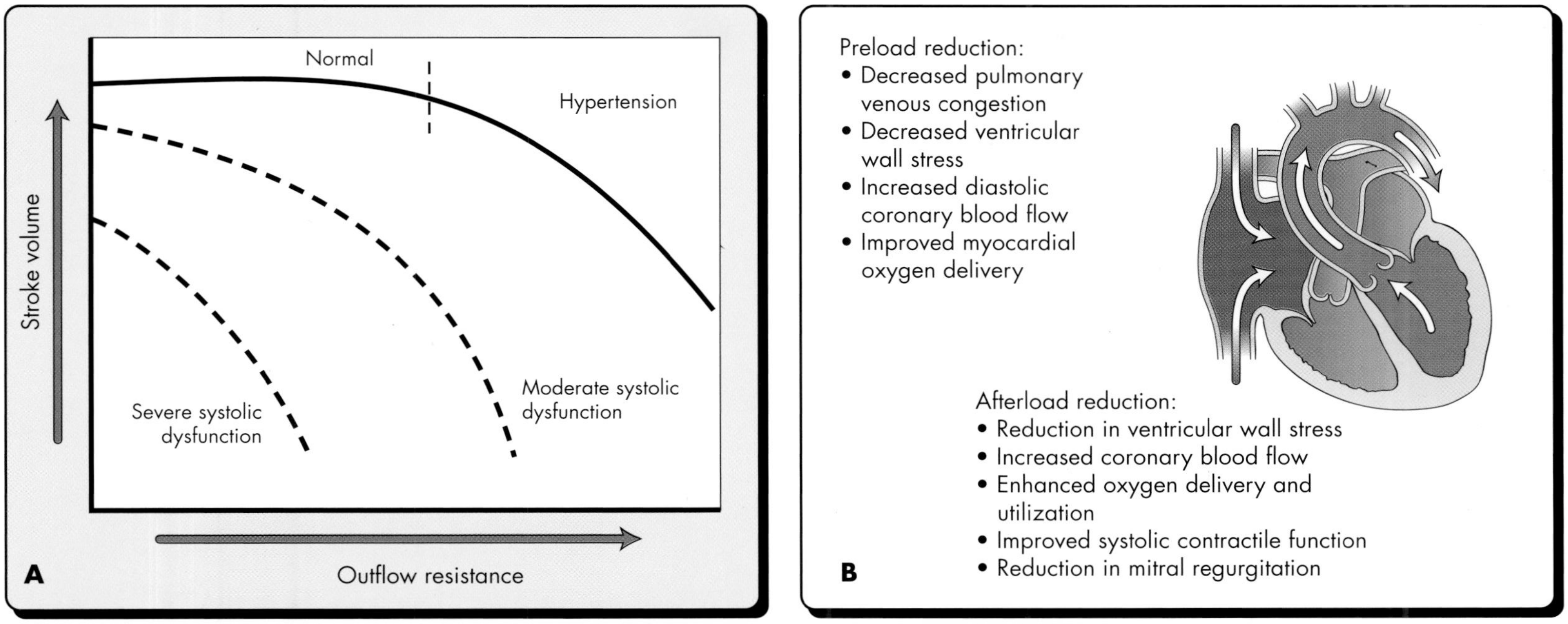

Preload reduction:
- Decreased pulmonary venous congestion
- Decreased ventricular wall stress
- Increased diastolic coronary blood flow
- Improved myocardial oxygen delivery

Afterload reduction:
- Reduction in ventricular wall stress
- Increased coronary blood flow
- Enhanced oxygen delivery and utilization
- Improved systolic contractile function
- Reduction in mitral regurgitation

Panel A axis labels: Stroke volume (y-axis), Outflow resistance (x-axis), with curves labeled Normal, Hypertension, Moderate systolic dysfunction, Severe systolic dysfunction.

A

B

Figure 2-20. Principles of vasodilator therapy. **A,** In normal patients there is little influence of ventricular outflow resistance on stroke volume. In hypertensive patients, however, there is some reduction in stroke volume as ventricular outflow resistance achieves very high levels. In contrast, in patients with both moderate and severe systolic ventricular function, stroke volume is greatly influenced by outflow resistance (afterload). Arterial vasodilators reduce outflow resistance and result in improved myocardial performance. This increase in stroke volume may offset a reduction in arterial systolic blood pressure that is seen with arterial vasodilation. Perfusion to vital organs and extremities may be improved with the improved myocardial performance. **B,** Vasodilator therapy is associated with a reduction in mortality in patients with congestive heart failure [33–35]. In early congestive heart failure, the heart compensates for reductions in contractile function by an increase in heart rate and by increases in intravascular volume and pressure. The net result is improvement of myocardial performance versus preload. As heart failure worsens, further increases in heart rate and intravascular volume lose effectiveness. At this point, symptoms of congestive heart failure are seen. Although vasodilators are frequently divided into arterial and venous vasodilators, most agents have a mixed pharmacologic profile. Preload reduction may be achieved by decreasing in intravascular volume (*eg,* diuretics) or by increasing venous capacitance (*eg,* venodilators). Preload reduction may result in decreased pulmonary venous congestion, decreased ventricular wall stress, increased diastolic coronary blood flow secondary to the reduced intraventricular pressures, and improved myocardial oxygen delivery. Afterload reduction improves hemodynamics in patients with congestive heart failure. There is a reduction in ventricular wall stress which leads to improvements in both oxygen supply and demand. Increases occur in coronary blood flow secondary to the decreases in left ventricular end-diastolic pressure. Mechanics of myocardial contraction are improved. (Panel A *adapted from* Cohn and Franciosa [33]; with permission.)

VASODILATOR DRUGS USED IN THE TREATMENT OF HEART FAILURE

Drug	Mechanism	Preload Reduction	Afterload Reduction	Usual Dose
Renin-angiotensin system antagonists				
Captopril	Inhibition of renal systemic and tissue generation of angiotensin II by ACE; decreased metabolism of bradykinin	++	++	6.25–50 mg po q8h
Enalapril		++	++	2.5–10 mg po q12h
Enalaprilat				0.5–2.0 mg IV q12h
Quinapril		++	++	10–80 mg po qd
Lisinopril		++	++	2.5–20 mg po q12–24h
Ramipril		++	++	1.25–5 mg po qd
Losartan	Blockade of angiotensin II (AT$_1$) receptors	++	++	25–50 mg q12h
Nitrovasodilators				
Nitroglycerin	Nitric oxide donors	+++	+	0.2–10 µg/kg/min IV
Isosorbide Dinitrate		+++	+	5–6 mg transdermal 10–60 mg qid
Nitroprusside		+++	+++	0.1–3 µg/kg/min IV
Direct vasodilators				
Hydralazine	Unclear	+	+++	10–100 po q6h
Nicorandil	Increased K$^+$ channel conductance and other mechanisms	++	+++	10–40 mg bid
Minoxidil		+	+++	5–10 mg qd
Diazoxide		+	+++	1–3 mg/kg q4–24h
Calcium channel blocking drugs				
Nifedipine	Inhibition of L-type voltage-sensitive Ca^{2+} channels	+	+++	10–30 mg po tid
Amiodipine		+	+++	5–10 mg po qd
Felodipine		+	+++	5–10 mg po qd
Phosphodiesterase inhibitors				
Amrinone	Inhibition of type III cAMP phosphodiesterase(s) and other mechanisms	++	++	0.5 mg/kg, then 2–10 µg/kg/min IV
Milrinone		++	++	50 µg/kg, then 0.25–1 µg/kg/min IV
Vesnarinone				60 mg qd
Sympathomimetics				
Dobutamine	Myocardial and vascular β-adrenergic agonist	+	++	2–20 µg/kg/min
Dopamine	Selective renal arterial vasodilation	-	--	≤ 2 µg/kg/min
Sympatholytics				
Prazosine (and other quinazoline derivatives)	α-Adrenergic receptor antagonist	+++	++	1–5 mg po q12h
Phentolamine	Nonselective α-adrenergic blockade	++	++	0.5–1.0 mg/min IV
Labetalol	β-Adrenergic and α$_1$-adrenergic blockade	+	++	100–400 mg bid po
Carvedilol	Additional mechanisms	+	++	12.5–50 mg po bid
Bucindolol*		+	++	Not determined

* Investigational and not approved by the US Food and Drug Administration at the time of this writing.

Figure 2-21. Vasodilator drugs used in the treatment of heart failure. ACE—angiotensin converting enzyme; cAMP—cyclic adenosine monophosphate; IV—intravenous. +—relative agonist effect; -—relative inhibition. (*Adapted from* Kelly and Smith [36]; with permission.)

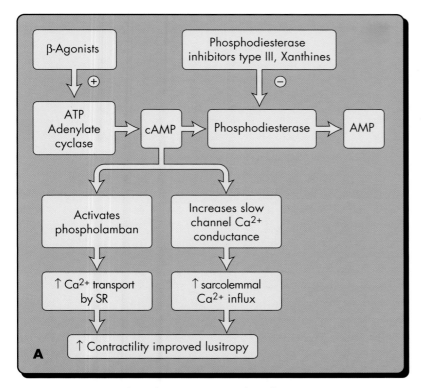

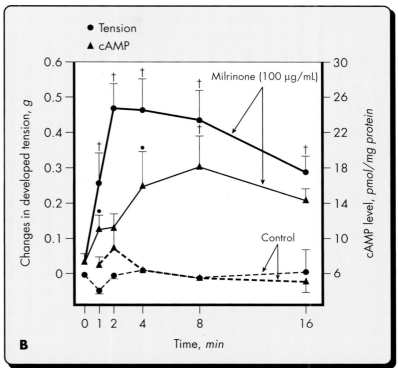

Figure 2-22. Cyclic adenosine monophosphate (cAMP). **A,** cAMP is an important component of the energy requiring processes of myocardial performance, specifically inotropy and energy-dependent diastolic relaxation (lusitropy). cAMP may be increased by direct action from β-agonists, or by inhibition of phosphodiesterase. The cAMP increases the conduction of calcium through voltage-dependent channels during depolarization. There is an inward shift of calcium resulting in increases in intracellular calcium levels and increased calcium release from the sarcoplasmic reticulum (SR) increasing contractility. cAMP also activates a phospholamban, one of the regulatory proteins of the sarcoplasmic reticulum. Activation of phospholamban increases the calcium reuptake into the SR, reducing intracellular ionized calcium [Ca^{2+}]$_i$, and returning the cell to the resting state. This intracellular calcium cycling results in improved energy-dependent diastolic relaxation seen when phosphodiesterase-inhibiting (PDE-I) agents are given. **B,** Studies in animals have demonstrated a link between cAMP levels and developed tension of myocardial contractility. Milrinone is a PDE-I that causes a significant rise in cAMP over a time course comparable to the development of increased muscle tension in isolated guinea pig papillary muscle. Further proof of this mechanism lies in the fact that carbachol, a muscarinic antagonist that acts to inhibit adenylyl cyclase, the enzyme for production of myocardial cAMP, reverses milrinone's effects [37]. These findings support the hypothesis of muscle contraction being mediated by intracellular cAMP mechanisms. AMP—adenosine monophosphate; ATP—adenosine triphosphate. (Panel A *modified from* Grossman [38]; with permission; panel B *from* Alousi and coworkers [39]; with permission.)

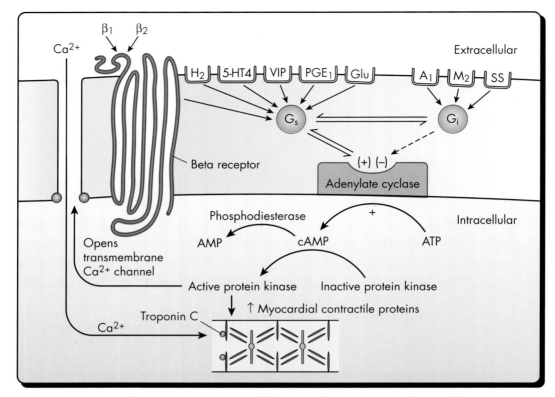

Figure 2-23. β-Adrenergic receptors. In the human heart, contractility and heart rate are regulated by numerous receptor systems all acting on the generation of cyclic adenosine monophosphate (cAMP). This generation of cAMP comes about via stimulation of G protein–mediated activity within the cell membrane. There are two G proteins, one of which is stimulatory (G_s) and one inhibitory (G_i). β-Receptor stimulation accounts for the greatest contribution of G protein–mediated cAMP generation and resultant improvements in contractility and heart rate. β-Receptor numbers in any tissue may decrease with chronic stimulation (down-regulation) or increase with chronic blockade (up-regulation). An example of chronic stimulation is chronic congestive heart failure [40]. Stimulation of the β-receptor causes dramatic interaction in the G_s and G_i regulatory proteins. These alterations result in stimulation of adenylate cyclase, which promotes the production of cAMP intracellularly. cAMP in turn activates protein kinases, which open energy dependent, receptor-operated calcium channels allowing calcium entry into the cell. This calcium becomes available for sequestration into the sarcoplasmic reticulum as well as release of calcium allowing binding to troponin C and subsequent activation of the actin-myosin complex. A_1—adenosine A_1 receptors; AMP—adenosine monophosphate; ATP—adenosine triphosphate; $β_1,β_2$—*beta$_1$- and $β_2$-adrenergic receptors; Ca^{2+}—calcium; G_1—inhibitory guanine nucleotide binding proteins; G_s—stimulatory guanine nucleotide binding proteins; Glu—glucagon receptors; H_2—histamine receptors; 5-HT$_4$—5-hydroxytryptamine type 4 receptors; M_2—muscarinic M_2 receptors; PGE$_1$prostaglandin E$_1$ receptors; SS—somatostatin receptors; VIP—vasoactive intestinal peptide receptors; +—activation; —inhibition. (*Modified from* Brodde and coworkers [41]; with permission.)

PHYSIOLOGIC EFFECTS OF β_1 AND β_2 RECEPTOR STIMULATION

Physiologic Effect	β_1 Response	β_2 Response
Cardiac		
Increased heart rate	++	++
Increased contractility		
Atrium	+	++
Ventricle	++	++
Increased automaticity and conduction velocity		
Nodal tissue	++	++
His-Purkinje	++	++
Arterial relaxation		
Coronary		++
Skeletal muscle		++
Pulmonary		+
Abdominal		+
Renal	+	+
Venous relaxation		++
Smooth muscle relaxation		
Tracheal and bronchial		+
Gastrointestinal		+
Bladder		+
Uterus		+
Splenic capsule		+
Ciliary muscle		+
Metabolic renin release	++	
Lipolysis	++	+
Insulin secretion		+
Glycogenolysis, gluconeogenesis		++
Cellular K^+ uptake		+
ADH secretion (pituitary)	+	

Figure 2-24. Physiologic effects of β_1- and β_2-receptor stimulation. There are three types of β-receptors identified in human cellular membranes. β-Receptors were originally classified into β_1- and β_2-receptors by Lands in 1967 [42]. In 1983 Tan *et al.* [43] postulated the existence of an atypical β-adrenergic receptor in rat adipose tissues and this subsequently has been classified into the β_3-receptor. In the human heart β_1 and β_2 receptors coexist. There is no evidence that β_3-receptors are present in the human heart [44]. In the right and left atria β_1- and β_2-receptor stimulation can lead to maximum positive inotropic effects, whereas in the right and left ventricles only β_1 receptor stimulation causes maximum positive inotropic effects [45,46]. In vivo experiments confirm that β_2-receptors can contribute to positive chronotropic and inotropic effects of β-receptor agonists [47]. β_3-receptor stimulation is associated with thermogenesis and carbohydrated fat metabolism. ADH—antidiuretic hormone. (*Modified from* Lefkowitz and coworkers [48].) +—presence of effect; ++—strong presence of effect.

PHARMACODYNAMIC EFFECTS OF EPINEPHRINE, NOREPINEPHRINE, AND ISOPROTERENOL

Agent	Receptor affinity	Physiologic action	Absorption, Fate, Excretion	Adverse effects	Indications	Dosage
Epinephrine	β_1 +++ β_2 ++ α_1 +++	Increases inotropy, ↑ heart rate, shortened systolic period, ↑ MVO_2, ↑CO Potent vasopressor Central redistribution of blood flow; cutaneous and renal vasoconstriction Bronchial muscle relaxation ↑ Glucose availability and uptake, ↑ free fatty acids, lactate in blood, ↑ K^+ Accelerates blood coagulation	Hepatic metabolism by COMT and MAO IV, aerosol, subcutaneous	Restlessness, tremor, dizziness, palpitations Arrhythmias Cerebral hemorrhage	Bronchospasm Cardiac arrest, resuscitation Low-output syndromes Local vasoconstriction	SQ: 0.3–0.5 mg IV bolus: 0.01 mg/kg–1 mg Infusion: 20–100 ng/kg/min
Norepinephrine	β_1 +++ β_2 0 α_1 +++	Cardiac output unchanged or decreased ↑ Total peripheral resistance Compensatory vagal reflex may slow heart rate ↓ Mesenteric, hepatic, renal blood flow ↑ Glucose levels	Same as epinephrine Norepinephrine constitutes 10% to 20% of catecholamines in adrenal medulla; and as much as 97% in pheochromocytomas IV, subcutaneous	Similar to epinephrine Severe hypertension Profound vasoconstriction and reduced blood flow	Blood pressure control during certain acute hypotensive states (ie, spinal anesthesia, sympathectomy, myocardial infarction, septicemia, drug reactions, blood transfusion reaction) Adjunct to other drugs or cardiac arrest, profound hypotension	Infusion: 10–50 ng/kg/min
Isoproterenol	β_1 +++ β_2 +++ α_1 —	↑ Heart rate, ↑ inotropy, ↑ cardiac output ↓ Peripheral vascular resistance, ↓ diastolic blood pressure Smooth muscle relaxation Relief of bronchoconstriction Insulin secretion stimulated Free fatty acid release	COMT Parenteral aerosol, IV, or subcutaneous	Palpatations, tachycardia, headache, flushed skin Cardiac ischemia, arrhythmias in patients with coronary artery disease	Heart block Cardiac arrest Bronchospasm Adjunct to fluid, other therapy for treatment of hypovolemia and septic shock, low-cardiac-output syndrome, CHF, cardiogenic shock	Bolus: 0.02–0.06 mg Infusion: 0.5–5 µg/min

Figure 2-25. Pharmacodynamic effects of epinephrine, norepinephrine, and isoproterenol on the heart. Epinephrine and norepinephrine are endogenous catecholamines and both are potent β- and α-receptor stimulants. Isoproterenol is a synthetic catecholamine with strong β-adrenergic action and little α-receptor agonism. These drugs are primarily indicated for support of the acutely compromised cardiovascular system. Epinephrine acts directly as a β_1-receptor stimulant increasing heart rate and myocardial contractility.

Norepinephrine is a chemical mediator stored in postganglionic adrenergic nerve cells. Cardiac output is unchanged or may be decreased and total peripheral resistance is elevated with norepinephrine administration. Blood pressure will rise. Blood flow may be reduced in the kidney, liver, and skeletal muscle. Coronary blood flow, however, may be enhanced by two mechanisms: 1) coronary vasodila-tion by direct adrenergic receptor stimulation, and 2) increases in coronary perfusion pressure secondary to elevated central aortic blood pressure. Norepinephrine is not associated with vasodilation of skeletal muscle bed. Isoproterenol is a potent nonselective β-adrenergic agonist with no α-agonist properties. Isoproterenol has profound β_2-effects on skeletal muscle resulting in vasodilation and lowering of peripheral vascular resistance in the vascular beds. Diastolic pressure typically falls and systolic pressure remains unchanged or may rise. Cardiac output is increased by positive inotropic and chronotropic effects. Isoproterenol has a profound effect on heart rate and is indicated in patients with bradycardia or heart block. CHF—congestive heart failure; CO—cardiac output; COMT—catechol-O-methyltransferase; IV—intravenous; MAO—monoamine oxidase; MVO_2—myocardial oxygen consumption; SQ—subcutaneous.

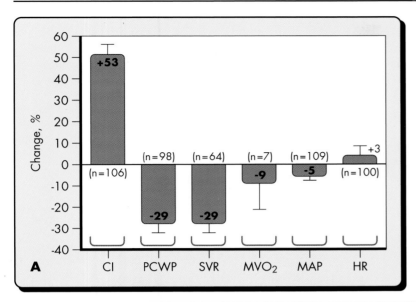

Figure 2-26. Physiologic effects of phosphodiesterase inhibitors. Phosphodiesterase inhibitors have multiple effects on cardiovascular physiology that are beneficial to patients with acute or chronic heart failure. Phosphodiesterase inhibitors increase myocardial contractility, increase lusitropy, and have vasodilating properties that reduce impedance to ventricular ejection. There may also be a reduction in ventricular wall stress, and reduced filling pressures with phosphodiesterase inhibiting agents. **A,** Several hemodynamic parameters are observed following the intravenous administration of amrinone to patients with heart failure. There is an overall improvement in cardiac index (CI) with associated reductions in pulmonary capillary wedge pressure (PCWP), systemic vascular resistance (SVR), myocardial oxygen consumption (MVO_2), and mean arterial pressure (MAP). There is little to no effect on heart rate (HR) [49]. **B,** Phosphodiesterase inhibiting agents are positive inotropic agents with vasodilator activity that is different in structure and mode of action from either digitalis glycosides or catecholamines. Milrinone is approximately 10-fold more potent than amrinone and the typical loading dose is 50 µg/kg administered over 10 minutes with an infusion rate ranging from 0.25 to 1.0 µg/kg/min. Amrinone is administered by an intravenous (IV) loading dose of 0.5 to 0.75 mg/kg given over 2 to 3 minutes followed by an infusion of 2 to 10 µg/kg/min. The drugs are contraindicated in patients who demonstrate hypersensitivity or who are known to be hypersensitive to bisulfites. Amrinone is associated with clinically significant thrombocytopenia in about 10% of patients, whereas thrombocytopenia is rare with milrinone. In some patients, milrinone may increase ventricular ectopy, including nonsustained ventricular tachycardia. CHF—congestive heart failure.

B. PHARMACOLOGY OF AMRINONE AND MILRINONE

Variable measured	Amrinone (IV)	Milrinone (IV)
Loading dose, mg/kg (per approved product labeling)	1.5 (0.72 × 2)	0.050
Loading dose (maximally effective)	3.0	0.075
Infusion rate, µg/kg/min (labeling)	5–10	0.375–0.75
Incompatible with dextrose solutions	Yes	No
Average half-life in CHF patients (h)	5–8	2–3
Incidence of thrombocytopenia	2.6%	0.4%
Incidence of ventricular tachycardia/fibrillation	0.8%	3.6%

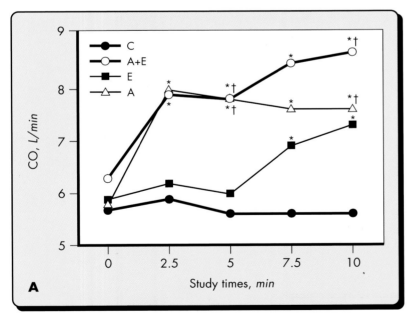

Figure 2-27. Benefits of combined β-agonist and phosphodiesterase inhibitor-agonist and (PDE-I) therapy. β-Adrenergic agonists and phosphodiesterase inhibiting agents may provide beneficial effects when administered together. **A,** These two agents work via different mechanisms; however, both result in enhanced intracellular levels of cyclic adenosine monophosphate. Amrinone (A) and epinephrine (E) improve overall cardiovascular performance in patients after cardiopulmonary bypass. Amrinone 0.5 mg/kg was found to be as effective as epinephrine 30 ng/kg/min at improving myocardial function after separation from cardiopulmonary bypass. *Asterisk* denotes significantly increased CO compared with placebo ($P<0.05$). The *dagger* denotes A and A + E groups were significantly different than C at 5 minutes and 10 minutes.
(Continued on next page)

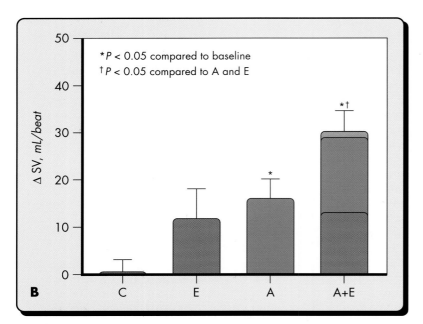

*P < 0.05 compared to baseline
†P < 0.05 compared to A and E

Figure 2-27. (*Continued*) **B,** The combination of amrinone and epinephrine improved ventricular function in an additive fashion. Oxygen delivery increased with the combination and this was associated with less increase in left ventricular stroke work. Right ventricular ejection fraction improved significantly with amrinone and amrinone-epinephrine (A + E), and this may be partially due to reductions in pulmonary vascular resistance [50]. C—control (placebo); CO—cardiac output; SV—stroke volume.

DOPAMINE AND DOBUTAMINE

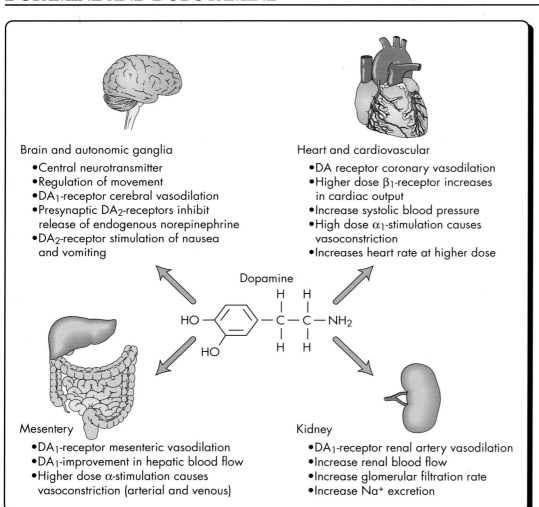

Brain and autonomic ganglia
- Central neurotransmitter
- Regulation of movement
- DA_1-receptor cerebral vasodilation
- Presynaptic DA_2-receptors inhibit release of endogenous norepinephrine
- DA_2-receptor stimulation of nausea and vomiting

Heart and cardiovascular
- DA receptor coronary vasodilation
- Higher dose β_1-receptor increases in cardiac output
- Increase systolic blood pressure
- High dose α_1-stimulation causes vasoconstriction
- Increases heart rate at higher dose

Dopamine

Mesentery
- DA_1-receptor mesenteric vasodilation
- DA_1-improvement in hepatic blood flow
- Higher dose α-stimulation causes vasoconstriction (arterial and venous)

Kidney
- DA_1-receptor renal artery vasodilation
- Increase renal blood flow
- Increase glomerular filtration rate
- Increase Na^+ excretion

Figure 2-28. Effects of dopamine. Dopamine is the third endogenous catecholamine and is the immediate metabolic precursor of norepinephrine and epinephrine. Dopamine activates dopamine 1 and 2 (DA_1 and DA_2) receptors and β- and α-adrenergic receptors in a dose-dependent fashion. The DA_1-receptors, located postsynaptically, are stimulated with low-dose dopamine in the range of 0.2 to 3.0 µg/kg/min. The effects of DA_1-receptors are vasodilation in the renal, mesenteric, coronary, and cerebral arterial blood vessels. DA_1-receptor vasodilation leads to improved renal blood flow. There is an increase in glomerular filtration rate. There is also an inhibition of tubular sodium reabsorption [51]. Dopamine infusion rates exceeding 3 µg/kg/min progressively stimulate β_1-receptors. β-receptor stimulation is associated with increases in cardiac output, heart rate, and systolic blood pressure. Continued elevation of dopamine administration exceeding 6 µg/kg/min may cause α-adrenergic stimulation and subsequent vasoconstriction and elevation of systolic blood pressure [52].

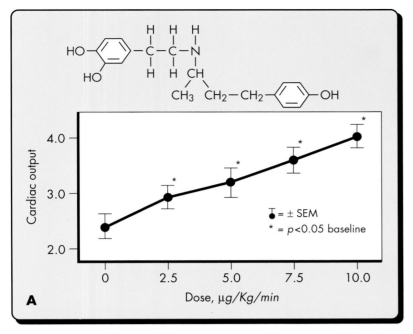

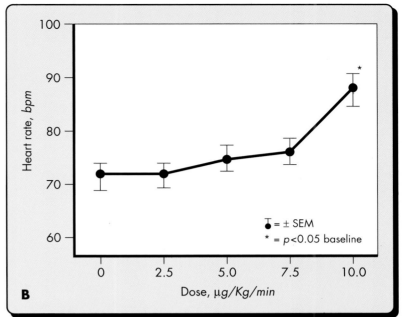

Figure 2-29. Effects of dobutamine on cardiac output (**A**) and heart rate (**B**). Dobutamine is a synthetic sympathomimetic amine that exists as a racemic mixture of two stereoisomers in which α-adrenergic activity is present in the levoisomer and β activity in the dextroisomer. In the lower dose range, β-adrenergic receptors dominate. Dobutamine increases cardiac output and will reduce ventricular diastolic pressure. There is little effect on vascular tone; however, total peripheral resistance may be slightly reduced. In patients with chronic congestive heart failure there is little tachycardia and few arrhythmias. Infusions are started at 2 μg/kg/min and may be titrated upward, usually not exceeding 20 μg/kg/min. Dobutamine will increase myocardial oxygen consumption by increasing contractility [53]. Dobutamine does not stimulate renal dopamine receptors and there is no associated increase in renal cortical blood flow as seen with low-dose dopamine. Much of the work done on dobutamine was performed in patients with chronic congestive heart failure. Surgical patients may exhibit a different hemodynamic profile secondary to the absence of β-receptor downregulation, myocardial catecholamine alteration, and metabolic disturbance. (*From* Leier and coworkers [54]; with permission.)

α-ADRENERGIC RECEPTORS

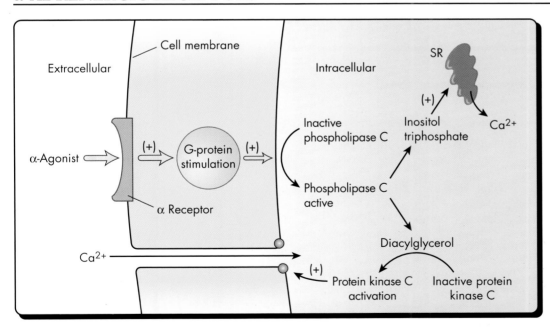

Figure 2-30. α-Adrenergic receptors. Two adrenergic receptors, α and β, were first described in 1948 by Ahlquist and they were classified according to the order of potency by which they are affected by sympathetic agonists and antagonists [55]. The α-receptors have subsequently been divided into α_1 and α_2 subtypes. α-Adrenergic agonists bind to a receptor on the cell membrane, which stimulates a G-protein–mediated message. There is stimulation of phospholipase C, which results in the production of two intracellular messengers: inositol triphosphate and diacylglycerol. Protein kinase C is activated by the diacylglycerol, which leads to an influx of calcium into the cell as well as increased sensitivity of contractile proteins to calcium. Inositol triphosphate stimulates release of calcium from the sarcoplasmic reticulum (SR) [56]. α-Receptors are responsible for mediating peripheral vasomotor tone, coronary vasoconstriction, myocardial contractility, and some central nervous system function. Postsynaptic vascular α_1-adrenergic receptors mediate vasoconstriction. Presynaptic α_2-adrenergic receptors are involved in a negative feedback mechanism, inhibiting the release of norepinephrine. α_1-Adrenergic agonists are useful in the treatment of some patients with hypotension or shock. Norepinephrine, phenylephrine, and methoxamine are direct-acting vasoconstrictors via the α_1 receptor. Mephentermine and metaraminol act both directly and indirectly at the α_1-adrenergic receptor, *ie*, a portion of their effect is mediated through release of endogenous norepinephrine.

CALCIUM

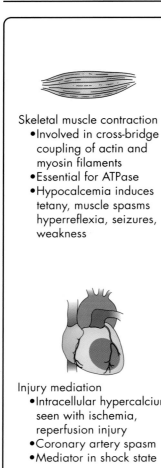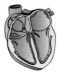

Skeletal muscle contraction
- Involved in cross-bridge coupling of actin and myosin filaments
- Essential for ATPase
- Hypocalcemia induces tetany, muscle spasms hyperreflexia, seizures, weakness

Vascular tone
- Hypocalcemia results in hypotension
- Calcium supplementation after CPB increases SVR without increase in CI

Cardiac contraction and relaxation
- Hypocalcemia results in decreased myocardial contraction [0.8mm]
- Ca²⁺ administration in hypocalcemia increases cardiac output; transient or no effect in eucalcemic patients

Ca²⁺
Ionized calcium
1.0 – 1.25 mmol/L

Injury mediation
- Intracellular hypercalcium seen with ischemia, reperfusion injury
- Coronary artery spasm
- Mediator in shock state

Effects on catecholamines
- Preadministration of calcium inhibits catecholamine inotropic action
- Little or no effect on phosphodiesterase inhibitors or α-adrenergic agonists (phenylephrine)
- May cause catecholamine resistance by blunting cAMP production

Myocardial conduction
- Heart rate generation
- Pacemaker activity
- Action potential generation
- Prolongation of QT interval with hypocalcemia

Figure 2-31. Effects of calcium. Calcium is a vital regulatory element essential for multiple physiologic functions. Both smooth muscle and skeletal muscle contraction and relaxation depend on intracellular calcium. Calcium regulates the interaction between the contractile proteins actin and myosin. Calcium is also essential for proper myocardial conduction and heart rate generation. The extracellular to intercellular gradient for free calcium is approximately 10,000 to 1. Ionized calcium levels range from 1.0 to 1.25 mmol/mL. ATPase—adenosinetriphosphatase; cAMP—cyclic adenosine monophosphate; CI—cardiac index; CPB—cardiopulmonary bypass; SVR—systemic vascular resistance.

REFERENCES

1. Ardehali A, Ports TA: Myocardial oxygen supply and demand. *Chest* 1990, 98:699–705.

2. Royster RL: Intraoperative administration of inotropes in cardiac surgery patients. *J Cardiothorac Anesth* 1990, 4, No. 6(Suppl 5):17–28.

3. Ryan TJ, Anderson JL, Antman EM, *et al.*: ACC/AHA guidelines for the management of patients with acute myocardial infarction: a report of the American College of Cardiology/American Heart Association Task Force on Practice Guidelines (Committee on Management of Acute Myocardial Infraction). *J Am Coll Cardiol* 1996, 28:1328–1428.

4. Overdyk FJ, Gramling-Babb PM, Handy JR Jr, *et al.*: Thoracic epidural anesthesia as the last option for treating angina in a patient before coronary artery bypass surgery. *Anesth Analg* 1997, 84:213–215.

5. Chirkov YY, Naujalis JI, Sage RE, Horowitz JD: Antiplatelet effects of nitroglycerin in healthy subjects and in patients with stable angina. *J Cardiovasc Pharmacol* 1993, 21:384–389.

6. Thadani U: Nitrate therapy and unstable angina. In *Unstable Angina*. Edited by Bleifield W, Hamm CW, Braunwald E, Berlin: Springer-Verlag; 1990:203–213.

7. Opie LH: *Drugs for the Heart*, edn 4. Philadelphia: WB Saunders; 1995.

8. Robertson RM, Robertson D: Drugs used for the treatment of myocardial ischemia. In *Goodman and Gilman's The Pharmacological Basis of Therapeutics*. Edited by Hardman JG, Limbird LE. New York: McGraw-Hill; 1996:759–779.

9. Gallagher JD, Moore RA, Jose AB, *et al.*: Prophylactic nitroglycerin infusions during coronary artery bypass surgery. *Anesthesiology* 1986, 64:785–789.

10. Dodds TM, Stone JG, Coromilas J, *et al.*: Prophylactic nitroglycerin infusion during noncardiac surgery does not reduce perioperative ischemia. *Anesth Analg* 1993, 76:705–713.

11. Thomson IR, Mutch WA, Culligan JD: Failure of intravenous nitroglycerin to prevent intraoperative myocardial ischemia during fentanyl-pancuronium anesthesia. *Anesthesiology* 1984, 61:385–393.

12. Coriat P, Daloz M, Bousseau D, *et al.*: Prevention of intraoperative myocardial ischemia during noncardiac surgery with intravenous nitroglycerin. *Anesthesiology* 1984, 61:193–196.

13. Eagle KA, Brundage BH, Chaitman BR, *et al.*: Guidelines for perioperative cardiovascular evaluation for noncardiac surgery. Report of the American College of Cardiology/American Heart Association Task Force on Practice Guidelines. Committee on Perioperative Cardiovascular Evaluation for Noncardiac Surgery. *Circulation* 1996, 93:1278–1317.

14. Campbell WB, Johnson AR, Callahan KS, Graham RM: Anti-platelet activity of β-adrenergic antagonists: inhibition of thromboxane synthesis and platelet aggregation in patients receiving long-term propranolol treatment. *Lancet* 1981, 2:1382–1384.

15. Royster RL, Zvara DA: Anti-ischemic drug therapy. In *Cardiac Anesthesia*, edn 4. Edited by Kaplan JA. Philadelphia: WB Saunders, in press.

16. Turi ZG, Braunwald E: The use of β-blockers after myocardial infarction. *JAMA* 1983, 249:2512–2516.

17. Mangano DT, Browner WS, Hollenberg M, *et al.*: Association of perioperative myocardial ischemia with cardiac morbidity and mortality in men undergoing noncardiac surgery. *N Engl J Med* 1990, 323:1781–1788.

18. Mangano DT, Browner WS, Hollenberg M, *et al.*: Long-term cardiac prognosis following noncardiac surgery. *JAMA* 1992, 268:233–239.

19. Browner WS, Li J, Mangano DT: In-hospital and long-term mortality in male veterans following noncardiac surgery. *JAMA* 1992, 268:228–232.

20. Siliciano D, Mangano DT: Postoperative myocardial ischemia: mechanisms and therapies. In *Opioids in Anesthesia II*. Edited by Estafanous FG. Boston: Butterworth-Heinemann, 1991:164–177.

21. Mangano DT, Layug EL, Wallace A, Tateo I: Effect of atenolol on mortality and cardiovascular morbidity after noncardiac surgery. *N Engl J Med* 1996, 335:1713–1720.

22. Barbier GH, Shettigar UR, Appunn DO: Clinical rationale for the use of an ultra-short acting β-blocker: esmolol. *Int J Clin Pharmacol Ther* 1995, 33:212–218.

23. Sperelakis N: Properties of calcium-dependent slow action potentials, and their possible role in arrhythmias. In *Calcium Antagonists and Cardiovascular Disease*. Edited by Opie LH, Krebs R. New York: Raven Press; 14;1984:277–291.

24. Sperelakis N: Cyclic AMP and phosphorylation in regulation of Ca^{++} influx into myocardial cells and blockade by calcium antagonistic drugs. *Am Heart J* 1984, 107:347–357.

25. Weiner DA: Calcium antagonists in the treatment of ischemic heart disease: angina pectoris. *Coron Artery Dis* 1994, 5:14–20.

26. Singh BN, Josephson MA, Nademanee KN: Calcium channel blockers in therapeutics. In *Cardiology: An Illustrated Text/Reference*, vol 1. Edited by Chaterjee K, Cheitlin MD, Karliner J, *et al.* Philadelphia: JB Lippincott; 1991:2.105–2.122.

27. Gersh BJ, Braunwald E, Rutherford JD: Chronic coronary artery disease. In *A Textbook of Cardiovascular Medicine*, edn 5. Edited by Braunwald E. Philadelphia: WB Saunders; 1997:1289–1365.

28. Kelly RA, Smith TW: The Pharmacologic Treatment of Heart Failure. In *Goodman and Gilman's The Pharmacologic Basis of Therapeutics*, edn. 9. Edited by Hardman JG, Limbird L. New York: McGraw-Hill, 1996:809–838.

29. Royster RL: Myocardial dysfunction following cardiopulmonary bypass: recovery patterns, predictors of inotropic need, theoretical concepts of inotropic administration. *J Cardiothorac Vasc Anesth* 1993, 7(Suppl 2):19–25.

30. Royster RL, Butterworth JF IV, Prough DS, *et al.*: Perioperative and intraoperative predictors of inotropic support and long-term outcome in patients having coronary artery bypass grafting. *Anesth Analg* 1991, 72:729–736.

31. Weathering W: An account of the fox glove and some of its medical uses, with practical remarks on dropsy and other diseases. In *Classics of Cardiology*. Edited by Willius FA, Keys TE. New York: Dover; 1941:1–231.

32. Netter FH: Heart. In The *CIBA Collection of Medical Illustrations*. Edited by Yonkman FF. Ciba: Summit, New Jersey; 1978:106.

33. Cohn JN, Franciosa JA: Vasodilator therapy of cardiac failure. *N Engl J Med* 1977, 297:27–31.

34. Cohn JN, Archibald DG, Ziesche S, *et al.*: Effect of vasodilator therapy on mortality in chronic congestive heart failure: results of Veteran's Administration Cooperative Study. *N Engl J Med* 1986, 314:1547–1552.

35. Consensus Trial Study Group: Effects of enalapril on mortality in severe congestive heart failure: results of the Cooperative North Scandinavian Enalapril Survival Study. *N Engl J Med* 1987, 316:1429–1435.

36. Kelly RA, Smith TW: The Pharmacologic Treatment of Heart Failure. In *Goodman and Gilman's Pharmacologic Basis of Therapeutics*, edn 9. Edited by Hardman JG, Limbird L. New York: McGraw-Hill, 1996:809–838.

37. Endoh M, Yanagisawa T, Taira N, *et al.*: Effects of new inotropic agents on cyclic nucleotide metabolism and calcium transients in canine ventricular muscle. *Circulation* 1986, 73(Suppl 3):117–133.

38. Grossman W: Diastolic dysfunction in heart failure. *Circulation* 1990, 81(Suppl 3):1–7.

39. Alousi AA, Canter JM, Montenaro MJ, *et al.*: Cardiotonic activity of milrinone, a new potent cardiac bipyridine, on the normal and failing heart of experimental animals. *J Carrdiovasc Pharmacol* 1983, 5:792–803.

40. Benovic JL, Bouvier M, Karon MG, *et al.*: Regulation of adenylyl cyclase-coupled β-adrenergic receptors. *Annu Rev Cell Biol* 1988, 4:405–428.

41. Brodde OE, Hilleman S, Kunde K, *et al.*: Receptor systems affecting force of contraction in the human heart and their alterations in chronic heart failure. *J Heart Lung Transplant* 1992, 11:164–174.

42. Lands AM, Arnold A, McAuliff JP, *et al.*: Differentiation of receptor systems activated by sympathomimetic amines. *Nature* 1967, 214:597–598.

43. Tan S, Curtis-Prior PB: Characterization of the β-adrenoceptor of the adipose cell of the rat. *Int J Obes* 1983, 7:409–414.

44. Kaumann AJ: Is there a third heart β-adrenoceptor? *Trends Pharmacol Sci* 1989, 10:316–320.

45. Bristow MR, Hershberger RE, Port JD, *et al.*: β_1 and β_2-adrenergic receptor–mediated adenylate cyclase stimulation in nonfailing and failing human ventricular myocardium. *Mol Pharmacol* 1989, 35:295–303.

46. Kaumann AJ, Hall JA, Murray KJ, *et al.*: A comparison of the effects of adrenaline and noradrenaline on human heart: the role of β_1- and β_2-adrenoceptors in the stimulation of adenylate cyclase and contractile force. *Eur Heart J* 1989, 10(Suppl B):29–37.

47. Brodde OE: Beta-adrenoceptors in cardiac disease. *Pharmacol Ther* 1993, 60:405–430.

48. Lefkowitz RJ, Hoffman BB, Taylor P: Neurotransmission: the autonomic and somatic motor nervous systems. In *Goodman and Gilman's The Pharmacological Basis of Therapeutics*, edn 9. Edited by Hardman JG, Limbird LE. New York: McGraw-Hill; 1996:105–139.

49. Grossman W: *Contemporary Issues in Heart Failure: the Therapy of Acute Heart Failure*. Little Falls, NJ: Health Learning Systems, Inc., 1993:1–28.

50. Royster RL, Butterworth JF IV, Prielipp RC, *et al.*: Combined inotropic effects of amrinone and epinephrine after cardiopulmonary bypass in humans. *Anesth Analg* 1993, 77:662–672.

51. Hilberman M, Maseda J, Stinson EB, *et al.*: The diuretic properties of dopamine in patients after open-heart operation. *Anesthesiology* 1984, 61:489–494.

52. Higgins TL, Chernow B: Pharmacotherapy of circulatory shock. *Dis Mon* 1987, 33:309–361.

53. Weinstein JS, Baim DS: The effects of acute dobutamine administration on myocardial metabolism and energetics. *Heart Failure* 1986, 1:110–116.

54. Leier CV, Heban PT, Huss P, *et al.*: Comparative systemic and regional effects of dopamine and dobutamine in patients with cardiomyopathic heart failure. *Circulation* 1978, 58:466–475.

55. Ahlquist RP: A study of adrenotropic receptors. *Am J Physiol* 1948, 153:586–600.

56. Zaloga GP, Prielipp RC, Butterworth JF IV, Royster RL: Pharmacologic cardiovascular support. *Crit Care Clin* 1993, 9:335–362.

Preoperative Cardiac Evaluation

Lee A. Fleisher

The preoperative evaluation of the patient with cardio-vascular disease undergoing noncardiac or cardiac surgery has received a great deal of attention over the past two decades. The goal of this research has been to identify those patients at greatest risk for perioperative complications. Particularly with the respect to noncardiac surgery, information regarding cardiovascular status is rarely complete. Frequently, the decision to perform expensive preoperative diagnostic test depends on the utility of the information obtained. Two recent guidelines have been produced, with slightly different approaches. The American Heart Association and American College of Cardiology have published guidelines on the perioperative cardiovascular evaluation for noncardiac surgery [1]. Based on the available evidence and expert opinion, the panel suggests that further diagnostic evaluation be predicated on the patient's clinical risk factors, the surgical procedure, and exercise capacity. The goal of this guideline is to establish the necessary information to appropriately manage the high-risk patient. The American College of Physicians has developed an evidence-based approach for preoperative risk stratification [2]. This guideline emphasizes the use of clinical risk indices and further diagnostic testing only in vascular surgery patients at high clinical risk. In either case, the decision to perform coronary angiography and revascularization should be limited to those patients in whom it is indicated independent of the surgical procedure and must take into account local institutional factors such as the rate of morbidity and mortality for both vascular and coronary revascularization procedures [3].

The emphasis for evaluating the cardiovascular patient undergoing cardiac surgery is different from noncardiac surgery. In this circumstance, there is ample information regarding cardiovascular function and anatomy necessary for determination of the surgical procedure. Recently, risk indices have been developed that provide a means to adjust patients' risk across different centers or provide the clinician with a probability of survival. With the emphasis on outcomes and the use of surgical report cards, the ability to demonstrate that the results of cardiac surgery at a particular institution are equal or superior to other institutions has taken on an even greater importance. In addition to the basic cardiovascular information, comorbidities take on increased importance from the provider's perspective.

EVALUATION OF THE PATIENT UNDERGOING NONCARDIAC SURGERY

DETSKY'S MODIFICATION OF THE CARDIAC RISK INDEX

Variable	Point Score
Coronary artery disease	
Myocardial infarction ≤6 mo	10
Myocardial infarction >6 mo	5
Angina (Canadian Cardiovascular Society class)	
III	10
IV	20
Unstable angina <6 mo	10
Alveolar pulmonary edema	
Within 1 week	10
Ever	5
Valvular disease	
Suspected critical aortic stenosis	20
Dysrhythmia	
Rhythm other than sinus, with or without atrial ectopy	5
Presence of >5 PVCs/min at any time	5
Poor general medical status	5
Age >70 y	5
Emergency surgical procedure	10

Figure 3-1. Detsky's modification of the cardiac risk index. In 1977, Goldman and colleagues published their landmark article describing weighted risk factors for perioperative cardiovascular complication after noncardiac surgery in 1001 patients over the age of 40 [4]. Nine major risk factors were identified. Detsky *et al.* evaluated the original cardiac risk index and determined that modifications increased the predictive value of the risk indices [5]. Importantly, the Detsky index was developed in one data set and subsequently validated in another. An increasing number of points denotes higher clinical risk, with three broad categories to find. The recent American College of Physicians' guidelines for assessing and managing the perioperative risk of coronary artery disease associated with major noncardiac surgery uses the Detsky index as the starting point for the evaluation [2]. PVC—premature ventricular contraction. (*Adapted from* Detsky and coworkers [5]; with permission.)

TWO CLASSIFICATIONS OF CARDIOVASCULAR DISEASE

Class	New York Heart Association Functional Classification	Canadian Cardiovascular Society Functional Classification
I	Patients with cardiac disease but without resulting limitations of physical activity. Ordinary physical activity does not cause undue fatigue, palpitation, dyspnea, or anginal pain.	Ordinary physical activity, such as walking and climbing stairs, does not cause angina. Angina with strenuous or rapid or prolonged exertion at work or recreation.
II	Patients with cardiac disease resulting in slight limitation of physical activity. They are comfortable at rest. Ordinary physical activity results in fatigue, palpitation, dyspnea, or anginal pain.	Slight limitation of ordinary activity. Walking or climbing stairs rapidly, walking uphill, walking or stair climbing after meals, in cold, in wind, or when under emotional stress, or only during the few hours after awakening. Walking more than two blocks on the level and climbing more than one flight of ordinary stairs at a normal pace and in normal conditions.
III	Patients with cardiac disease resulting in marked limitations of physical activity. They are comfortable at rest. Less than ordinary physical activity causes fatigue, palpitation, dyspnea, or anginal pain.	Marked limitation of ordinary physical activity. Walking one to two blocks on the level and climbing more than one flight of normal conditions.
IV	Patient with cardiac disease resulting in inability to carry on any physical activity without discomfort. Symptoms of cardiac insufficiency or of the anginal syndrome may be present even at rest. If any physical activity is undertaken, discomfort is increased.	Inability to carry on any physical activity without discomfort—anginal syndrome *may be* present at rest.

Figure 3-2. Several classifications of cardiovascular disease have been developed. The Canadian Cardiovascular Society Classification is a means of assessing the cardiovascular status based on the extent of physical activity [6]. A higher number (I to IV) is associated with a greater degree of physical impairment. In contrast, the New York Heart Association Classification scheme focuses on the functional status of the heart and the presence of congestive heart failure [7]. Therefore, information from these two indices is complementary. (*From* Goldman and coworkers [8]; with permission.)

SELECTED STUDIES ON REINFARCTION IN PATIENTS WITH A PRIOR MI

Time from Prior MI to Date of Operation, *mo*	Tarhan *et al.* [9], *n* (%)	Rao *et al.* [10], *n* (%)	Shah *et al.* [11], *n* (%)
0–3	3/8 (37)	3/52 (5.8)	1/23 (4.3)
4–6	3/19 (16)	2/86 (2.3)	0/18 (4.3)
>6	22/322 (5.6)	9/595 (1.5)	10/174 (5.7)
Age indeterminate			2/60 (3.3)

Figure 3-3. Selected studies on reinfarction in patients with a prior myocardial infarction (MI). Initially, a recent infarction (≤ 3 months) was associated with a marked increase in perioperative reinfarction (37%). There was a steady decrease in the incidence of reinfarction from 4 to 6 months, and after 6 months. Subsequently, Rao *et al.* [10] studied patients with a recent MI and used pulmonary artery catheters and prolonged recovery in an intensive care unit. The incidence of reinfarction dramatically decreased from previous studies, although a gradient based on time from previous infarction continued to exist. Most recently, Shah *et al.* [11] evaluated the rate of reinfarction and demonstrated a similar low incidence of morbidity in the group with a very recent MI, but the highest rate in the group with an MI greater than 6 months previously.

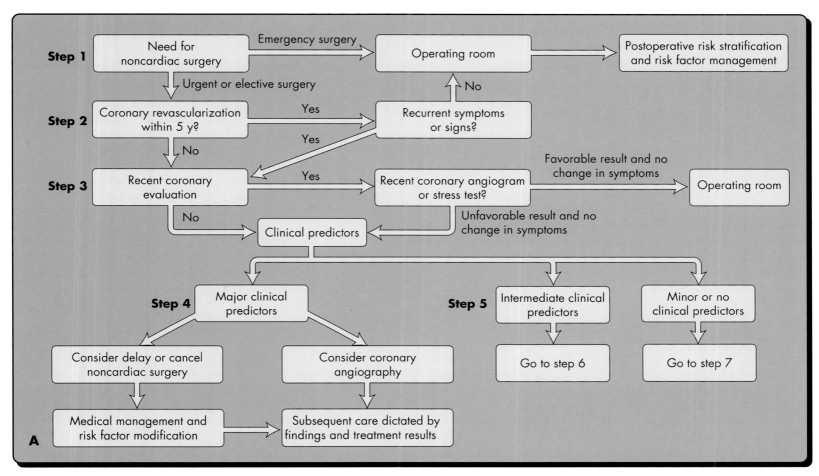

Figure 3-4. The American Heart Association/American College of Cardiology Task Force on Perioperative Evaluation of Cardiac Patients undergoing Noncardiac Surgery has proposed an algorithm for decisions regarding the need for further evaluation. This repre sents one of multiple algorithms proposed in the literature. It is based on expert opinion, and incorporates eight steps. First, the clinician must evaluate the urgency of the surgery and the appropriateness of a formal preoperative assessment (**A**).

(*Continued on next page*)

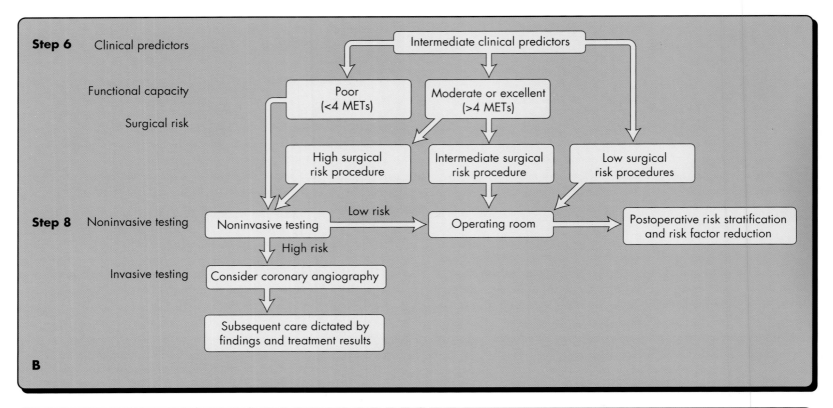

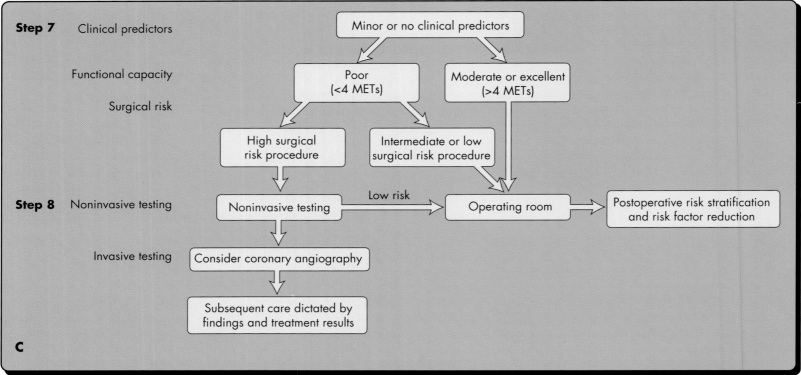

Figure 3-4. (*Continued*) Next, he or she must determine whether the patient has had a previous revascularization procedure or coronary evaluation. Those patients with unstable coronary syndromes should be identified, and appropriate treatment should be instituted. The decision to have further testing depends on the interaction of the clinical risk factors, surgery-specific risk, and functional capacity (**B** and **C**). MET—metabolic equivalent. (*Adapted from* Eagle and coworkers [1]; with permission.)

CLINICAL PREDICTORS OF INCREASED PERIOPERATIVE CARDIOVASCULAR RISK (MI, CHF, DEATH)

Major	Intermediate
Unstable coronary syndrome	Mild angina pectoris (Canadian Class I or II)
Recent MI* with evidence of important ischemic risk by clinical symptoms or noninvasive study	Prior MI by history or pathologic Q waves
Unstable or severe† angina (Canadian Class III or IV) [6]	Compensated or prior CHF
Decompensated CHF	Diabetes mellitus
Significant arrhythmias	**Minor**
High-grade atrioventricular block	Advanced age
Symptomatic ventricular arrhythmias in the presence of underlying heart disease	Abnormal ECG (left ventricular hypertrophy, left bundle branch block, ST-T abnormalities)
Supraventricular arrhythmias with uncontrolled ventricular rate	Rhythm other than sinus (*eg*, atrial fibrillation)
Severe valvular disease	Low functional capacity (*eg*, inability to climb one flight of stairs with a bag of groceries)
	History of stroke
	Uncontrolled systemic hypertension

* The American College of Cardiology National Database Library defines *recent MI* as greater than 7 days but less than or equal to 1 month (30 days).
† May include "stable" angina in patients who are unusually sedentary.

Figure 3-5. Clinical predictors of increased perioperative cardiovascular risk (myocardial infarction [MI], congestive heart failure [CHF], or death) adapted from the American Heart Association/American College of Cardiology guidelines for perioperative cardiovascular evaluation for noncardiac surgery. Three categories of predictors were identified: major, intermediate, and minor. The major predictors are unstable syndromes and are based on prospective cohort studies and general cardiologic knowledge. For the purpose of the guidelines, a recent MI is defined as greater than 7 days but less than or equal to 30 days. Intermediate risk factors have been found to be strong independent predictors of perioperative risk in several studies of predominantly vascular patients. Minor risk factors are those that have not been specifically identified as predictors of perioperative risk in multiple trials but have been associated with an increased risk of coronary artery disease. (*Adapted from* Eagle and coworkers [1].)

CARDIAC RISK* STRATIFICATION FOR NONCARDIAC SURGICAL PROCEDURES

High	Intermediate	Low†
(Reported cardiac risk often > 5%)	(Reported cardiac risk generally < 5%)	(Reported cardiac risk generally < 1%)
Emergent major operations, particularly in the elderly	Carotid endarterectomy	Endoscopic procedures
Aortic and other major vascular	Head and neck	Superficial procedure
Peripheral vascular	Intraperitoneal and intrathoracic	Cataract
Anticipated prolonged surgical procedures associated with large fluid shifts and/or blood loss	Orthopedic	Breast
	Prostate	

* Combined incidence of cardiac death and nonfatal myocardial infarction.
† Do not generally require further preoperative cardiac testing.

Figure 3-6. Cardiac risk stratification for noncardiac surgical procedures. This table is adapted from the American Heart Association/American College of Cardiology guidelines for perioperative cardiovascular evaluation for noncardiac surgery. Surgery is stratified by the estimated combined risk of cardiac death and nonfatal myocardial infarction. The data are based on the estimated incidence reported in the literature. It is important to acknowledge that the incidence of morbidity varies between institutions and among surgeons. Therefore, a category of anticipated prolonged surgery is included in the high-risk group. Further cardiovascular testing is rarely needed in the low-risk surgical group. (*From* Eagle and coworkers [1].)

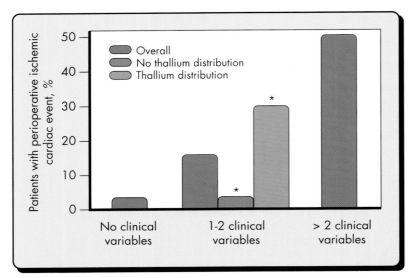

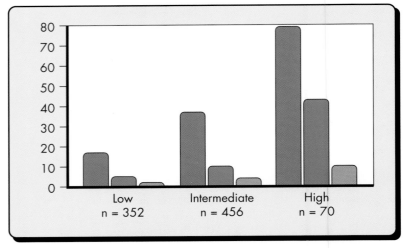

Figure 3-7. Importance of clinical risk factors. Eagle *et al.* [12] identified five clinical predictors of risk: ventricular ectopic activity (VEA) being treated, Q waves on electrocardiography, angina, age greater than 70, and diabetes, which predicted increased perioperative risk in 200 patients undergoing major vascular surgery. In determining the value of further noninvasive diagnostic testing, patients with no risk factors had an extremely low perioperative cardiac morbidity and mortality, and therefore further diagnostic testing did not provide any additional discriminatory value. Similarly, patients with three or more clinical predictors had such high perioperative morbidity and mortality that noninvasive testing was of minimal value and coronary angiography was suggested as the test of choice. Diagnostic testing only provided discriminatory value in those patients with one or two clinical predictors. *Asterisk* indicates P < 0.05 for the additive value of thallium imaging. (*Adapted from* Eagle and coworkers [12].)

Figure 3-8. Relationship between clinical predictors and angiographic findings in patients undergoing vascular surgery. Paul and coworkers [13] retrospectively reviewed patients who received coronary angiography at the Cleveland Clinic and determined the presence of clinical risk factors defined by Eagle and coworkers [12]: angina, age greater than 70, ventricular ectopic activity being treated, diabetes, and Q waves on preoperative electrocardiogram. Paul demonstrated that increasing clinical risk was associated with an increasing probability of severe, multivessel, or critical coronary artery disease. In multivariate analysis, diabetes and age were not independent predictors of risk. Importantly, the absence of clinical predictors associated with documented coronary artery disease (angina, myocardial infarction, or congestive heart failure) identified a cohort with a 94% probability of minimal or noncritical coronary artery disease. This supports the contention that clinical predictors can be used for risk stratification. *Purple bars* represent proportions of patients with severe multivessel disease; *aqua bars*, critical three-vessel or left main coronary disease; *gold bars*, left main coronary artery stenosis greater than or equal to 70%. (*From* Paul and coworkers [13].)

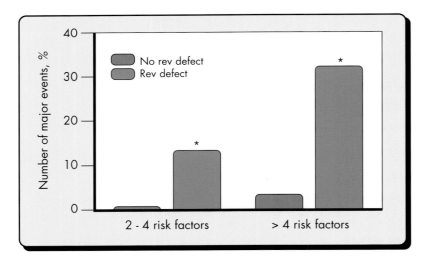

Figure 3-9. Additive value of noninvasive testing demonstrated in a double blind manner. Vanzetto *et al.* [14] studied 517 consecutive aortic surgery patients, in the only study in which selective testing was performed in an *a priori* manner and the clinicans were unaware of the results of the noninvasive test. Dipyridamole thallium imaging was performed on those patients who had at least two clinical risk factors for coronary artery disease. Neither the caregivers nor the individual assessing cardiac morbidity was aware of the results of the thallium imaging. Patients with zero or one risk factor had very low perioperative morbidity. The incidence of perioperative cardiac morbidity increased with an increasing number of clinical risk factors, and the presence of redistribution in patients with at least two risk factors was associated with a significantly worse outcome than those patients with normal scans. This study was cited by the American College of Physicians guidelines as strong evidence to support the use of noninvasive imaging in risk stratification before vascular surgery [2]. *Asterisk* indicates P < 0.05 for the additive value of thallium imaging. (*Adapted from* Vanzetto and coworkers [14].)

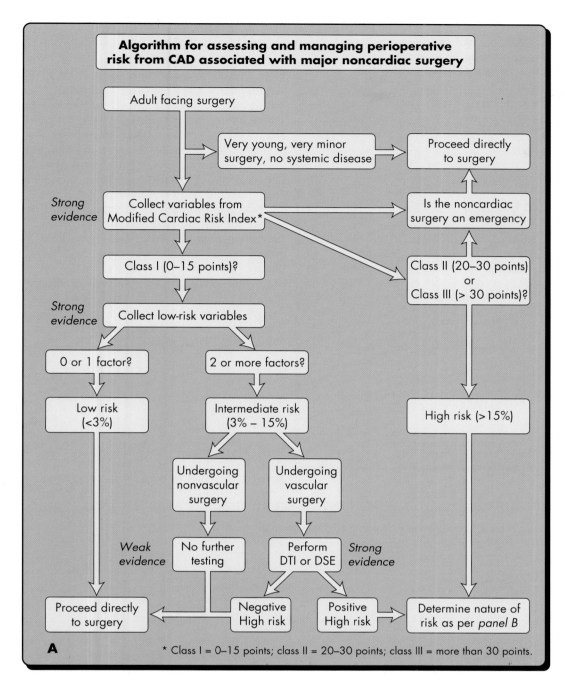

Algorithm for assessing and managing perioperative risk from CAD associated with major noncardiac surgery

Adult facing surgery

Strong evidence — Collect variables from Modified Cardiac Risk Index*

Very young, very minor surgery, no systemic disease → Proceed directly to surgery

Class I (0–15 points)?

Is the noncardiac surgery an emergency

Strong evidence — Collect low-risk variables

Class II (20–30 points) or Class III (> 30 points)?

0 or 1 factor?   2 or more factors?

Low risk (<3%)   Intermediate risk (3% – 15%)   High risk (>15%)

Undergoing nonvascular surgery   Undergoing vascular surgery

Weak evidence — No further testing   Perform DTI or DSE — *Strong evidence*

Proceed directly to surgery ← Negative High risk   Positive High risk → Determine nature of risk as per *panel B*

A   * Class I = 0–15 points; class II = 20–30 points; class III = more than 30 points.

Figure 3-10. The American College of Physicians Guidelines for assessing and managing the perioperative risk from coronary artery disease (CAD) associated with major noncardiac surgery [2]. The commentary in *italics* beside the boxes represents the strength of evidence to support each decision process in the algorithm. **A,** An evidence-based analysis of the literature accompanied the algorithm in a paper by Palda and Detsky [2]. Initially, patients are assessed using the Detsky modification of the cardiac risk index to determine if they are class I (low risk) or class II or III (high risk). If they are class I, clinical predictors such as those identified by Eagle [12] are collected to determine if they represent low or high clinical risk. Only those patients with several clinical predictors are then determined to be at intermediate perioperative risk. Those patients with an intermediate risk and undergoing vascular surgery should be considered for noninvasive imaging with dipyridamole thallium imaging or dobutamine stress echocardiography. No further testing is suggested in those patients undergoing nonvascular surgery.

(*Continued on next page*)

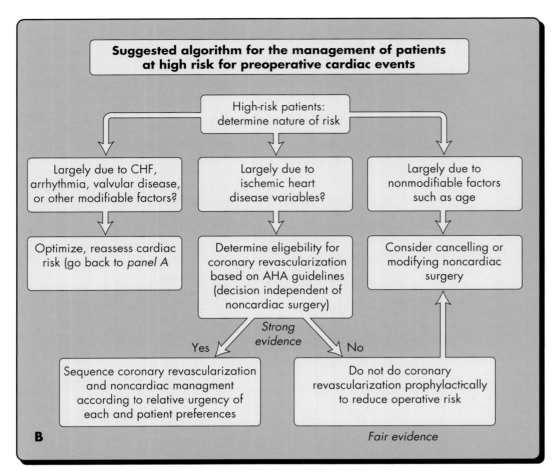

Figure 3-10. (*Continued*) **B,** If the noninvasive testing is positive or the patient is at high clinical risk (Detsky index criteria) then it is important to determine the nature of the risk. If the risk is largely due to ischemic heart disease, then it is important to determine if the patient would be eligible for coronary revascularization based on American Heart Association (AHA) guidelines independent of noncardiac surgery. If the risk is of nonischemic origin then the ideal choice is to optimize and reassess. Finally, if risk is due to largely nonmodifiable factors then either canceling the case or modifying the noncardiac surgery should be considered. The author suggests that β-blockers be considered in all high risk patients, based on data from Mangano *et al.* [15]. CHF—congestive heart failure; DSE—dobutamine stress echocardiography; DTI—dipyridamole thallium imaging. (*From* American College of Physicians [2]; with permission.

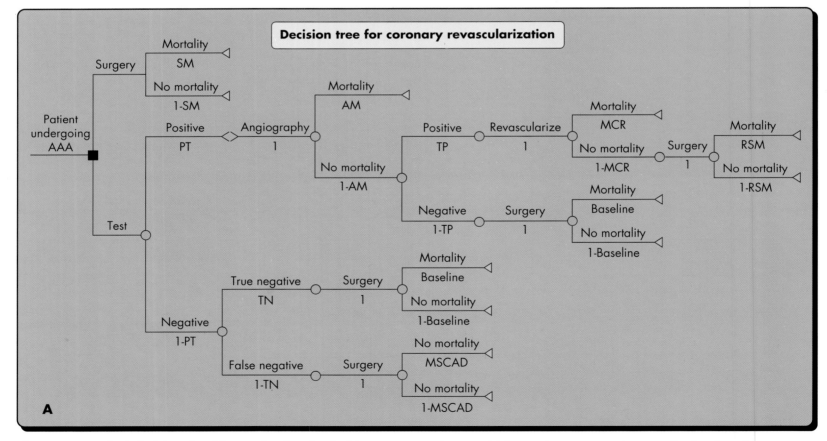

Figure 3-11. **A,** A decision algorithm evaluating the decision between vascular surgery alone or coronary artery revascularization before vascular surgery. There are currently no randomized trials to address the optimal strategy. By outlining the multiple decision points at which a patient can sustain mortality by choosing to undergo coronary revascularization first, the optimal strategy for preoperative evaluation can be demonstrated. Specifically, variation in mortality at each decision point can change the optimal strategy.

(*Continued on next page*)

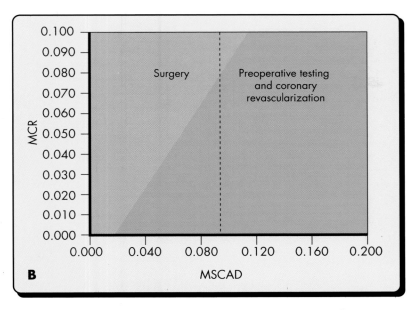

Figure 3-11. (*Continued*) B, A two-way sensitivity analysis demonstrating the optimal preoperative strategy of surgery alone or coronary revascularization before vascular surgery. As the probability of mortality from coronary revascularization increases, then vascular surgery alone is the preferred strategy. In contrast, as the probability of mortality from aortic surgery in patients with significant coronary artery disease increases, then coronary revascularization before vascular surgery is the optimal strategy. The average mortality for vascular surgery in patients with significant coronary artery disease is 9.5%, suggesting that the strategy with the lowest mortality is very sensitive to local morbidity and mortality. However, if long-term mortality is included in the model, the coronary revascularization might prove to be more beneficial. AAA—abdominal aortic aneurysm; AM—mortality from coronary angiography; MCR—mortality for coronary revascularization; Baseline—baseline cardiac mortality for AAA surgery; DTI—dipyridamole thallium imaging; MSCAD—cardiac mortality related to AAA surgery in patients with significant uncorrected coronary artery disease; PT—probability of a positive DTI test; RSM—cardiac mortality related to AAA surgery in patients who have undergone coronary revascularization; SM—cardiac mortality related to AAA surgery if no testing or revascularization is performed; TN—probability that a negative DTI test is a true negative; TP—true positive. (*Adapted from* Fleisher and coworkers [3]; with permission.)

EVALUATION OF THE PATIENT UNDERGOING CARDIAC SURGERY

OPERATIVE MORTALITY

Clinical characteristics
    Age
    Sex
Angina classification
    Canadian Cardiovascular Society Class I–IV
    Unstable angina
Manifestations of heart failure
    History of heart failure
    Pulmonary rales
    Use of digitalis
    Use of diuretics
    Congestive heart failure score (0–4)
Coronary artery anatomy
    Number of vessels with ≥ 70% stenosis
    Left main coronary artery stenosis
        (none < 50%, mild 50%–74%, moderate 75%–89%, severe
        ≥ 90%)
Left ventricular function
    Cardiac enlargement of chest roentgenogram (slight, moderate,
        marked)
    Cardiothoracic ratio ≥ 0.50
    Left ventricular end-diastolic pressure
    Ejection fraction
    Wall motion score (5–30)
    Myocardial jeopardy index (0–2)
Surgery
    Priority of surgery (elective, urgent, emergent)
    Aneuysmectomy and/or plication
    Mitral valve replacement

Figure 3-12. Clinical and angiographic predictors of operative mortality from the Collaborative Study in Coronary Artery Surgery [16]. The Coronary Artery Surgery Study (CASS) was a collaborative study begun in 1974 to compare surgical (coronary artery bypass graft [CABG]) with medical therapy for coronary artery disease. The study included both a randomized and nonrandomized component in which the decision to undergo revascularization was based on physician and patient preference. Importantly, the indications for CABG were not well defined, and many patients underwent revascularization of a single stenosis. A total of 6630 patients in both arms underwent isolated CABG between 1975 and 1978. Women had a significantly higher mortality than men, with mortality increasing with advancing age in men, but not significantly with women. Increasing severity of angina, manifestations of heart failure, and number and extent of coronary artery stenoses all correlated with higher mortality, whereas ejection fraction was not a predictor. Urgency of surgery was a very strong predictor of outcome, with those patients requiring emergent surgery in the presence of a 90% left main coronary artery stenosis sustaining a 40% mortality. (*From* Kennedy and coworkers [16].)

ASSOCIATIONS BETWEEN PATIENT AND CLINICAL VARIABLES AND IN-HOSPITAL MORTALITY

Variable	Multivariate analysis	
	Odds ratio	P
Patient age, y		
< 55	1.0	0.0001
55–59	1.5	(trend)
60–64	2.0	
65–69	2.6	
70–74	3.4	
≥ 75	4.7	
Patient sex (female vs male)	1.2	0.460
Body surface area (m^2)		
≥ 2.00	1.0	0.009
1.80–1.99	1.3	(trend)
1.60–1.79	1.8	
< 1.60	2.4	
Charlson comorbidity score		
0	1.0	0.002
1	1.5	(trend)
≥ 2	2.3	
Prior coronary artery bypass grafting (yes vs no)	3.6	0.0001
Ejection fraction		
≥ 60%	1.0	0.013
50%–59%	1.4	(trend)
40%–49%	1.6	
< 40%	1.9	
Left ventricular end-diastolic pressure (mm Hg)		
≤14	1.0	0.005
15–18	1.3	(trend)
19–22	1.6	
> 22	2.1	
Priority of surgery		
Elective	1.0	0.001
Urgent	2.1	(trend)
Emergency	4.4	
Left main coronary artery stenosis		
< 50%	1.0	0.929
50%–89%	1.0	(trend)
≥ 90%	1.0	
No. of diseased coronary vessels		
One	1.0	0.166
Two	1.3	(trend)
Three	1.6	

Figure 3-13. Multivariate predictor of in-hospital mortality with coronary artery bypass graft (CABG). In an effort both to compare data across centers and to define surgical risk, multiple investigators began developing risk models. O'Connor et al. [17] used data collected from 3055 patients undergoing isolated CABG at five clinical centers between 1987 and 1989. A regression model was developed in a training set and subsequently validated in a test set. Independent predictors of mortality included patient's age, body surface area, comorbidity score, prior CABG, ejection fraction, left ventricular end-diastolic pressure, and priority of surgery. The Charlson comorbidity score was developed and validated for predicting risk for mortality in cancer patients but has been used in other clinical scenarios. The odds ratio for increased in-hospital mortality is shown, with advanced age (≥ 75 years), reoperation, and emergency surgery conferring the greatest risk. (*From* O'Connor and coworkers [17]; with permission.)

A. PARSONNET INDEX OF RISK FACTORS FOR PATIENTS UNDERGOING CABG

Risk factor	Assigned weight
Female gender	1
Morbid obesity (≥ 1.5 × ideal weight)	3
Diabetes (unspecified type)	3
Hypertension (systolic BP > 140 mm Hg)	3
Ejection fraction, %: (actual value when available)	
Good (≥ 50)	0
Fair (30–49)	2
Poor (< 30)	4
Age, y:	
70–74	7
75–79	12
≥ 80	20
Reoperation	
First	5
Second	10
Preoperative IABP	2
Left ventricular aneurysm	5
Emergency surgery following PTCA or catheterization complications	10
Dialysis dependency (PD or Hemo)	10
Catastrophic states (*eg*, acute structural defect, cardiogenic shock, acute renal failure)*	10–50†
Other rare circumstances (*eg*, paraplegia, pacemaker dependency, congenital HD in adult, severe asthma)*	2–10†
Valve surgery	
Mitral	5
PA pressure ≥ 60 mm Hg	8
Aortic	5
Pressure gradient >120 mm Hg	7
CABG at the time of valve surgery	2

* On the actual worksheet, these risk factors require justification.
† Values were predictive of increased risk of operative mortality in univariate analysis.

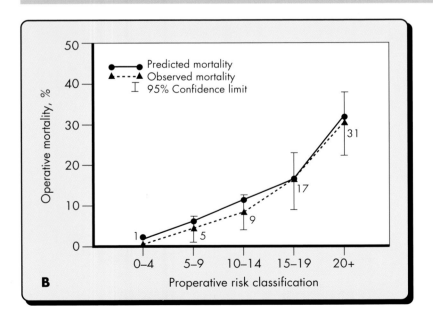

B

Figure 3-14. Uniform stratification of risk for coronary artery bypass graft (CABG) by Parsonnet and colleagues [18]. Fourteen risk factors were identified following univariate regression analysis of 3500 consecutive operations. **A,** An additive model was constructed and prospectively evaluated in 1332 open heart procedures. The presence of each of the defined risk factors was associated with a given number of points, with catastrophic states and advanced age conferring the greatest risk. **B,** Five categories of risk were identified, based on the total number of points. Numbers by the *triangles* indicate actual mortality in the observed groups. Increasing risk category was associated with increasing mortality rates at the Newark Beth Israel Medical Center. The Parsonnet index is frequently used as a benchmark for comparison among institutions. BP—blood pressure; HD—heart disease; Hemo—hemodialysis; IABP—intra-aortic balloon pump; PA—pulmonary artery; PD—peritoneal dialysis; PTCA—percutaneous transluminal coronary angioplasty. (Part A *adapted from* Parsonnet and coworkers [18]; with permission.)

A. FINAL MULTIVARIATE MODEL FOR IDENTIFICATION OF CABG PATIENT EXPERIENCING ONE OR MORE PERIOPERATIVE COMPLICATIONS

Variable	Relative risk*
Intercept	—
Prior heart surgery	1.98
Creatinine	1.24
NYHA functional class	1.27
Surgical priority	1.29
Age	1.24
Preoperative IABP	1.81
Peripheral vascular disease	1.32
CHF	1.35
COPD	1.27
Cerebral vascular disease	1.22
Diabetes	1.18

B. FINAL MULTIVARIATE MODEL FOR IDENTIFICATION OF VALVE AND OTHER CARDIAC SURGERY PATIENTS EXPERIENCING ONE OR MORE PERIOPERATIVE COMPLICATIONS

Variable	Relative risk*
Intercept	—
Age	1.61
Surgical priority	1.54
Peripheral vascular disease	1.75
Prior heart surgery	1.58
Active endocarditis	2.10
Cardiomegaly	1.41
Mitral valve replacement	1.53
Creatinine	1.14
All other procedures	1.41
Great vessel repair	1.05

Figure 3-15. Multivariate model for identification of coronary artery bypass graft (CABG) patients experiencing one or more perioperative complications [19]. Numerous models of cardiac risk have been developed, each of which has an inherent bias based upon the referral pattern of the institution in which the indices were developed. Hammermeister *et al.* analyzed perioperative complications in 10,634 patients undergoing a diverse group of cardiac surgery procedures in Veterans Administration Hospitals. Multivariate models to predict the relative risk for experiencing one or more perioperative complications after CABG (**A**) or valvular surgery (**B**). *Asterisk* indicates that the relative risks assume a dichotomous variable, except for creatinine (1.0 mg/dL increment), 1-unit increment in functional class, change from elective to urgent or urgent to emergent surgery, and 10-year increment in age. The importance of elevated creatinine and peripheral vascular disease may reflect their prevalence in the population studied compared with other series. CHF—congestive heart failure; COPD—chronic obstructive pulmonary disease; IABP—intra-aortic balloon pump; NYHA—New York Heart Association. (*From* Hammermeister and coworkers [19]; with permission.)

CLINICAL SEVERITY SCORING SYSTEM

Preoperative factors	Score
Emergency case	6
Serum creatinine	
≥ 141 and ≤ 167 µmol/L	1
(≥ 1.6 and ≤ 1.8 mg/dL)	
≥ 168 µmol/L (≥ 1.9 mg/dL)	4
Severe left ventricular dysfunction	3
Reoperation	3
Operative mitral valve insufficiency	3
Age ≥ 65 and ≤ 74 y	1
Age ≥ 75 y	2
Prior vascular surgery	2
Chronic obstructive pulmonary disease	2
Anemia (hematocrit ≤ 0.34)	2
Operative aortic valve stenosis	1
Weight ≤ 65 kg	1
Diabetes, on oral or insulin therapy	1
Cerebrovascular disease	1

Figure 3-16. Clinical severity score for coronary artery bypass graft (CABG) developed at the Cleveland Clinic [20]. A multivariate logistic regression model to predict perioperative risk was developed in 5051 patients and subsequently validated in a cohort of 4069 patients. Each independent predictor was assigned a weight or score, with increasing morbidity and mortality associated with an increasing total score. Many of the strongest (highest score) risk factors are identical to those described in previous studies. Importantly, the morbidity was lower than the predicted 99.4% confidence interval at scores of 2, 5, 6 and 7 through 9. The morbidity was actually higher in the validation set than observed for the developed set for clinical severity scores greater than or equal to 10, although it was still within the confidence limits of the predicted rate. This demonstrates the potential problems of prospectively applying any of the scoring systems, because perioperative management may change over time. (*From* Higgins and coworkers [20]; with permission.)

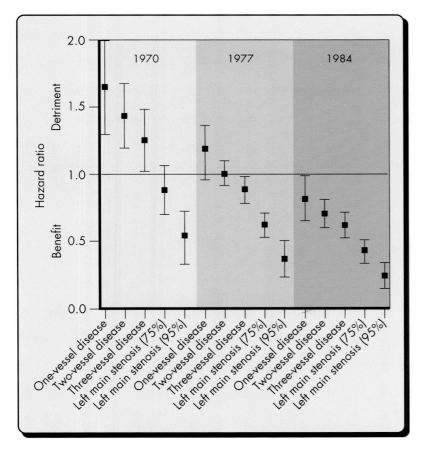

Figure 3-17. Comparison of medical and surgical average event-free survival hazard ratios for patients treated in 1970, 1977, and 1984 according to coronary anatomy [21]. This observational study from Duke University involved 5824 patients followed for 20 years. Event-free survival was more favorable with surgery compared with medical treatment (hazard ratio < 1) with increasing severity of coronary artery disease. During the earliest era, there was actually a detriment to surgery for patients without left main coronary artery disease, whereas surgery in patients with less severe disease was associated with improved survival during the most modern period (1984). Nonrandomized data such as this support the potential greater value of surgical interventions during the modern era. Yet, medical therapy has also improved during the past 10 years, and definitive answers regarding the optimal treatment of coronary artery disease will require further studies. *Center blocks* represent point estimates; *edge bars* represent 95% confidence limits of average hazard ratios. (*From* Mahlbaier and coworkers [21]; with permission.)

CORE PREOPERATIVE CABG AND LEVEL 1 VARIABLES

Information category	Core variables	Level 1 variables
Demographics	Age	Height
	Gender	Weight
Administrative		
History	Previous heart operation	PTCA on current admission
		Date of most recent myocardial infarction
		Angina history
Left ventricular function	Left ventricular ejection fraction	
Left main disease	% stenosis of left main coronary artery	
Other coronary disease	No. of major coronary arteries with stenosis >70%	
Other cardiac conditions		Serious ventricular arrhythmias
		Congestive heart failure
		Mitral regurgitation
Cardiovascular risk factors		Diabetes
		Cerebrovascular disease
		Peripheral vascular disease
Comorbid conditions		Chronic obstructive pulmonary disease
		Creatinine levels
Acuity/priority/hierarchy	Elective	
	Urgent	
	Emergent/ongoing ischemia	
	Emergent/hemodynamic instability	
	Emergent/salvage	

Figure 3-18. Identification of preoperative variables needed for risk adjustment of short-term mortality in seven separate databases [22]. In an effort to standardize the collection of data, a working group was established to develop a standard of practice for variables that should be captured by databases to assess coronary artery bypass graft (CABG) mortality. Currently, the Society of Thoracic Surgery (STS) has a multicenter database to which surgeons can send their data for collation and comparison with other institutions. As described in the other figures, numerous investigators have defined a number of variables associated with increased perioperative morbidity and mortality, some of which are included in the STS database, others of which are not. In an effort to establish a consensus and collect the highest quality and most important data, multiple databases were assessed and variables were ranked according to importance. The variables that should be included in all databases were considered as core and level 1 variables. PTCA—percutaneous transluminal coronary angioplasty. (*Adapted from* Jones and coworkers [22].)

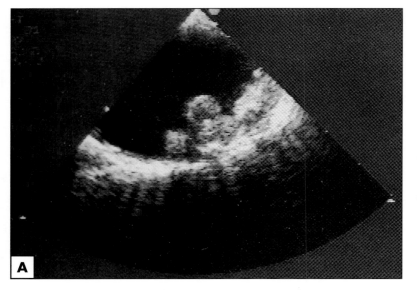

Figure 3-19. Assessment of aortic atheroma for prediction of perioperative neurologic dysfunction. Although cardiovascular morbidity and overall mortality are important outcomes, neurologic dysfunction occurs commonly after cardiac surgery. This is particularly true after valvular surgery or in the elderly. Neurologic complications can range from an overt stroke to minor neuropsychiatric dysfunction, and can have a profound impact on both the patient's quality of life and medical costs. Increasing evidence suggests that the presence and morphology of ascending aortic atheroma is the best predictor of perioperative neurologic dysfunction [23]. Transesophageal and epiaortic echocardiography have been used to demonstrate protruding atheroma. **A,** Transesophageal echocardiogram demonstrates a large atheroma protruding into the lumen.

(Continued on next page)

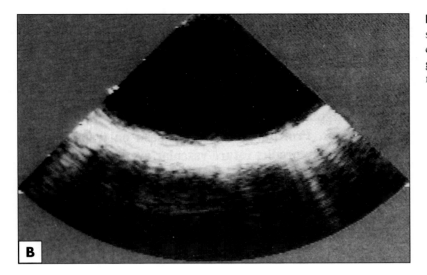

B

Figure 3-19. (*Continued*) **B**, Normal aortic arch. This has led several centers to perform either preoperative or intraoperative precordial, transthoracic, or epiaortic ultrasound as a method of guiding the surgeon in placement of the aortic cross-clamp or proximal graft sites. (*From* Tunick and coworkers [24]; with permission.)

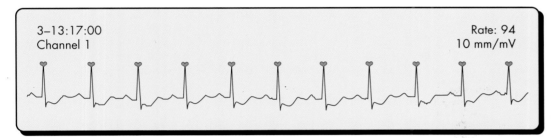

3–13:17:00
Channel 1

Rate: 94
10 mm/mV

Figure 3-20. Ambulatory electrocardiographic strip demonstrating significant ST-segment depression. The electrocardiogram is recorded on digitized magnetic tape in newer solid-state recorders. The presence of 1-mm horizontal or downsloping ST-segment depression (demon-

strated in the figure) or 2-mm ST-segment elevation is considered positive for silent myocardial ischemia. Preoperative Holter monitoring for silent myocardial ischemia has been advocated as a less expensive noninvasive means of assessing risk [25–27]. Although the positive predictive value of preoperative ischemia is similar to other noninvasive tests, a large majority of patients have baseline electrocardiographic abnormalities that preclude accurate analysis, and the test is not quantifiable to determine those at highest risk.

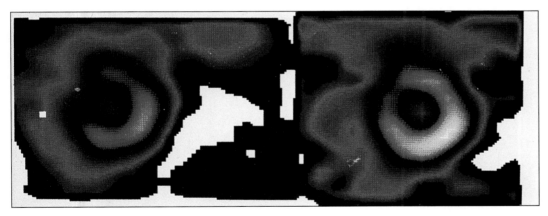

Figure 3-21. A dipyridamole-thallium single photon emission computed tomography image demonstrating a reversible defect. Dipyridamole works to increase flow to normal coronary arteries by blocking adenosine reuptake, and thereby redirecting flow away

from areas distal to a coronary artery stenosis. This results in a defect on initial imaging with thallium, which fills in on subsequent imaging if the myocardium is viable (redistribution defect). Those areas that are nonviable do not take up thallium, and demonstrate a persistent defect. A redistribution defect on dipyridamole-thallium imaging has been shown to identify patients at risk for developing perioperative cardiac events [27–30], although recent studies have demonstrated that the test loses its predictive accuracy when used in consecutive patients [31,32]. The figure demonstrates defects consistent with areas of low perfusion or ischemia, which fill on subsequent imaging.

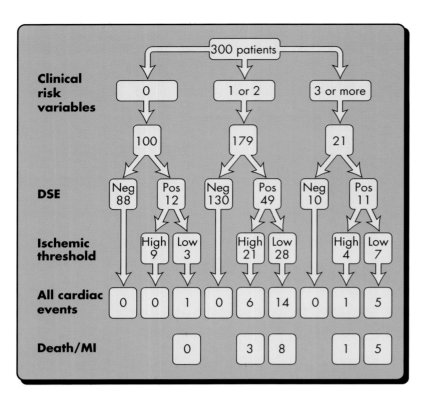

Figure 3-22. Predictive value of dobutamine stress echocardiography according to clinical risk stratification, the test results, and ischemic threshold for new regional wall motion abnormalities. Heart rate is increased by dobutamine, with the addition of atropine if maximal heart rate was less than 85% of predicted. The electrocardiogram is monitored continuously and echocardiography is used to monitor wall motion at defined points. The appearance of new or worsened regional wall motion abnormalities is considered a positive test. These represent areas at risk for myocardial ischemia. The advantage of this test is that it is a dynamic assessment of ventricular function. Dobutamine echocardiography has also been studied and found to have among the best positive and negative predictive values of all tests [33]. Poldermans *et al.* [34] demonstrated that the group at greatest risk were those who demonstrated regional wall motion abnormalities at low heart rates. Specifically, a high ischemic threshold occurred when the new regional wall motion abnormalities occurred at heart rates greater than 70% of maximal age-corrected heart rate. The test demonstrated the best discriminative value in those patients with at least one clinical variable, *eg*, age greater than 70 years, angina, diabetes requiring treatment, Q waves on the electrocardiogram, and a history of ventricular ectopic activity being treated. Many investigators believe that this test may offer the best prediction of risk in noncardiac surgery because it more accurately mimics the hyperdynamic state observed during the perioperative period. DSE—dobutamine-atropine stress test; MI—myocardial infarction; neg—negative test results; pos—positive test results. (*From* Poldermans and coworkers [34]; with permission.)

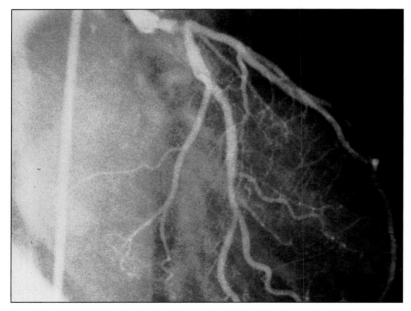

Figure 3-23. Coronary angiogram demonstrating a significant distal left main coronary artery stenosis. This patient had exertional angina and would be a candidate for coronary revascularization according to the American Heart Association/American College of Cardiology criteria [35]. Importantly, coronary angiography is an

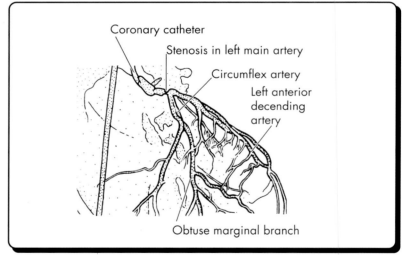

anatomic test and does not denote functional effects of a coronary stenosis. It is therefore the gold standard for coronary artery disease but does not necessarily correlate with the extent of symptoms. (*Courtesy of* Eric R. Powers.)

REFERENCES

1. Eagle K, Brundage B, Chaitman B, *et al.*: Guidelines for perioperative cardiovascular evaluation for noncardiac surgery. A report of the American Heart Association/American College of Cardiology Task Force on Assessment of Diagnostic and Therapeutic Cardiovascular Procedures. *Circulation* 1996, 93:1278–1317.

2. Palda VA and Detsky AS: Guidelines for assessing and managing the perioperative risk from coronary artery disease associated with major noncardiac surgery. *Ann Intern Med* 1997, 127:313–328.

3. Fleisher LA, Skolnick ED, Holroyd KJ, Lehmann HP: Coronary artery revascularization before abdominal aortic aneurysm surgery: a decision analytic approach. *Anesth Analg* 1994, 79:661–669.

4. Goldman L, Caldera DL, Nussbaum SR, *et al.*: Multifactorial index of cardiac risk in noncardiac surgical procedures. *N Engl J Med* 1977, 297:845–850.

5. Detsky A, Abrams H, McLaughlin J, *et al.*: Predicting cardiac complications in patients undergoing non-cardiac surgery. *J Gen Intern Med* 1986, 1:211–219.

6. Campeau L: Grading of angina pectoris (letter). *Circulation* 1975, 54:522–523.

7. The Criteria Committee of the New York Heart Association: *Nomenclature and Criteria for Diagnosis: Diseases of the Heart and Blood Vessels.* Boston: Little, Brown; 1964.

8. Goldman L, *et al.*: Comparative reproducibility and validity of systems for assessing cardiovascular function. *Circulation* 1981, 64:1227.

9. Tarhan S, Moffitt EA, Taylor WF, Giuliani ER: Myocardial infarction after general anesthesia. *JAMA* 1972, 220:1451–1454.

10. Rao TK, Jacobs KH, El-Etr AA: Reinfarction following anesthesia in patients with myocardial infarction. *Anesthesiology* 1983, 59:199–505.

11. Shah KB, Kleinman BS, Sami H, *et al.*: Reevaluation of perioperative myocardial infarction in patients with prior myocardial infarction undergoing noncardiac operations. *Anesth Analg* 1990, 71:231–235.

12. Eagle KA, Coley CM, Newell JB, *et al.*: Combining clinical and thallium data optimizes preoperative assessment of cardiac risk before major vascular surgery. *Ann Intern Med* 1989, 110:859–866.

13. Paul SD, Eagle KA, Kuntz KM, *et al.*: Concordance of preoperative clinical risk with angiographic severity of coronary artery disease in patients undergoing vascular surgery. *Circulation* 1996, 94:1561–1566.

14. Vanzetto G, Machecourt J, Blendea D, *et al.*: Additive value of thallium single-photon emission computed tomography myocardial imaging for prediction of perioperative events in clinically selected high cardiac risk patients having abdominal aortic surgery. *Am J Cardiol* 1996, 77:143–148.

15. Mangano DT, Layug EL, Wallace A, Tateo I: Effect of atenolol on mortality and cardiovascular morbidity after noncardiac surgery: Multicenter Study of Perioperative Ischemia Research Group. *N Engl J Med* 1996, 335:1713–1720.

16. Kennedy JW, Kaiser GC, Fisher LD, *et al.*: Clinical and angiographic predictors of operative mortality from the Colloborative Study in Coronary Artery Surgery (CASS). *Circulation* 1981, 63:793–802.

17. O'Connor G, Plume S, Olmstead E, *et al.*: Multivariate prediction of in-hospital mortality associated with coronary artery by-pass graft surgery. *Circulation* 1992, 85:2110–2118.

18. Parsonnet V, Dean D, Bernstein A: A method of uniform stratification of risk for evaluating the results of surgery in acquired adult heart disease. *Circulation* 1989, 79:I3–I12.

19. Hammermeister K, Burchfiel C, Johnson R, Grover F: Identification of patients at greatest risk for developing major complications of cardiac surgery. *Circulation* 1990, 82:IV380–IV389.

20. Higgins T, Estafanous F, Loop F, *et al.*: Stratification of morbidity and mortality outcome by preoperative risk factors in coronary artery bypass patients. *JAMA* 1992, 267:2344–2348.

21. Muhlbaier LH, Pryor DB, Rankin JS, *et al.*: Observational comparison of event-free survival with medical and surgical therapy in patients with coronary artery disease. 20 years of follow-up. *Circulation* 1992, 86:II198–II204.

22. Jones RH, Hannan EL, Hammermeister KE, *et al.*: Identification of preoperative variables needed for risk adjustment of short-term mortality after coronary artery bypass graft surgery. The Working Group Panel on the Cooperative CABG Database Project. *J Am Coll Cardiol* 1996, 28:1478–1487.

23. Hammon JW Jr, Stump DA, Kon ND, *et al.*: Risk factors and solutions for the development of neurobehavioral changes after coronary artery bypass grafting. *Ann Thorac Surg* 1997, 63:1613–1618.

24. Tunick PA, Rosenzweig BP, Katz ES, *et al.*: High risk for vascular events in patients with protruding aortic atheromas: a prospective study. *J Am Coll Cardiol* 1994, 23:1085–1090.

25. Raby KE, Goldman L, Creager MA, *et al.*: Correlation between perioperative ischemia and major cardiac events after peripheral vascular surgery. *N Engl J Med* 1989, 321:1296–1300.

26. Fleisher L, Rosenbaum S, Nelson A, Barash P: The predictive value of preoperative silent ischemia for postoperative ischemic cardiac events in vascular and nonvascular surgical patients. *Am Heart J* 1991, 122:980–986.

27. Fleisher LA, Rosenbaum SH, Nelson AH, *et al.*: Preoperative dipyridamole thallium imaging and Holter monitoring as a predictor of perioperative cardiac events and long term outcome. *Anesthesiology* 1995, 83:906–917.

28. Boucher CA, Brewster DC, Darling RC, *et al.*: Determination of cardiac risk by dipyridamole-thallium imaging before peripheral vascular surgery. *N Engl J Med* 1985, 312:389–394.

29. Cutler BS, Leppo JA: Dipyridamole thallium 201 scintigraphy to detect coronary artery disease before abdominal aortic surgery. *J Vasc Surg* 1987, 5:91–100.

30. Eagle KA, Singer DE, Brewster DC, *et al.*: Dipyridamole-thallium scanning in patients undergoing vascular surgery: optimizing preoperative evaluation of cardiac risk. *JAMA* 1987, 257:2185–2189.

31. Baron JF, Mundler O, Bertrand M, *et al.*: Dipyridamole-thallium scintigraphy and gated radionuclide angiography to assess cardiac risk before abdominal aortic surgery. *N Engl J Med* 1994, 330:663–669.

32. Mangano DT, London MJ, Tubau JF, *et al.*: Dipyridamole thallium-201 scintigraphy as a preoperative screening test: a reexamination of its predictive potential. Study of Perioperative Ischemia Research Group. *Circulation* 1991, 84:493–502.

33. Poldermans D, Fioretti PM, Forster T, *et al.*: Dobutamine stress echocardiography for assessment of perioperative cardiac risk in patients undergoing major vascular surgery [see comments]. *Circulation* 1993, 87:1506–1512.

34. Poldermans D, Arnese M, Fioretti PM, *et al.*: Improved cardiac risk stratification in major vascular surgery with dobutamine-atropine stress echocardiography. *J Am Coll Cardiol* 1995, 26:648–653.

35. ACC/AHA guidelines and indications for coronary artery bypass graft surgery. A report of the American College of Cardiology/American Heart Association Task Force on Assessment of Diagnostic and Therapeutic Cardiovascular Procedures (Subcommittee on Coronary Artery Bypass Graft Surgery). *Circulation* 1991, 83:1125–1173.

Ischemic Heart Disease

B. Hugh Dorman

Ischemic heart disease continues to represent a major health problem in the United States, afflicting an estimated 7–8 million individuals [1]. Approximately 1 million patients with cardiac disease have surgery annually, which can be associated with a significant incidence of perioperative morbidity. Based on recent studies, at least 50,000 patients have a perioperative myocardial infarction each year. Patients with a prior myocardial infarction who undergo surgery have an increased risk for perioperative myocardial reinfarction, ranging from 2% to 35%. Mortality among patients with preexisting coronary artery disease who sustain a perioperative myocardial reinfarction has been reported to range from 36% to 70%. Thus, ischemic heart disease represents a formidable challenge to the anesthesiologist during both cardiac and noncardiac surgery, and should increase in magnitude in the future as older and more medically debilitated patients undergo surgery.

Myocardial ischemia occurs when coronary blood flow is not sufficient to meet oxidative substrate demands of the myocardium. The pathophysiology of myocardial ischemia is multifactorial, including a reduction in oxygen supply owing to coronary stenosis from fixed atherosclerotic disease, vasospasm, thrombosis, or a combination of fixed and dynamic narrowing of the coronary arteries [2–4]. Increases in myocardial oxygen demand can also create an unfavorable balance of myocardial oxygen supply and demand, and precipitate ischemia. The management of ischemic heart disease stems from an understanding of the determinants of myocardial oxygen supply and demand and the physiology of coronary blood flow.

The diagnosis of coronary artery disease preoperatively is usually accomplished with a positive history followed by exercise stress testing. Coronary catheterization with contrast ventriculography provides valuable information on the extent and distribution of obstructive coronary lesions, and on ventricular function from measurement of ejection fraction, intracavitary pressures, and abnormal wall motion. Other preoperative studies that can provide useful information in the patient with ischemic heart disease include echocardiography to visualize wall motion abnormalities and determine ejection fraction, nuclear imaging techniques to detect areas of abnormal perfusion or prior infarction, and first-pass radionuclide angiography or multiple unit gated acquisition scans to detect ventricular volumes, ejection fraction, abnormal pulmonary blood flow, and cardiac output. Thus, valuable information can be obtained preoperatively from a variety of noninvasive and invasive studies to delineate the extent of coronary artery disease, exercise tolerance and left ventricular function, which can be used to assess prognosis and construct an anesthetic management plan.

Intraoperatively, the most sensitive and earliest indicator of myocardial ischemia is provided by transesophageal echocardiography [5,6]. Regional wall motion abnormalities and wall thinning during systole are characteristic of myocardial ischemia and occur prior to electrocardiographic changes. ST-segment depression on the electrocardiogram is a common manifestation of subendocardial ischemia, whereas new-onset ST-segment elevation typically represents transmural myocardial ischemia and is usually associated with acute coronary occlusion without well-developed collateral flow. Abrupt elevations in the pulmonary artery or pulmonary capillary wedge pressure with large A waves reflecting decreased ventricular compliance or pathologic V waves representing mitral regurgitation due to papillary muscle dysfunction are also indicators of myocardial ischemia that can be diagnosed with the Swan-Ganz catheter. Finally, the blood pressure–heart rate ratio has been proposed to be a useful predictor of myocardial ischemia [7]. It is evident that the anesthesiologist has a variety of monitoring capabilities that can result in rapid intraoperative diagnosis of myocardial ischemia, allowing for early intervention.

The treatment of ischemic heart disease is dependent on the severity of symptoms and the setting in which the diagnosis is made. Acute onset of myocardial ischemia with evolving myocardial injury can be treated with thrombolytic agents or percutaneous transluminal coronary angioplasty (PTCA). Coronary atherectomy and intracoronary stents are techniques that have been recently developed in an attempt to decrease the incidence of restenosis following coronary dilatation [8,9]. Coronary artery bypass graft (CABG) is frequently performed in patients with multivessel coronary disease, in patients whose anatomy is not amenable to PTCA, in patients in which thrombolytic therapy or PTCA is not successful, or in patients whose angioplasty is complicated by intimal or branch-point dissection and subsequent coronary occlusion. Intra-aortic balloon pump (IABP) counterpulsation is useful to stabilize patients in cardiogenic shock due to myocardial ischemia prior to cardiac catheterization or CABG. The IABP increases coronary blood flow during diastole and unloads the left ventricle during systole by mass displacement of blood in the proximal segment of the descending aorta.

Intraoperatively, the treatment of myocardial ischemia is primarily by pharmacologic intervention. It is important to aggressively treat intraoperative hemodynamic abnormalities temporally related to the onset of ischemia that could precipitate imbalances of myocardial oxygen supply and demand. The mainstay of anti-ischemic drug therapy is nitroglycerin. β-Adrenergic antagonists have also proved useful in the treatment of myocardial ischemia by reducing myocardial oxygen consumption, increasing diastolic coronary blood flow, and inhibiting platelet aggregation. Finally, calcium channel antagonists exert an anti-ischemic effect by coronary artery dilatation, a reduction in myocardial oxygen demand by decreasing contractility, and the prevention of sympathetically mediated coronary vasoconstriction. Proper management of myocardial ischemia intraoperatively depends on early recognition and diagnosis, an understanding of myocardial oxygen supply and demand dynamics, appropriate hemodynamic control, and optimal anti-ischemic drug therapy. The objectives of this chapter, therefore, are to provide an improved understanding of the etiology, pathophysiology, diagnosis, and treatment of ischemic heart disease, especially in the perioperative setting.

PRIMARY DETERMINANTS OF MYOCARDIAL OXYGEN SUPPLY AND DEMAND

Oxygen supply	Oxygen demand
Coronary blood flow	Contractility
Heart rate	Heart rate
Coronary varscular resistance	Wall tension
Blood oxygen content	Afterload
Oxygen saturation	LVEDP (preload)
Hematocrit	Minor determinants
PaO$_2$	Sarcomere shortening
Oxygen-hemoglobin dissociation (pH;	Basal metabolic requirement
2,3-DPG; temperature)	

Figure 4-1. Primary determinants of myocardial oxygen supply and demand. Coronary blood flow is defined as coronary perfusion pressure (aortic diastolic pressure minus left ventricular end diastolic back pressure) divided by coronary vascular resistance. Left ventricular-end diastolic back pressure was once defined as either left ventricular end-diastolic pressure (LVEDP) or coronary sinus pressure (whichever was higher), but may be several mm Hg greater than either pressure [10]. Heart rate can affect both oxygen supply and demand; increases in heart rate potentiate myocardial oxygen demand and can reduce subendocardial perfusion by shortening diastole. Wall tension is defined as intracavitary ventricular pressure times intracavitary radius divided by ventricular wall thickness, and is directly proportional to both afterload and preload. LVEDP can therefore affect both myocardial oxygen requirement and delivery of oxygen to the myocardium; an increase in LVEDP increases wall tension and reduces coronary blood flow. 2,3-DPG—2,3-diphosphoglycerate.

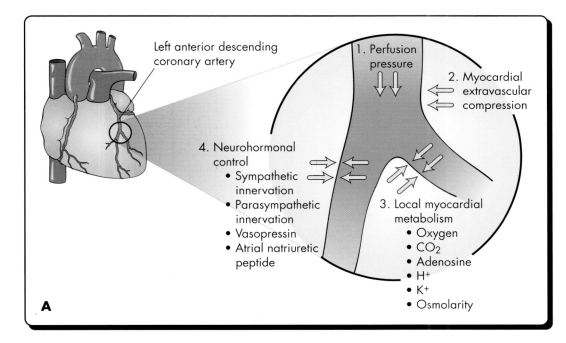

A

Figure 4-2. Physiology of coronary blood flow. The four primary determinants of coronary blood flow include perfusion pressure (*1*), myocardial extravascular compression (*2*), local myocardial metabolism (*3*), and neurohormonal influences (*4*) (**A**). Coronary blood flow is proportional to the pressure gradient that exists across the coronary circulation, but is modulated by numerous factors. Resistance to coronary perfusion secondary to extravascular compression is greatest in the left ventricle; compression of intramyocardial arteries results in a majority of left ventricular coronary perfusion in diastole when intramyocardial pressure is lowest. Myocardial metabolism is the major determinant of coronary blood flow, coupling myocardial oxygen demand (MVO$_2$) to blood flow due to either substrate depletion or metabolic byproduct accumulation [11]. Finally, neurohormonal influences can modulate coronary vascular resistance and assist in correlating coronary blood flow to local and global demand.

(*Continued on next page*)

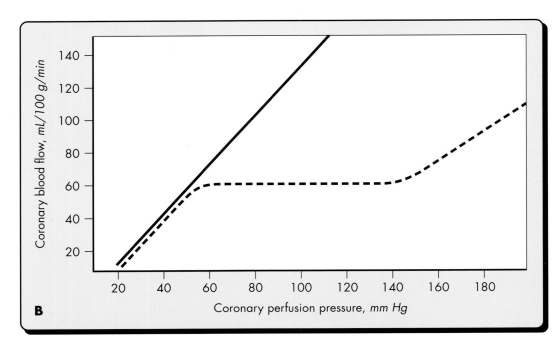

Figure 4-2. (*Continued*) Coronary blood flow is an example of an autoregulated system, such that tissue blood flow remains constant (**B**) over a wide range of perfusion pressures (60 to 140 mm Hg) at a fixed MVO$_2$. Since oxygen extraction by the myocardium is so efficient (myocardial venous oxygen tension equals 15 to 20 mm Hg), an increase in oxygen availability occurs primarily by increases in coronary blood flow. Coronary flow reserve is the difference between autoregulated flow (*dotted line*) and nonautoregulated, maximal flow (*solid line*), and represents the additional capacity of the coronary arteriolar vasculature to dilate in response to decreased luminal diameter or increased MVO$_2$. As autoregulation fails owing to more pronounced obstruction of a coronary artery, coronary reserve becomes exhausted and flow becomes pressure dependent.

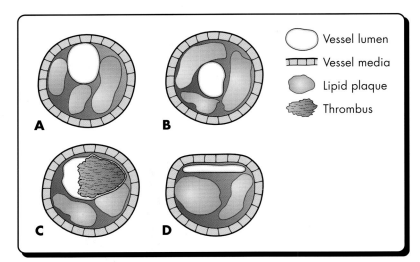

Figure 4-3. Coronary artery stenosis. Cross-sectional illustrations of various presentations of coronary atherosclerotic disease. Coronary artery stenosis is primarily the result of an accumulation of fibrous plaque containing lipid-laden macrophages, due to advanced atherosclerotic disease. In significant coronary stenosis approximately 75% of the lesions are eccentric (**A**), bounded in part by a portion of normal muscular arterial wall that can vary in diameter and alter vascular resistance. Only 25% of coronary plaques are concentric (**B**), with the vessel lumen surrounded completely by fibrous plaque. Although severe acute coronary ischemia is often precipitated by plaque rupture and thrombus formation (**C**), segments of normal wall in diseased arteries may respond abnormally and constrict inappropriately to various stimuli [12]; such abnormal response of stenotic coronary arteries appears to be the result of endothelial dysfunction and may lead to dynamic stenosis (**D**) due to coronary vasoconstriction. (*Adapted from* Brown and coworkers [13].)

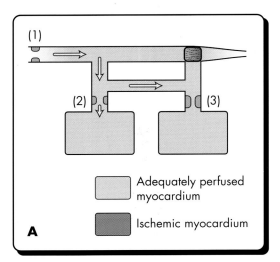 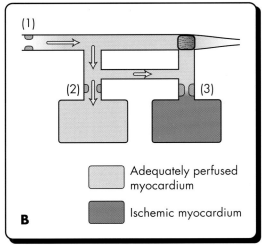

23% of patients with ischemic heart disease [4] and includes the presence of a vascular bed distal to a severe stenosis (*3*), maximally dilated without coronary reserve, which is dependent on collateral flow from a parallel vascular bed that is also stenotic but has intact autoregulation (*2*). At rest (**A**), myocardium distal to the severe stenosis (*3*) receives adequate collateral flow to match metabolic demand. However, with exercise (**B**) or pharmacologically induced vasodilatation (adenosine, dipyridamole), dilation of the vascular bed with intact autoregulation (*2*) occurs to increase distal flow. Dilation of arteries distal to (*2*) will increase flow to local myocardium, but will reduce perfusion pressure throughout the vascular bed distal to (*1*), and can result in a redistribution of blood flow away from the myocardium distal to the severe stenosis (*3*).

Figure 4-4. Coronary steal. An increase in myocardial blood flow in one area that reduces flow in another is called "coronary steal." Anatomy conducive to coronary steal occurs in up to

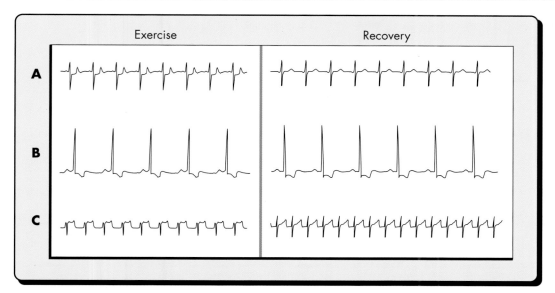

Figure 4-5. Exercise stress testing. The evaluation of ischemic heart disease in a patient with a positive history frequently involves exercise stress testing to help diagnose and determine the severity of coronary artery disease. Exercise test protocols cause a progressive increase in myocardial work, necessitating an increase in coronary blood flow to meet myocardial oxygen demand. Because coronary vascular reserve is limited in patients with coronary atherosclerotic disease, impairment of adequate myocardial blood flow during periods of increased demand allows for measurement of ischemia, dysrhythmias, and cardiac pump dysfunction. The primary method to determine ischemia is with measurement of ST-segment displacement using exercise electrocardiography. Three major types of ST-segment displacement have been described: type I—ST depression with an initial upsloping of the ST segment that may progress to a flat segment, with progressive J point depression (**A**) that quickly resolves early in the immediate postexercise period; type II—ST-segment depression with a flat or downsloping segment occurring during exercise, with a progressively more abnormal response for several minutes during recovery (**B**); and type III—ST-segment elevation (**C**) occurring in 3% to 5% of patients. Although type II generally carries the worst prognosis for multivessel, severe disease, ST-segment elevation in a non-Q wave, noninfarct lead may represent transmural myocardial ischemia and a severe ischemic response. Stress testing has increased prognostic value when the ST-segment depression is greater than 1.0 mm, persists into the recovery phase, and is associated with either hypotension, arrhythmias, angina, or less than predicted increases in heart rate [14].

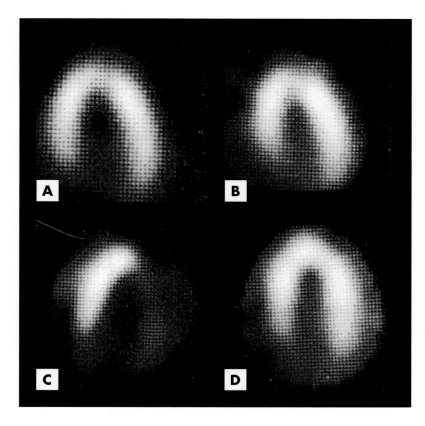

Figure 4-6. Myocardial perfusion imaging. Myocardial single photon emission computed tomography (SPECT) using thallium-201 for diagnosis of myocardial ischemia. Myocardial perfusion scanning with exercise can help demonstrate the extent, reversibility, and location of coronary artery disease and the quantity of myocardium at risk for infarction. Myocardial perfusion scintigraphy with thallium-201 is significantly more accurate for the detection of coronary artery disease than the exercise electrocardiogram [15]. **A** and **B**, Horizontal long-axis tomographic reconstructions in the absence of coronary perfusion defects show thallium extracted by normal myocardium during periods of stress (Brüce treadmill protocol) (*panel A*) and during the recovery period (*panel B*), providing a horseshoe configuration around the central ventricular cavity. **C** and **D**, In contrast, in the patient with significant coronary artery disease, gated SPECT images of the left ventricle at peak stress (*panel C*) reveals marked decreased perfusion in the inferolateral wall, which dramatically improves and normalizes at rest (*panel D*). Findings are consistent with extensive stress-induced ischemia in the distribution of the circumflex coronary artery.

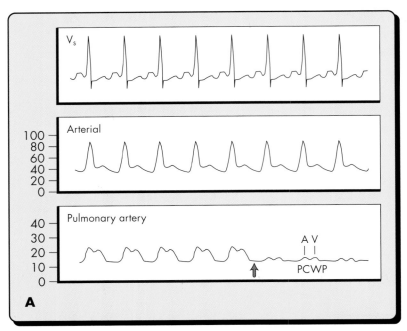

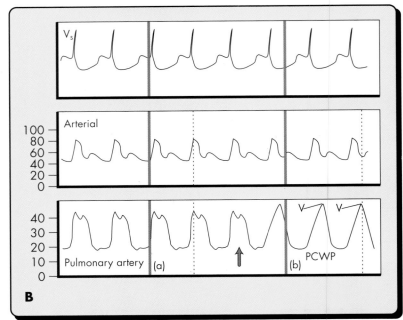

Figure 4-7. The utility of the pulmonary artery catheter in the diagnosis of intraoperative myocardial ischemia. Electrocardiographic, arterial, pulmonary artery, and pulmonary capillary wedge pressure (PCWP) tracings from a patient before (**A**) and during (**B**) an intraoperative episode of acute myocardial ischemia. Prior to ischemia (**A**), the patient has a normal-appearing electrocardiographic (ECG) trace without ST-segment changes, a relatively low pulmonary artery pressure, and a normal-appearing PCWP tracing (*balloon inflated at the arrow*) with typical A and V waves. In contrast, during an episode of myocardial ischemia (**B**), ST depression is apparent in the ECG tracing

with attendant reductions in arterial blood pressure. The pulmonary artery pressure is elevated and a prominent V wave appears in the pulmonary capillary wedge tracing. The giant V wave represents acute mitral regurgitation secondary to papillary muscle ischemia. Although the V wave resembles the pulmonary artery waveform, the two can be differentiated by the relationship to the electrocardiographic QRS complex and the arterial waveform. The pulmonary artery waveform peaks concurrently with the arterial trace and the electrocardiographic T wave (a), while the V wave is delayed, peaking after the arterial waveform and the T wave of the ECG (b).

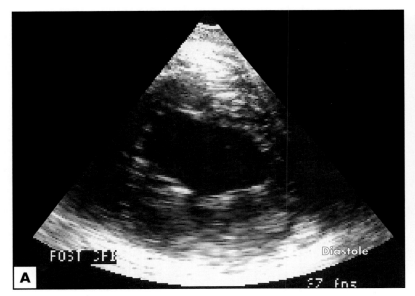

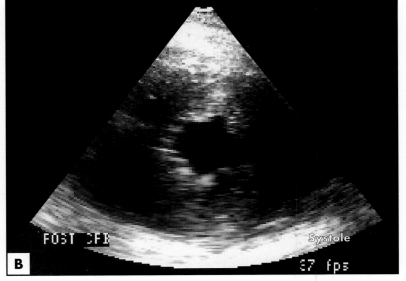

Figure 4-8. The utility of transesophageal echocardiography (TEE) in the diagnosis of intraoperative ischemia. For detection of myocardial ischemia by TEE, myocardial wall motion abnormalities and alterations in wall thickening are assessed. Clinical studies have shown that echocardiographic assessment of wall motion abnormalities provides a more sensitive and earlier indicator of myocardial

ischemia than abnormalities detected by electrocardiography or pulmonary artery catheter [5,6,16]. In the left ventricular (LV) short-axis view of well-perfused myocardium without coronary artery disease (**A** and **B**), inward wall motion during systole occurs throughout all wall segments and the LV wall shows a normal increase in thickness.

(*Continued on next page*)

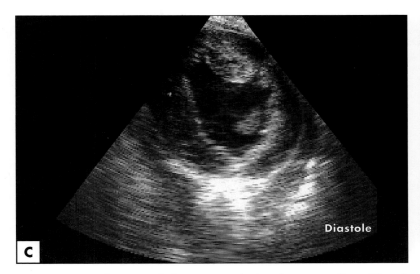

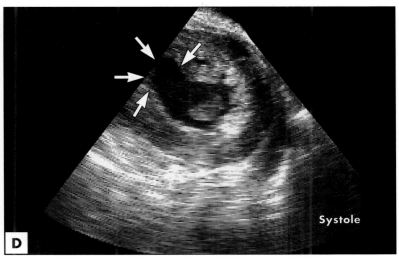

Figure 4-8. (*Continued*) In contrast, ischemic myocardium (**C** and **D**) shows regional wall motion abnormalities ranging from hypokinesis to dyskinesis in the affected segments and there is a reduction in thickness, or actual thinning, of the ischemic tissue during systole. As shown in *panel D*, the posterior-septal wall is dyskinetic (*arrows*), and does not move inward with systole. Although wall thinning appears to be a more specific indicator of ischemia than wall motion abnormalities, the epicardium cannot always be clearly visualized and, therefore, regional wall motion changes provide a more consistent marker of myocardial ischemia.

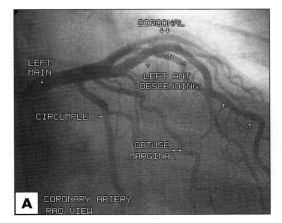

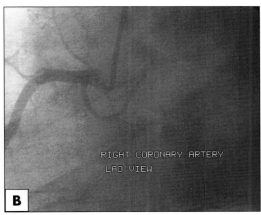

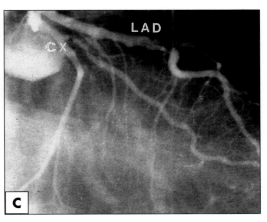

Figure 4-9. Cardiac catheterization for diagnosis of ischemic heart disease. Coronary arteriograms illustrating normal coronary anatomy (**A** and **B**) and coronary artery disease (**C**). The left coronary artery system is shown in *panel A* from a right anterior oblique (RAO) view. The left main coronary artery bifurcates into the circumflex (CX) and left anterior descending (LAD) arteries; both septal perforators and diagonal branches arise from the LAD, while marginal branches arise from the CX. In *panel B* the right coronary artery (RCA) is shown from a left anterior oblique (LAO) view. In greater than 80% of patients the posterior descending artery (PDA) originates from the RCA (right dominant system) and supplies the inferior aspect of the left ventricle and inferior one third of the ventricular septum. Selective coronary angiography of the left coronary artery in the RAO view is seen in *panel C*. A very high grade lesion is noted in the proximal LAD accompanied by a long, high-grade lesion at the origin of the first posterolateral branch of the CX. The actual reduction in cross-sectional area associated with coronary stenosis is greater than the degree of stenosis or diameter reduction assessed by coronary angiograms in two dimensions; a 75% diameter reduction corresponds to a 90% cross-sectional area reduction. In addition to characterization of the magnitude and severity of atherosclerotic coronary artery disease, cardiac catheterization can also help identify dynamic coronary vascular lesions, such as spasm and thrombosis, and can define the sequelae of ischemic heart disease such as ventricular dysfunction, aneurysms, septal defects, and ischemic mitral regurgitation [17].

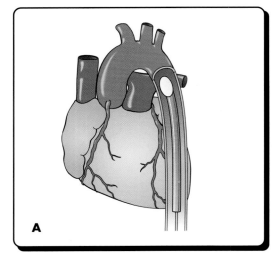

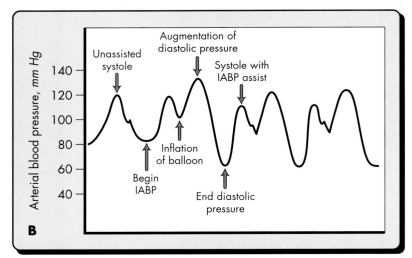

Figure 4-10. Intra-aortic balloon pump (IABP). Use of the IABP to stabilize a patient with unstable angina before coronary artery bypass grafting. Temporary hemodynamic stabilization and improvement of myocardial ischemia prior to definitive mechanical procedures can be obtained with the IABP. The IABP is inserted percutaneously via the femoral artery into the thoracic aorta and positioned with the balloon just distal to the left subclavian artery (**A**). Arterial waveforms observed during IABP assist (**B**). The balloon is inflated immediately following closure of the aortic valve, which augments diastolic aortic pressure and coronary perfusion. Deflation of the balloon occurs just prior to the onset of systole to improve systolic unloading and reduce impedance to left ventricular (LV) ejection. The reduction in LV afterload reduces myocardial oxygen demand, while the augmented diastolic pressure increases coronary perfusion and improves myocardial oxygen supply. Cardiac output is typically increased with improvements in systemic perfusion.

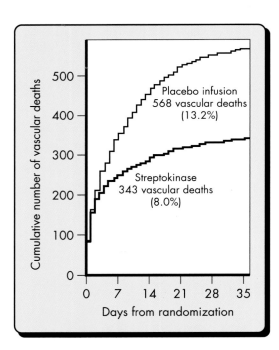

Figure 4-11. Thrombolytic therapy in ischemic heart disease. Pharmacologic agents for lysing coronary thrombi, such as streptokinase and tissue plasminogen activation (tPA), work by converting plasminogen to the active enzyme plasmin. Thrombolytic therapy in acute myocardial infarction (AMI) recanalizes thrombotic occlusions and restores coronary flow, resulting in a reduction in infarct size and improved myocardial function and patient survival (shown in the figure). The most dramatic improvement in patient survival with AMI occurs when thrombolytic agents are administered within 2 hours of symptoms; however, a beneficial effect on survival is still apparent when they are administered within 6 to 12 hours from the onset of ischemic symptoms [18]. Thrombolytic therapy during AMI is of relatively greater benefit in patients with anterior ST-segment elevation, bundle branch block, systolic blood pressure less than 100 mm Hg, or a history of diabetes. Both tPA and streptokinase have been successfully used during AMI; however, an accelerated tPA regimen with immediate intravenous heparin appears to result in the lowest 30-day mortality, highest graft patency and best regional and global left ventricular function [19]. Although the routine use of percutaneous transluminal coronary angioplasty (PTCA) after thrombolytic therapy in the treatment of AMI has not proved beneficial, PTCA may be more effective than thrombolytic treatment as an initial therapy in patients with AMI and cardiogenic shock, or in patients with an elevated risk of intracerebral hemorrhage (age > 65 years, weight < 70 kg, hypertensive on presentation). (*From* Second International Study of Infarct Survival [1SIS-2] Collaborative Group [20].)

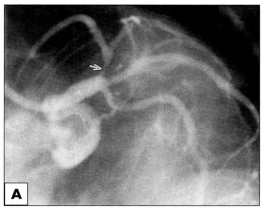 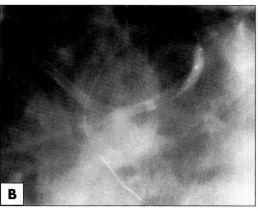 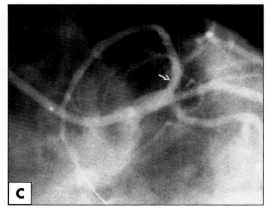

Figure 4-12. Percutaneous transluminal coronary angioplasty (PTCA) for treatment of coronary artery stenosis. A preangioplasty angiogram of the left coronary artery in the left anterior oblique view with caudal angulation reveals an 80% stenosis (*arrow*) at the ostium of the left anterior descending (LAD) coronary artery (**A**). A guidewire has been passed through the stenotic lesion and the balloon inflated across the stenotic region (**B**). Following removal of the balloon there is no residual stenosis (**C**, *arrow*). PTCA has the highest success rate (> 85%) with fewest complications (2%) on type "A" coronary lesions that are discrete (< 10 mm length), concentric, accessible lesions with a smooth contour and nonangulated segments, without calcification, thrombosis, total occlusion, major branch involvement, or an ostial location. In contrast, PTCA procedures with type "C" lesions have lower success rates (< 6%) and higher complication rates (21%), and consist of diffuse (length > 2 cm) or totally occluded lesions (> 3 months) with excessive tortuosity, angulated segments (> 90 degrees) that involve major side branches or degenerated vein grafts. In recent years PTCA procedures have enjoyed improved success rates, especially in male patients with chronic stable angina, preserved ventricular function (ejection fraction > 40%), and type "A" lesions [21,22]. Despite recent advances in PTCA procedures, coronary artery bypass graft appears to be more appropriate than PTCA for patients with left main disease, two- or three-vessel disease with left ventricular dysfunction, patients with a single remaining conduit that serves as the only source for coronary perfusion, or patients with anatomy not suitable for PTCA, including diffuse coronary involvement or chronic total occlusion.

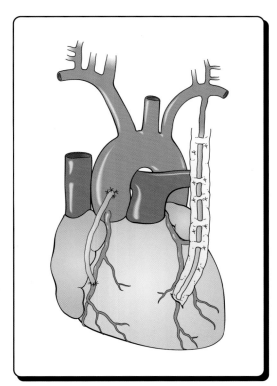

Figure 4-13. Coronary artery bypass graft surgery (CABG) for treatment of ischemic heart disease Revascularization of the right coronary artery via a saphenous vein graft and internal mammary artery (IMA) grafting to the left anterior descending (LAD) coronary artery is illustrated. The IMA graft, which has minimal development of intimal hyperplasia, is a superior conduit for bypass grafting with greater than 90% patency at 10 to 12 years, compared with a 40% to 60% patency rate for saphenous vein grafts [23]. The benefit from CABG is most evident in patients with the most complete revascularization, with approximately 75% of patients free from an ischemic event, sudden death, myocardial infarction, or recurrent angina 5 years after CABG, and 50% symptom-free 10 years postoperatively. The indications for surgical versus medical treatment of the patient with ischemic heart disease are still debated. However, CABG has been shown to improve survival in large, randomized trials in patients with left main coronary artery disease, in patients with two- or three-vessel disease with proximal LAD involvement, and in patients with two- or three-vessel disease with left ventricular dysfunction. Thus, CABG is currently being performed in an increasing number of older, higher risk patients with unstable angina, multivessel disease, poor ventricular function, and comorbid conditions, including hypertension, diabetes and peripheral vascular disease, because of improved survival with surgery in this subpopulation of patients. Such aggressive surgical intervention may change the overall surgical mortality of 2.2% for elective first-time CABG observed over the past decade.

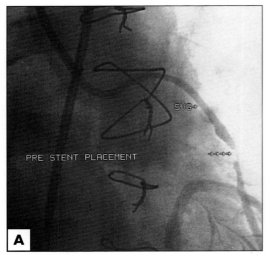
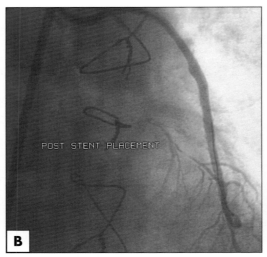
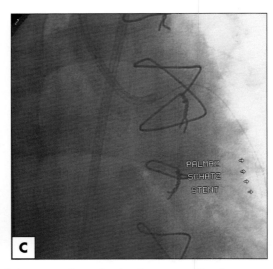

Figure 4-14. New devices in interventional cardiology. New devices for interventional cardiology have evolved to bypass limitations inherent with balloon angioplasty, including a high rate of restenosis and lower success rates with coronary lesions that are totally occluded, tortuous, calcified, or situated in saphenous vein grafts. One of the most commonly used new devices includes intracoronary stents. **A,** A saphenous vein graft (SVG) with a high grade stenosis (*arrows*), with patency restored following placement of an intracoronary stent (**B**). **C,** The Palmaz Schatz stent (*arrows*) is seen within the SVG. Intracoronary stents are used as a scaffold to support and maintain patency of a diseased artery or vein graft, reducing recoil and restenosis [24]. Although stents appear to be useful as a primary revascularization procedure with a reduced incidence of restenosis and as a "bail-out" procedure following abrupt vessel closure with balloon angioplasty, the thrombogenicity of metallic stents can result in acute thrombotic closure or distal embolization, and aggressive prophylactic anticoagulation regimens carry a risk for hemorrhagic complications. Other new interventional tools include coronary atherectomy devices that remove atheromatous material from coronary lesions (success rate, 82% to 88%) by either incising the plaque with a spinning blade (directional and extraction atherectomy), or abrading the plaque with rotational atherectomy techniques [25]. Laser angioplasty is another new methodology that directly ablates coronary plaques using thermal, acoustic, and photo dissociation mechanisms, but has an increased risk for major complications, including coronary dissection and perforation [26]. Large, prospective clinical trials are clearly needed to ascertain the efficacy and safety of these new interventional modalities compared with conventional balloon angioplasty techniques.

INTRAOPERATIVE HEMODYNAMIC ABNORMALITIES AND MYOCARDIAL ISCHEMIA

Abnormal hemodynamic profile	Treatment
Hypertension, tachycardia	IV nitroglycerin IV β-blockade Increased anesthetic depth Labetalol
Hypertension, normal heart rate	IV nitroglycerin Increased anesthetic depth SL nifedipine IV nicardipine IV β-blockade for reflex tachycardia
Normotension, tachycardia	R/O arrhythmia Check volume status, hematocrit Check anesthetic depth (change technique?) IV β-blockade IV nitroglycerin
Hypotension, tachycardia	R/O arrhythmia Check volume status, hematocrit ⎫ Check contractile function ⎬ Specific, directed treatment Calculate SVR ⎭ Check anesthetic depth IV α-agonist to support coronary perfusion pressure IV β-blockade once normotensive (with adequate contractile function) IV nitroglycerin once normotensive
Hypotension, bradycardia	R/O arrhythmia (ie, junctional rhythm) Check volume status ⎫ Check contractile function ⎬ Specific, directed treatment Calculate SVR ⎭ IV ephedrine IV atropine IV epinephrine (infusion vs low-dose bolus) IV nitroglycerin once normotensive
Hypotension, normal heart rate	Check volume status ⎫ Check contractile function ⎬ Specific, directed treatment Calculate SVR ⎭ IV α-agonist for reduced SVR Volume and/or inotrope to correct specific abnormality IV nitroglycerin once normotensive

Figure 4-15. Intraoperative hemodynamic abnormalities and myocardial ischemia. Although a majority of episodes of intraoperative myocardial ischemia are not directly associated with hemodynamic changes, there are a number of hemodynamic abnormalities that can compromise the myocardial oxygen supply-demand relationship and directly precipitate ischemia [27]. Deleterious hemodynamic abnormalities that are temporally associated with ischemia (*see* table) should be promptly diagnosed and treated. In the setting of an acute change in hemodynamic profile intraoperatively, the adequacy of oxygenation, ventilation, and volume status must be quickly confirmed and an arrhythmia or surgical factor (acute blood loss, cardiac manipulation) must be considered. Ideally, invasive cardiac monitoring with a pulmonary artery catheter or transesophageal echocardiography allows for prompt investigation of the cause of any hemodynamic alteration and appropriate, directed therapy. For example, hypotension can compromise coronary perfusion and can be secondary to a reduction in preload, afterload, contractile function, or an arrhythmia; appropriate management of volume status, systemic vascular resistance, inotropy, anesthetic depth, and heart rate and rhythm is necessary for optimal treatment of deleterious hemodynamic changes and subsequent resolution of intraoperative myocardial ischemia. Although nitroglycerin is the mainstay of treatment for ischemic heart disease, coronary perfusion pressure must be maintained and heart rate needs to be strictly controlled, since tachycardia has been shown to be directly associated with the development of ischemia [27]. IV—intravenous; R/O—rule out; SL—sublingual; SVR—systemic vascular resistance. (*Adapted from* Kaplan [28]; with permission.)

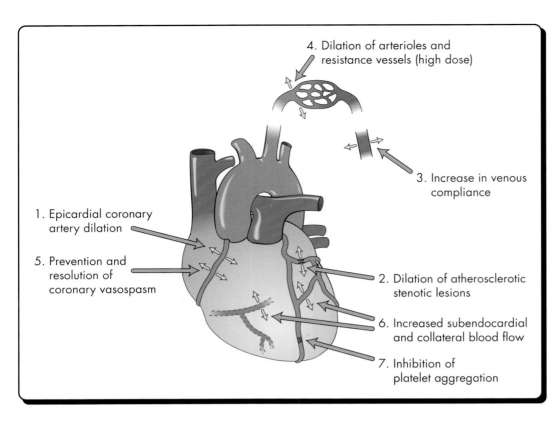

4. Dilation of arterioles and resistance vessels (high dose)

3. Increase in venous compliance

1. Epicardial coronary artery dilation

5. Prevention and resolution of coronary vasospasm

2. Dilation of atherosclerotic stenotic lesions

6. Increased subendocardial and collateral blood flow

7. Inhibition of platelet aggregation

Figure 4-16. Beneficial effects of nitroglycerin in ischemic heart disease. Nitroglycerin is a potent dilator of epicardial coronary arteries, with a more pronounced effect on smaller coronary arteries. Atherosclerotic stenoses also dilate with nitroglycerin, provided that a normal segment of endothelium is present. The reduction in preload from increased venous compliance and the decrease in afterload with high doses of nitroglycerin contribute to a reduction in myocardial oxygen demand. The improvement of blood flow to the subendocardium, the myocardium with the highest ischemia risk, is secondary to both improved collateral flow and a decreased resistance to blood flow in the setting of a reduced left ventricular end diastolic pressure [29]. Vasospasm of both native coronary arteries and internal mammary artery grafts can be prevented by nitroglycerin. The usefulness of nitroglycerin in ischemic heart disease also stems from the inhibition of platelet aggregation, mediated by the nitroglycerin metabolite nitric oxide and related nitroso compounds, resulting in an increased platelet cyclic guanosine monophosphate [30].

BENEFICIAL EFFECTS OF β-BLOCKERS IN ISCHEMIC HEART DISEASE

Reduction in myocardial oxygen consumption
Prolonged myocardial diastolic perfusion period
Decreased infarct size and morbidity associated with myocardial infarction
Decreased mortality following myocardial infarction
Treatment of cardiac arrhythmias

Figure 4-17. Beneficial effects of β-blockers in ischemic heart disease. β-Antagonists are commonly prescribed for patients with coronary artery disease. The primary benefit of β-blockade stems from the reduction in myocardial oxygen consumption [31]. This is accomplished by β_1-receptor antagonism, resulting in reductions in heart rate, cardiac index, stroke index, blood pressure, and tension-time index. β-Blockers may also augment myocardial oxygen supply by prolonging the diastolic perfusion period, increasing collateral flow with redistribution to ischemic areas and promoting oxygen dissociation from hemoglobin. β-Blockers administered during an evolving myocardial infarction appear to reduce the extent of infarction and associated morbidity if given within 4 to 6 hours after the onset of symptoms. Numerous trials have illustrated the improvement in patient survival after myocardial infarction with chronic administration of β-blockers. Although β-blockers have been commonly used in rate reduction of atrial fibrillation and flutter via slowing of atrioventricular nodal conduction, β-antagonists are also efficacious in the treatment of ventricular arrhythmias in awake patients with coronary artery disease or during the perioperative period when catecholamine levels are elevated.

BENEFICIAL EFFECTS OF CALCIUM CHANNEL BLOCKERS IN ISCHEMIC HEART DISEASE

	Coronary blood flow	Subendocardial/subepicardial blood flow	Platelet aggregation	Arterial vasodilation	Inotropy*	Chronotropy*
Verapamil	↑↑	↑↑	↓↓	↑	↓↓	↓↓
Diltiazem	↑↑↑	↑↑	↓↓	↑	↓	↓↓
Nifedipine	↑↑↑↑	↑↑	↓↓	↑↑↑↑	←→	←→
Nicardipine	↑↑↑↑	↑↑	↓↓	↑↑↑↑	←→	←→

* Intact animal with compensatory baroreceptor reflexes intact.
↑–increase; ↓–decrease; ←→–minimal or no effect.

Figure 4-18. Beneficial effects of calcium channel blockers in ischemic heart disease. Although calcium channel antagonists cause increases in coronary blood flow, the most important effects with regard to treatment of ischemic heart disease appear to be the prevention and resolution of coronary vasoconstriction or spasm. A number of studies have shown that calcium channel antagonists can improve subendocardial coronary blood flow relative to subepicardial flow and enhance collateral flow distal to stenotic lesions. The inhibition of platelet aggregation also plays an important role in the treatment of myocardial ischemia by calcium channel blockers, and appears to be mediated by preventing the calcium-induced release of platelet aggregatory factors [32]. The negative inotropic and chronotropic properties contribute to the anti-ischemic effects of both verapamil and diltiazem, primarily by reducing myocardial oxygen demand. Although nifedipine and nicardipine are also potent, direct negative inotropic and chronotropic agents in isolated myocardial tissue, reflex activation of the sympathetic nervous system in the whole animal owing to marked arterial dilatation offsets the intrinsic negative effects on contractility and heart rate; the addition of a β-blocker to nifedipine and nicardipine therefore, may improve the anti-anginal effect. Finally, recent studies have suggested that chronic administration of calcium antagonists may have an antiatherogenic effect [33].

REFERENCES

1. Mangano DT: Perioperative cardiac morbidity. *Anesthesiology* 1990, 72:153–184.

2. Conti CR, Mehta JL: Acute myocardial ischemia: role of atherosclerosis, thrombosis, platelet activation, coronary vasospasm, and altered arachidonic acid metabolism. *Circulation* 1987, 75(Suppl V):V84–V95.

3. Davies MJ: A macro and micro view of coronary vascular insult in ischemic heart disease. *Circulation* 1990, 82(Suppl II):II38–II46.

4. Buffington CW, Davis KB, Gillispie S, Pettinger BS: The prevalence of steal-prone anatomy in patients with coronary artery disease: an analysis of the Coronary Artery Surgery Study registry. *Anesthesiology* 1988, 69:721–727.

5. Smith JS, Cahalan MK, Benefiel DJ, *et al.*: Intraoperative detection of myocardial ischemia in high risk patients: electrocardiography versus two-dimensional transesophageal echocardiography. *Circulation* 1985, 72:1015–1021.

6. Leung JM, O'Kelly B, Browner WS, *et al.*: Prognostic importance of postbypass regional wall-motion abnormalities in patients undergoing coronary artery bypass graft surgery. *Anesthesiology* 1989, 71:16–25.

7. Buffington CW: Hemodynamic determinants of ischemic myocardial dysfunction in the presence of coronary stenosis in dogs. *Anesthesiology* 1985, 63:651–662.

8. Ellis SG, DeCesare NB, Pinkerton CA, *et al.*: Relation of stenosis morphology and clinical presentation to the procedural results of directional coronary atherectomy. *Circulation* 1991, 84:644–653.

9. Serruys PW, Strauss BH, Beatt KJ, *et al.*: Angiographic follow-up after placement of a self-expanding coronary-artery stent. *N Engl J Med* 1991, 324:13–17.

10. Klocke FJ, Mates RE, Canty JM, Ellis AK: Coronary pressure-flow relationships. controversial issues and probable implications. *Circ Res* 1985, 56:310–323.

11. Broten TP, Romson JL, Fullerton DA, *et al.*: Synergistic action of myocardial oxygen and carbon dioxide in controlling coronary blood flow. *Circ Res* 1991, 68:531–542.

12. Werns SW, Walton JA, Hsia HH, *et al.*: Evidence of endothelial dysfunction in angiographically normal coronary arteries of patients with coronary artery disease. *Circulation* 1989, 79:287–291.

13. Brown BG, Bolson EL, Dodge HT: Dynamic mechanism in human coronary stenosis. *Circulation* 1984, 70:917–922.

14. Gianrossi R, Detrano R, Mulvihill D, *et al.*: Exercise-induced ST depression in the diagnosis of coronary artery disease: a meta-analysis. *Circulation* 1989, 80:87–98.

15. Bailey IK, Griffith LS, Rouleau J, *et al.*: Thallium-201 myocardial perfusion imaging at rest and during exercise: comparative sensitivity to electrocardiography in coronary artery disease. *Circulation* 1977, 55:79–87.

16. VanDaele ME, Sutherland GR, Mitchell MM, *et al.*: Do changes in pulmonary capillary wedge pressure adequately reflect myocardial ischemia during anesthesia? *Circulation* 1990, 81:865–871.

17. Johnson LW, Lozner EC, Johnson S: Coronary arteriography 1984–1987: A report of the Registry of the Society for Cardiac Angiography and Intervention—results and complications. *Cathet Cardiovasc Diagn* 1989, 17:5–12.

18. Weaver WD: Time to thrombolytic treatment: factors affecting delay and their influence on outcome. *J Am Coll Cardiol* 1995, 25:3S–9S.

19. The Gusto Investigators: An international randomized trial comparing four thrombolytic strategies for acute myocardial infarction. *N Engl J Med* 1993, 329:673–682.

20. Second International Study of Infarct Survival (ISIS-2) Collaborative Group: Randomized trial of intravenous streptokinase, oral aspirin, both, or neither among 17, 187 cases of suspected acute myocardial infarction. *Lancet* 1988, 1:349–360.

21. Ellis SG, Cowley MJ, Whitlow PL, *et al.*: Prospective case-control comparison of percutaneous transluminal coronary revascularization in patients with multivessel disease treated in 1986–1987 versus 1991: Improved in-hospital and 12-month results. Multivessel Angioplasty Prognosis Study (MAPS) Group. *J Am Coll Cardiol* 1995, 25:1137–1142.

22. Mark DB, Nelson CL, Califf RM, *et al.*: Continuing evolution of therapy for coronary artery disease. Initial results from the era of coronary angioplasty. *Circulation* 1994, 89:2015–2025.

23. Cameron A, Davis KB, Green G, Schaff HV: Coronary bypass surgery with internal-thoracic-artery grafts: Effects on survival over a 15 year period. *N Engl J Med* 1996, 334:216–219.

24. Fischman DL, Leon MB, Baim DS, *et al.*: A randomized comparison of coronary-stent placement and balloon angioplasty in the treatment of coronary artery disease. *N Engl J Med* 1994, 331:496–501.

25. Topol EJ, Leya F, Pinkerton CA, *et al.*: A comparison of directional atherectomy with coronary angioplasty in patients with coronary artery disease. *N Engl J Med* 1993, 329:221–228.

26. Litvack F, Eigler N, Margolis J, *et al.*: Percutaneous excimer laser coronary angioplasty: results in the first consecutive 3000 patients. *J Am Coll Cardiol* 1994, 23:323–329.

27. Slogoff S, Keats AS: Does chronic treatment with calcium entry blocking drugs reduce perioperative myocardial ischemia? *Anesthesiology* 1988, 68:676–680.

28. O'Connor JP, Ramsey JG, Wynands JE, Kaplan JA, *et al.* Anesthesia for Myocardial Revascularization. In *Cardiac Anesthesia*, edn 3. Philadelphia: WB Saunders; 1993:587–628.

29. Parker JD: Nitrates and angina pectoris. *Am J Cardiol* 1993, 72:3C–8C.

30. Stamler JS, Loscalzo J: The antiplatelet effects of organic nitrates and related nitroso compounds in-vitro and in-vivo and their relevance to cardiovascular disorders. *J Am Coll Cardiol* 1991, 18:1529–1536.

31. Parker JD, Testa MA, Jimenez AH, *et al.*: Morning increase in ambulatory ischemia in patients with stable coronary artery disease: importance of physical activity and increased cardiac demand. *Circulation* 1994, 89:604–614.

32. Ware JA, Johnson PC, Smith M, Salzman EW: Inhibition of human platelet aggregation and cytoplasmic calcium response by calcium antagonists: studies with aequorin and quin 2. *Circ Res* 1986, 59:39–42.

33. Waters D, Lesperance J: Interventions that beneficially influence the evolution of coronary atherosclerosis: the case for calcium channel blockers. *Circulation* 1992, 86(Suppl III):111–116.

5

Cardiac Valvular Disease

John T. Apostolakis and Robert M. Savage

Cardiac valvular disorders can have a profound effect on the function of the heart and on the hemodynamic responses to anesthesia and surgery. An understanding of the limitations imposed by valvular lesions and the ensuing pathophysiologic responses facilitates safe and effective management of the surgical patient. Left ventricular pressure *vs* volume tracings obtained for the full cardiac cycle provide a convenient way of representing the pathophysiology of valvular diseases. These diagrams can be used to illustrate preload reserve, afterload mismatch, the consequences of hypertrophy in response to volume and pressure loads, and decompensation in heart failure. The anesthetic plan for the patient with valvular disease should include appropriate management of preload, afterload, rate, rhythm, and contractility, and the monitoring necessary to accomplish this. The choice of specific anesthetic agents and techniques is based on the desired effect on hemodynamic parameters as well as the demands of the surgical procedure. Following surgical correction of these valvular lesions, there will be an alteration of these hemodynamic goals according to the patient's remaining unique pathophysiology.

Aortic valve stenosis imposes a very large afterload increase on the ventricle. Extreme left ventricular pressures are required to maintain cardiac output across the stenosed orifice. Consequently, much more work must be done by the ventricle to pump a given volume. These high ventricular pressures result in high ventricular wall stress. The attendant pathophysiologic response is concentric myocardial hypertrophy. Aortic valve replacement will acutely reduce left ventricular afterload toward normal, but the requirements for management of concentric hypertrophy remain. Additionally, adequate, myocardial protection under cardiopulmonary bypass can be difficult. Transesophageal echocardiography is of great benefit in the diagnosis and grading of aortic stenosis, assessment of left ventricular performance and adequacy of compensation for the valvular lesion, and in assessing prosthetic valve function.

Hypertrophic obstructive cardiomyopathy, although of different etiology than aortic valvular stenosis, shares many of the pathophysiologic consequences. Treatment goals are directed to maintaining a large enough end systolic volume to prevent this obstruction. Following correction of the left ventricular outflow tract (LVOT) obstruction and mitral regurgitation with myectomy and/or mitral valve replacement, diastolic dysfunction chronically persists in these patients.

It is useful to consider aortic regurgitation separately in the acute and chronic states. In both cases the demand placed on the ventricle is a volume load. In the case of chronic aortic regurgitation (AR), however, eccentric hypertrophy of the left ventriculer (LV) compensates very well for this added volume work load until late in the disease. Decompensation occurs when the wall thickness to radius ratio can no longer be preserved, resulting in afterload mismatch. The challenge is to time surgical replacement to occur just before ventricular decompensation begins. In acute AR there is no compensatory ventricular hypertrophy. Volume overload quickly results, with LV dilation causing malfunction of the mitral valve (MV) tensor apparatus, an inability of the MV leaflets to coapt, and mitral regurgitation. In acute AR surgery is often urgently required. For acute and chronic AR, management is directed toward preserving forward cardiac output.

As the lesion in mitral stenosis is proximal to the left ventricle, the morphologic changes and the effect on LV function are more subtle. Overall cardiac function is marked by a chronic underfilling of the left ventricle due to both loss of atrial kick and the limitations on flow rate into the ventricle, and by an intolerance to rapid heart rates, which exacerbate both left atrial pressures and inadequate ventricular filling. Management should be focused on preventing rapid heart rates, maintaining adequate preload to insure venous filling without exacerbating pulmonary edema, preservation of contractility with support as needed after bypass, and minimization of pulmonary vascular resistance.

Mitral regurgitation, like aortic regurgitation, is a disorder of volume overload that can be considered in acute and chronic forms. The chronically exposed ventricle will undergo eccentric hypertrophy. Unlike chronic AR, however, afterload can be considered reduced as a consequence of ejection during systole via the mitral valve as well as via the aortic valve. This feature tends to mask LV dysfunction until after mitral valve regurgitation (MVR) with restoration of afterload. Management goals are directed toward limiting regurgitation and preserving forward cardiac output. Phosphodiesterase III inhibitors may prove helpful in reducing both pulmonary and systemic vascular resistance while improving contractility. Echocardiography has proven very helpful in assessing valve function immediately after cardiopulmonary bypass, especially in the setting of the increasingly popular approach of repairing native valves. Mortality from operations for mitral regurgitation is higher than that for other left sided valvular lesions, possibly due to the new afterload stress imposed on the ventricle and association with a primary etiology of myocardial ischemia. Tricuspid regurgitation occurs as a primary disorder or, more commonly, as a sequella of chronic pulmonary hypertension. Secondary tricuspid regurgitation often is a sign of severe left sided valvular disease. Management is directed toward treatment of the primary valve lesion and reducing right ventricular afterload.

PATHOPHYSIOLOGY OF VALVULAR DISEASE

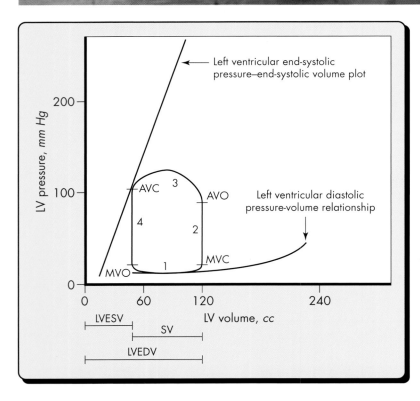

Figure 5-1. A typical left ventricular (LV) pressure-volume loop. Phase 1 represents diastolic filling between mitral valve opening (MVO) and mitral valve closure (MVC). This curve lies on the LV pressure-volume relationship, which reflects LV compliance. Phase 2 is isovolumic contraction, during which LV volume does not change whereas pressure rises. Phase 3 is the systolic ejection phase, occurring between aortic valve opening (AVO) and aortic valve closure (AVC). The volume at which ejection ends defines one point on the left ventricular end-systolic pressure (LVESP)–left ventricular end-systolic volume (LVESV) plot, a measure of contractility. It can be constructed by plotting several cardiac cycles at various left ventricular end-diastolic volume (LVEDVs) levels keeping afterload and contractility constant. Phase 4 is the isovolumic relaxation phase, occurring between AVC and MVO. SV is demonstrated. Ejection fraction is the ratio of stroke volume to LVEDV. The area within this loop represents the external work of the heart. (*Adapted from* Jackson and coworkers [13] with permission.)

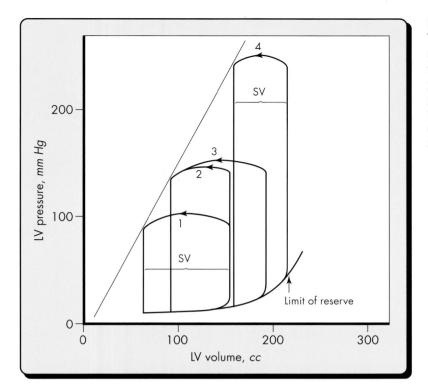

Figure 5-2. A pressure-volume loop illustrating preload reserve. The effect of an acute increase in afterload (loop 2) is a decrease in stroke volume (SV). To compensate, preload is increased (loop 3) thus restoring stroke volume at the expense of increased work. The preload available to accomplish this increased work is termed preload reserve. As afterload continues to increase so does preload until the limits of diastolic compliance are reached, preventing adequate increase in preload. This condition is referred to as afterload mismatch (loop 4). (*Adapted from* Ross [2]; with permission.)

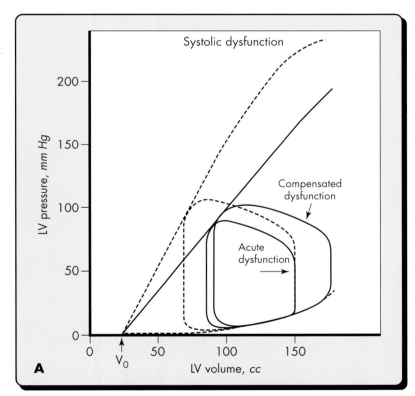

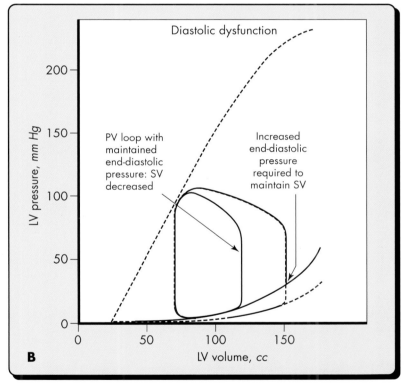

Figure 5-3. **A,** Effect of negative inotropy on a pressure-volume (PV) loop. The end-systolic pressure-volume point has been shifted to the right and down. Stroke volume (SV) is reduced. With compensation utilizing preload reserve, stroke volume is restored at the expense of ejection fraction. **B,** Effect of decreased left ventricular (LV) compliance. At a given LV end-diastolic pressure, LV end-diastolic volume is reduced, consequently stroke volume also falls. (*Adapted from* Lynch and Lake [3]; with permission.)

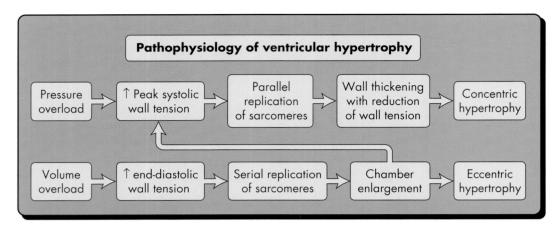

Pathophysiology of ventricular hypertrophy

Pressure overload → ↑ Peak systolic wall tension → Parallel replication of sarcomeres → Wall thickening with reduction of wall tension → Concentric hypertrophy

Volume overload → ↑ end-diastolic wall tension → Serial replication of sarcomeres → Chamber enlargement → Eccentric hypertrophy

Figure 5-4. Development of ventricular hypertrophy. In the pressure overloaded ventricle, elevated end-systolic wall stress provides the stimulus for wall thickening, which lowers end-systolic wall stress according to the LaPlace equation: stress = radius × pressure/ 2× thickness. In the volume-overloaded ventricle, elevated end-diastolic stress causes chamber enlargement, which elevates wall stress again, as demonstrated by the Laplace equation. This secondary stimulus causes some parallel sarcomere replication to restore the balance between radius and pressure. The result is eccentric hypertrophy. (*Adapted from* Grossman and coworkers [4]; with permission.)

EFFECTS OF PRESSURE OVERLOAD HYPERTROPHY

Positive
  Increases ventricular work
  Normalizes wall stress
  Normalizes systolic shortening
Negative
  Decreases ventricular diastolic distensibility
  Impairs ventricular relaxation
  Impairs coronary ventricular vasodilator reserve, leading to subendocardial ischemia

Figure 5-5. Consequences of concentric hypertrophy. (*From* Lorell and Grossman [5]; with permission.

CONSEQUENCES OF A LOW-COMPLIANCE VENTRICLE

Function sensitive to volume depletion
Dependence on atrial contraction for preload
Changes in ventricular filling pressure with small volume changes
PAOP underestimates LVEDP
Increased LVEDP reduces coronary perfusion pressure

Figure 5-6. Consequences of a low-compliance ventricle. LVEDP—left ventricular end-diastolic pressure. PAOP—pulmonary artery occlusion pressure. (*From* Barash and coworkers [6]; with permission.)

ETIOLOGY OF AORTIC VALVE STENOSIS

Congenital: bicuspid and unicuspid
Acquired
  Rheumatic
  Calcific (degenerative/autoimmune)
  Rare causes
    Obstructive infective vegetations
    Homozygous type II hyperlipoproteinemia
    Paget's disease of the bone
    Systemic lupus erythematosus
    Rheumatoid involvement
    Ochronosis (alkaptonuria)
    Irradiation

Figure 5-7. Etiology of aortic valve stenosis. (*From* Rahimtoola and coworkers [7]; with permission.)

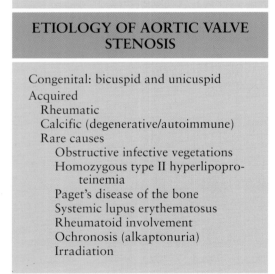
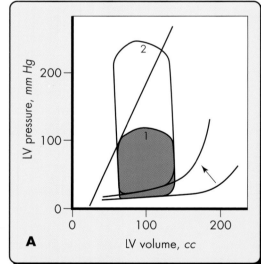
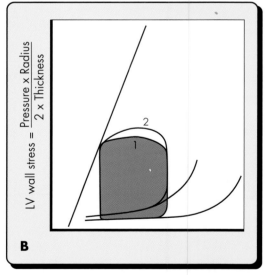

Figure 5-8. Pressure-volume loop in aortic stenosis (AS) (**A**). Compared with the normal heart (*loop 1*) the diastolic pressure-volume curve is shifted upward in AS, reflecting the decrease in left ventricular (LV) compliance from hypertrophy (*loop 2*). The stroke volume and ejection fraction are preserved, but at the cost of much greater external cardiac work, as reflected by the area within the loop (**B**). The apparent increase in contractility disappears when the loop is normalized for hypertrophy by plotting wall stress rather than pressure against volume. In fact contractility is not enhanced. H—ventricular wall thickness; P—pressure; R—radius. (*From* Ross [2]; with permission.)

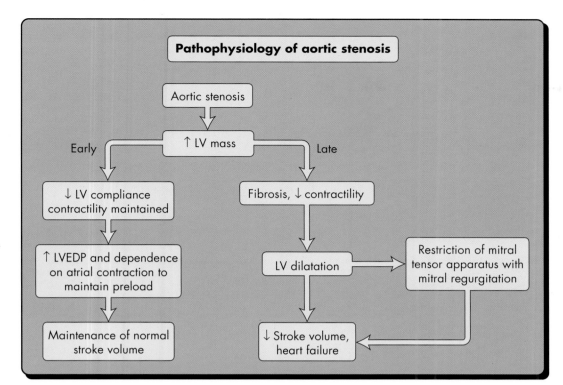

Figure 5-9. Pathophysiology of aortic stenosis. Initially concentric hypertrophy compensates well for the stress of outflow obstruction. Ultimately left ventricular (LV) dysfunction and heart failure ensue. LVEDP—left ventricular end-diastolic pressure. (*Adapted from* Thomas and Lowenstein [8]; with permission.)

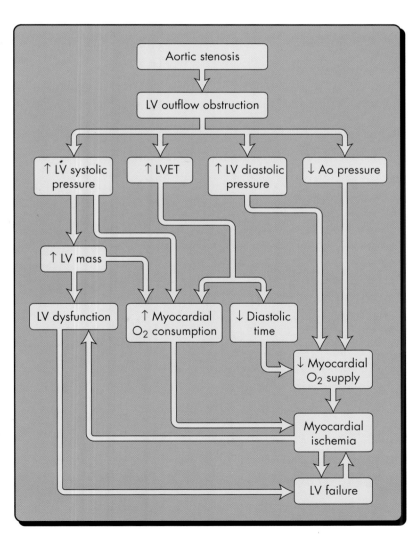

Figure 5-10. Pathphysiology of aortic stenosis (AS). A consequence of AS and compensatory concentric hypertrophy is an increased susceptibility to myocardial ischemia. AO—aortic; LV—left ventricular. LVET—left ventricular ejection time. (*From* Boudoulas and Gravanis [9]; with permission.)

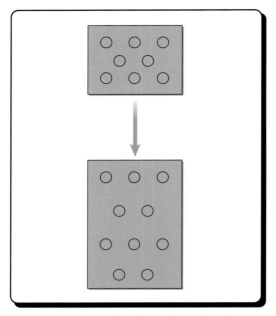

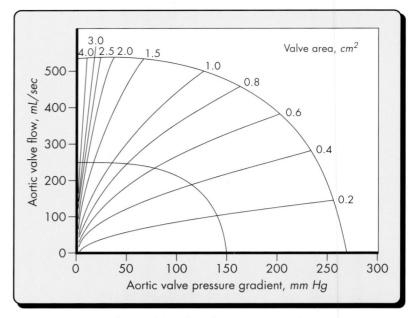

Figure 5-11. Pathophysiology of ischemia in aortic stenosis. Schematic representation of myocardial mass and capillary density in cross section. With concentric hypertrophy the increase in myocardial thickness is disproportionate to the growth in coronary vasculature, leaving patients at increased risk of ischemia. (*From* Marcus [10]; with permission.)

Figure 5-12. Relationship of cardiac output to the pressure gradient across the aortic valve in patients with aortic stenosis. For a given valve area, higher outputs are necessarily associated with greater pressure gradients. Conversely, as the left ventricle (LV) fails, the pressure gradient may drop, reflecting decreasing cardiac output. A decreased gradient may be an ominous sign. (*From* Grossman [11]; with permission.)

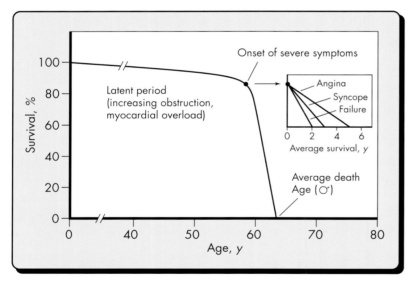

Figure 5-13. The onset of symptoms from aortic stenosis is associated with poor median survival times. (*From* Ross and Braunwald [12]; with permission.)

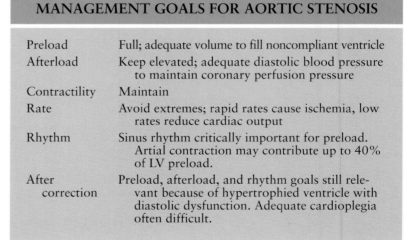

MANGEMENT GOALS FOR AORTIC STENOSIS	
Preload	Full; adequate volume to fill noncompliant ventricle
Afterload	Keep elevated; adequate diastolic blood pressure to maintain coronary perfusion pressure
Contractility	Maintain
Rate	Avoid extremes; rapid rates cause ischemia, low rates reduce cardiac output
Rhythm	Sinus rhythm critically important for preload. Artial contraction may contribute up to 40% of LV preload.
After correction	Preload, afterload, and rhythm goals still relevant because of hypertrophied ventricle with diastolic dysfunction. Adequate cardioplegia often difficult.

Figure 5-14. Management of aortic stenosis focuses on a hypertrophied ventricle with a fixed impedance to ejection. (*Adapted from* Wray Roth and coworkers [6].)

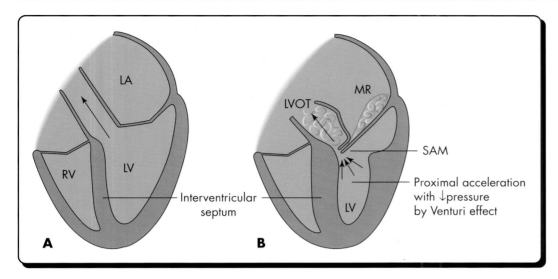

Figure 5-15. A, Normal ventricle during systole. B, Ventricle with hypertrophic obstructive cardiomyopathy. One pathway to this condition arises when a primary defect in myocardial contractility results in hypertrophy that is asymmetric, favoring the septum. This narrows the left ventricular outflow tract (LVOT). To maintain stroke volume the blood must flow faster through the narrower space. The Venturi effect (decreased pressure under valve leaflet and increased pressure above) may cause systolic anterior motion (SAM) of the coapted mitral valve, drawing it into the LVOT and causing a dynamic obstruction to outflow. Separation of the coapted leaflets results in a regurgitant jet. LA—left atrium; LV—left ventricle; MR—mitral regurgitation; RV—right ventricle. (*Adapted from* Levine [13]; with permission.)

Figure 5-16. Morphologic classification of hypertrophic obstructive cardiomyopathy. A number of different pathological processes can result in the same abnormal function. (*From* Savage and coworkers [14]; with permission.)

MORPHOLOGIC CLASSIFICATION OF HYPERTROPHIC OBSTRUCTIVE CARDIOMYOPATHY

Asymmetric hypertrophy
  Familial
  Sigmoid-shaped septum associated with elderly patients
  Apical variant-spadelike appearance
  Midventricular rings
  Miscellaneous
    Eisenmenger's complex with septal hypertrophy
    Septal sarcomas
    Left ventricular hypertrophy with lateral wall infarction
    Neonates of diabetic mothers
    Pulmonary hypertension and right ventricular hypertrophy
    Transient occurrence during fetal development
Symmetric hypertrophy
  Concentric hypertrophy with chronic hypertension
  Concentric hypertrophy with chronic aortic stenosis
  Miscellaneous abnormalities
    Cardiac amyloidosis
    Friedreich's ataxia
    Myxedema
    Glycogen storage diseases
    After mitral valve repair
    Lung transplantation (hypovolemia)
    Hepatic disease

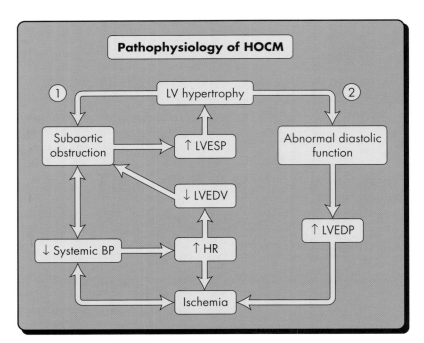

Figure 5-17. Pathophysiology of hypertrophic obstructive cardiomyopathy (HOCM). When loading conditions result in subaortic obstruction, a self-propagating "vicious cycle" can result, with possibly fatal consequences. BP—blood pressure; HR—heart rate; LV—left ventricle; LVEDP—left ventricular end-diastolic pressure; LVEDV—left ventricular end-diastolic volume; LVESP—left ventricular end-systolic pressure. (*Adapted from* Maron and coworkers [15]; with permission.)

LVOT OBSTRUCTION: PATHOPHYSIOLOGIC SUBSTRATES

Decreased diameter of LVOT

Small ventricular cavity
  Decreased left ventricular volume
    Hypovolemia
    Tachycardia
    Left ventricular hypertrophy and diastolic dysfunctions
Septal hypertrophy
Abnormal mitral valve apparatus or motion
  Anterior papillary muscle
  Redundancy of mitral valve leaflets
  Systolic anterior motion of mitral valve leaflets

Velocity of Blood Flow in LVOT

Hypercontractile
  Increased sympathetic tone
  Inotropes
Decreased afterload
  Exercise
  Drug induced
    Vasodilators
    β-2 agonists
    Inodilators
Systemic shunts
  Hepatic disease
  Arteriovenous malformations
  Pregnancy
Medical conditions
  Anemia
  Thyroid disease
  Pheochromocytoma
  Paget's disease
Hypovolemia
Pulmonary hypertension
Lung transplantation

Figure 5-18. Causes of dynamic left ventricular outflow tract (LVOT) obstruction. LVOT obstruction from systolic anterior motion (SAM) can result from 1) a decrease in LVOT diameter or 2) an increase in flow velocity through the LVOT. Either results in the Venturi effect responsible for SAM. Every LVOT diameter has a critical velocity at which SAM will potentially occur. (*Adapted from* Savage and coworkers [14]; with permission.)

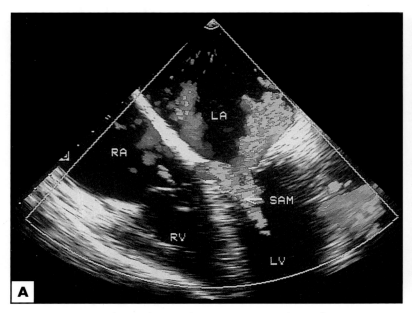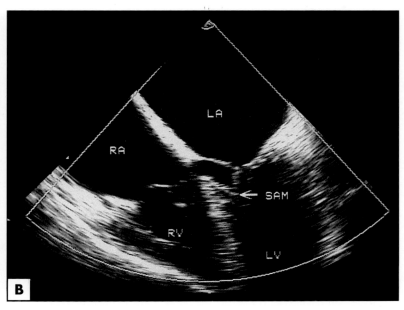

Figure 5-19. Echocardiographic appearance of systolic anterior motion (SAM) in mitral regurgitation (**A**, color Doppler image) and in left ventricular outflow tract obstruction (**B**). LA—left atrium; LV—left ventricle; RA—right atrium; RV—right ventricle. (*From* Savage [15]; with permission.)

MANAGEMENT GOALS FOR HOCM	
Preload	Full
Afterload	Increased
Contractility	Depress to maintain larger end-systolic volume
Rate	Keep low
Rhythm	Sinus rhythm critically important
Postmyectomy	Diastolic dysfunction remains. Maintain atrial rhythm, full volume; increased afterload for adequate myocardial perfusion

Figure 5-20. Management of hypertrophic obstructive cardiomyopathy (HOCM). Management goals can be summarized by a desire to keep left ventricular (LV) systolic volume large to minimize degree of obstruction. After cardiopulmonary bypass for myectomy, transesophageal echocardiography can be used to exclude the possibility of ventricular septal defect or to administer isoproterenol in an attempt to provoke systolic anterior motion. Management should also be adapted for a low compliance ventricle. (*Adapted from* Wray Roth and coworkers [6]; with permission.)

Figure 5-21. Etiology of aortic regurgitation. (*From* Rackley and coworkers [16]; with permission.)

ETIOLOGY OF CHRONIC AND ACUTE AORTIC REGURGITATION*

Chronic aortic regurgitation

Rheumatic fever

Syphilis

Aortitis (Takayasu)

Heritable disorders of connective tissue
  Marfan's syndrome
  Ehlers-Danlos syndrome
  Osteogenesis imperfecta

Congenital heart disease
  Bicuspid aortic valve
  Interventricular septal defect
  Sinus of Valsalva aneurysm

Arthritic diseases
  Ankylosing spondylitis
  Reiter's syndrome
  Rheumatoid arthritis
  Lupus erythematosus

Aortic root disease

Aorticoannuloectasia

Cystic medial necrosis of aorta

Hypertension

Arteriosclerosis

Myxomatous degeneration of valve

Infective endocarditis

Following prosthetic valve surgery

Associated with aortic stenosis

Acute aortic regurgitation

Rheumatic fever

Infective endocarditis

Congenital (rupture of sinus of Valsalva)

Acute aortic dissection

Following prosthetic valve surgery

Trauma

* Please note that certain disorders are capable of producing both acute and chronic regurgitation.

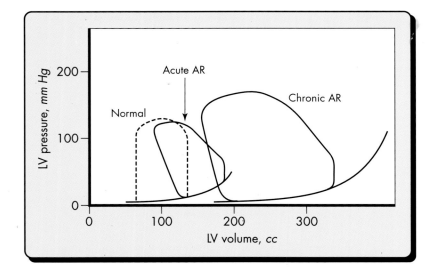

Figure 5-22. Pressure-volume loop (PV) for acute and chronic aortic regurgitation (AR). In acute AR the PV loop has been shifted to the right along the diastolic compliance curve. Left ventricular end-diastolic pressure (LVEDP) is considerably higher, indicating that the limits of compliance have been reached, and preload reserve is exhausted. Aortic valve opening occurs at a lower pressure due to lower aortic diastolic pressure. Isovolumic relaxation has been eliminated, because during diastole the ventricle is filling from either the mitral or regurgitant aortic valve. Stroke volume appears preserved, but some fraction of this flows back into the ventricle, so effective stroke volume is decreased. In chronic AR eccentric hypertrophy has caused a rightward shift of the diastolic compliance curve. LVEDP is not necessarily as high as the acute case, despite much larger left ventricular end-diastolic volume. Total stroke volume is very large, so effective stroke volume may be preserved. (*Adapted from* Jackson and coworkers [1]; with permission.)

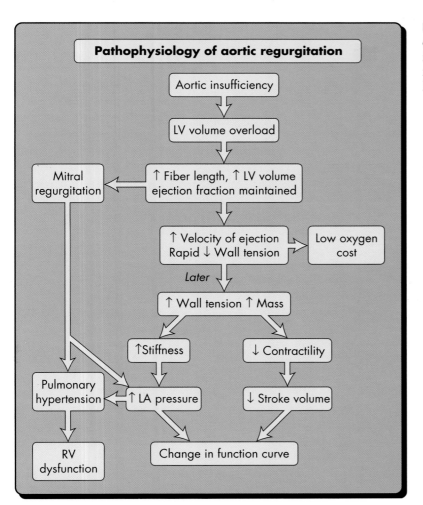

Pathophysiology of aortic regurgitation

Aortic insufficiency

LV volume overload

Mitral regurgitation ← ↑ Fiber length, ↑ LV volume ejection fraction maintained

↑ Velocity of ejection Rapid ↓ Wall tension → Low oxygen cost

Later ↓

↑ Wall tension ↑ Mass

↑Stiffness   ↓ Contractility

Pulmonary hypertension ← ↑ LA pressure   ↓ Stroke volume

RV dysfunction   Change in function curve

Figure 5-23. Pathophysiology of aortic regurgitation. Later in the condition, wall tension increases as parallel replication of sarcomeres fails to keep pace with chamber enlargement (*see* Fig. 5-4). The result is decompensation. LV—left ventricular; RV—right ventricular. (*From* Thomas and Lowenstein [8]; with permission.)

MANAGEMENT GOALS IN AORTIC REGURGITATION

Preload	Full enough for adequate venous filling
Afterload	Decreased to promote forward flow
Contractility	Maintain
Rate	Raise to increased cardiac output, maintain smaller chamber size
Rhythm	Usually not critically important
After correction	Treat for persistent mitral regurgitation, pulmonary hypertension, and RV dysfunction

Figure 5-24. Management goals in aortic regurgitation. RV—right ventricular. (*From* Wray Roth and coworkers [6]; with permission.)

CAUSES OF MITRAL STENOSIS

	Involved structures			
Cause	Leaflet	Chordae	Commissures	Other
Rheumatic fever	+	+	+	
Congenital	+	+	–	Single papillary muscle
Active infective endocarditis	+	–	–	Vegetation
Neoplasm	–	–	–	Mass, pulmonary vein obstruction
Massive annular calcification	+	–	–	Rigid annulus
Systemic lupus erythematosus	+	+	+	Verrucous vegetations may extend into papillary muscles
Methysergide therapy	+	+	–	Serotonin agonist/antagonist
Hunter-Hurler syndromes	–	–	–	Mucopolysaccharide deposits
Fabry's disease	–	–	–	Aramide trihexoxide deposits
Whipple's disease	–	–	–	PAS-positive macrophage deposits
Rheumatoid arthritis	+	+	+	PAS-positive plasma cell infiltrate

Figure 5-25. Etiology of mitral stenosis. Processes that cause mitral stenosis operate at the leaflets, chordae, or commissures. *Plus signs* indicate location of pathology. PAS—periodic acid–Schiff stain. (*From* Kawinishi and Rahimtoola [17]; with permission. © Shahbudin H. Rahimtoola.)

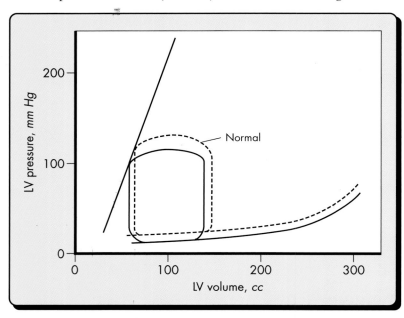

Figure 5-26. Pressure-volume loop for mitral stenosis. It is nearly indistinguishable from the normal loop operating at reduced preload, differing in a diastolic compliance curve that may be slightly shifted, reflecting thinning of a chronically underfilled ventricle. There is effectively little preload reserve available to adjust to a demand for greater output or greater afterload because of restrictions to left ventricular inflow (LV) inflow. (*Adapted from* Jackson and coworkers [1]; with permission.)

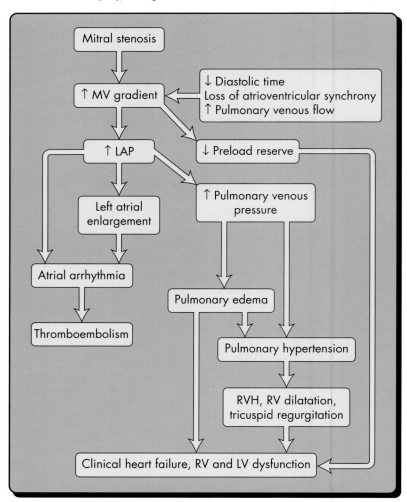

Figure 5-27. Pathophysiology of mitral stenosis. Increased left atrial pressures are needed to overcome the stenosed mitral orifice, resulting in left atrial enlargement, atrial fibrillation and elevated pulmonary pressures. Over time chronic elevation of pulmonary pressures can result in irreversible pulmonary hypertension, right ventricular dilation, and secondary tricuspid regurgitation. LAP—left atrial pressure; LV—left ventricular; MV—mitral valve; RV—right ventricular; RVH—right ventricular hypertrophy. (*Adapted from* Kawanishi and Rahimtoola [17]; with permission. © Shahbudin H. Rahimtoola.)

$$\text{MV Pressure gradient} = \left(\frac{\text{Flow rate across valve}}{\text{K·valve area (MVA)}}\right)^2$$

$$\text{Flow rate across valve} = \frac{\text{Stroke volume (SV)}}{\text{Diastolic time interval (DTI)}}$$

$$\text{MV pressure gradient} = \left(\frac{\text{SV}}{\text{DTI·K·MVA}}\right)^2$$

Figure 5-28. Effect of heart rate on pressure gradient. The Gorlin formula describes the relationship between flow, pressure gradient, and mitral valve area. It can be used to demonstrate the effect of heart rate changes on pressure gradient. Recall that systolic time interval is relatively fixed at about 0.25 sec, regardless of heart rate. Therefore, as heart rate increases, diastolic time interval must shorten, flow rate increases, and pressure gradient must increase. DTI—diastolic time interval; K—a constant; LA—left atrium; LV—left ventricle; MVA—mitral valve area; SV—stroke volume.

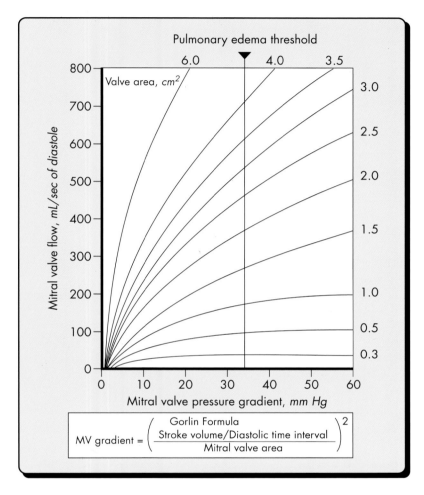

$$\text{MV gradient} = \left(\frac{\text{Gorlin Formula}}{\frac{\text{Stroke volume/Diastolic time interval}}{\text{Mitral valve area}}}\right)^2$$

Figure 5-29. Pathophysiology of mitral stenosis. A depiction of the relationship between the pressure gradient and flow across the mitral valve for various valve areas as dictated by the Gorlin formula. Transudation of fluid begins when capillary pressure exceeds plasma oncotic pressure, about 25 to 35 mm Hg. For valve areas below 1 cm², flow cannot increase much without the development of pulmonary edema. Hence there is little preload reserve. LA—left atrium; LV—left ventricle. (*From* Schlant [18]; with permission.)

Figure 5-30. Management of mitral stenosis. LV—left ventricle. (*Adapted from* Wray Roth and coworkers [6]; with permission.)

MANAGEMENT GOALS FOR MITRAL STENOSIS

Preload	Enough to maintain gradient; take care to avoid pulmonary edema
Afterload	Reduce right-side afterload as possible; avoid hypercarbia, hypoxia, acidosis
Contractility	Right ventricle may need support; left usually adequate
Rate	Slow to keep pressure gradient low
Rhythm	Usually atrial fibrillation. Control ventricular response
After correction	RV may need continued support due to severity of pulmonary hypertension; LV dysfunction may be uncovered

ETIOLOGY OF MITRAL REGURGITATION

Etiology of chronic MR	Mechanism	Echocardiographic appearance
Rheumatic 　Lupus erythematosus 　Anticardiolipin syndrome 　Carcinoid 　Ergot lesions 　After radiation	Retraction Thickening	Thickened chordae, leaflets Normal or restricted motion
Degenerative 　Marfan 　Ehlers-Danlos 　Phentermine-fenfluramine	Prolapsed leaflets Thickening	Prolapsing or flail leaflets Redundant tissue
Ischemic 　Myocardial disease 　Chronic ischemia 　Cardiomyopathies	Dilation of annulus Traction of anterior leaflet	Normal leaflets Reduced leaflet motion
Infiltrative disease 　Hypereosinophilia 　Endomyocardial fibrosis 　Hurler's disease	Thickening leaflet Loss of coaptation	Thickened leaflets Reduced motion
Congenital	Cleft leaflet Transposed valve	Cleft leaflet

Etiology of acute MR	Mechanism	Echocardiographic appearance
Traumatic	Ruptured chordae Ruptured papillary muscle	Flail leaflet Ruptured chordae
Infarction	Ruptured papillary muscle	Flail leaflet
Endocarditis	Destructive lesions	Perforation Flail leaflet

Figure 5-31. Etiology of mitral regurgitation (MR). (*Adapted from* Rahimtoola and coworkers [19]; with permission.)

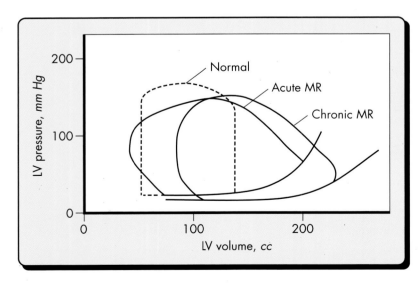

Figure 5-32. Pressure-volume loop for acute and chronic mitral regurgitation. In the acute disease, the loop is shifted to the right. Left ventricular end-diastolic pressure is high, limiting cardiac performance. There is little preload reserve. There is no isovolumic contraction, because blood flows across the regurgitant mitral valve. Isovolumic relaxation is foreshortened by the higher left atrial pressures. Forward stroke volume is reduced. With the eccentric dilation that accompanies chronic mitral regurgitation (MR), ejection fraction may be increased. Forward stroke volume is preserved in compensated disease. (*Adapted from* Jackson and coworkers [20]; with permission.)

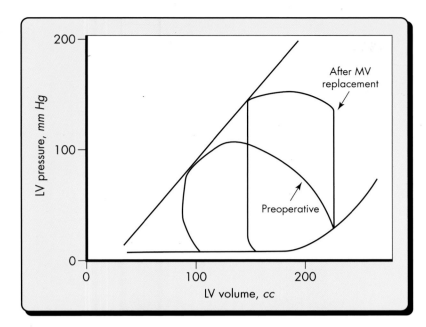

Figure 5-33. Pressure-volume loop for mitral regurgitation before and after surgical correction in a patient with left ventricular (LV) dysfunction. Preoperatively, ejection fraction appears normal because blood can flow out the low-impedance pathway offered by the regurgitant mitral valve (MV). After correction, this low-pressure chamber venting effect is eliminated, and a previously normal-appearing ventricle may suddenly exhibit more severe dysfunction on separation from bypass. (*Adapted from* Jackson [20]; with permission.)

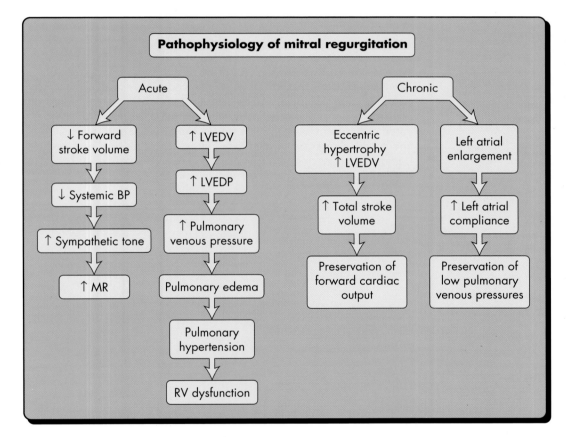

Figure 5-34. Pathophysiology of mitral regurgitation (MR). The left atrial enlargement that accompanies chronic MR functions to protect the pulmonary capillaries from elevated pressures until late in the condition, when pulmonary hypertension may develop. In acute MR, lacking compensatory enlargement of the LV and LA, preload reserve is quickly exhausted in an attempt to accommodate larger left ventricular end diostolic volumes, resulting in elevated filling pressures and pulmonary edema. Patients with acute or late chronic MR are at risk for right ventricular failure from pulmonary hypertension. BP—blood pressure; LVEDP—left ventricular end-diastolic pressure; LVEDV—left ventricular end-diastolic volume; RV—right ventricular.

MANAGEMENT GOALS FOR MITRAL REGURGITATION

Preload	Balance venous filling against pulmonary edema
Afterload	Decreased to reduce regurgitant fraction
Contractility	Maintain; may have hidden dysfunction
Rate	Fast to improve cardiac output and decrease ventricular size
Rhythm	Less critical; sometimes in atrial fibrillation
After correction	Effective afterload increased by loss of regurgitation. Reduce afterload, add inotrope if necessary. Treat pulmonary hypertension and RV dysfunction

Figure 5-35. Management of mitral regurgitation. Goals for management include promoting forward flow and reducing ventricular dilation. Patients may be at risk for right ventricular failure from chronic pulmonary hypertension, so it is important to avoid conditions that may increase pulmonary vascular resistance such as hypercarbia, hypoxia, and acidosis. RV—right ventricular. (*Adapted from* Wray Roth and coworkers [6]; with permission.)

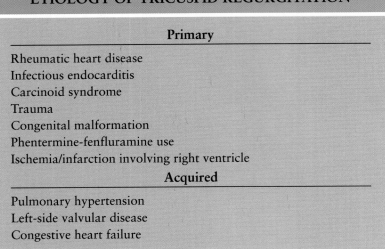

ETIOLOGY OF TRICUSPID REGURGITATION

Primary

Rheumatic heart disease
Infectious endocarditis
Carcinoid syndrome
Trauma
Congenital malformation
Phentermine-fenfluramine use
Ischemia/infarction involving right ventricle

Acquired

Pulmonary hypertension
Left-side valvular disease
Congestive heart failure

Figure 5-36. Etiology of tricuspid regurgitation. In primary tricuspid regurgitation, patients often have minimal symptoms, because the compliance of the right atrium and vena cava results in minimal pressure changes. (*Adapted from* Jackson and coworkers [21]; with permission.)

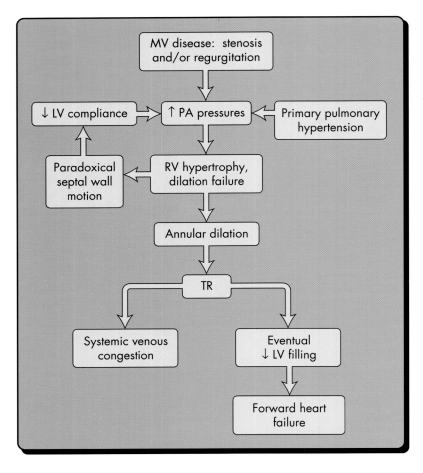

Figure 5-37. Pathophysiology of acquired tricuspid regurgitation (TR). Secondary TR is a more ominous condition because it heralds a failure of right ventricular adaptation to a pressure load. Classically, a pre-existing left-sided valve lesion causes chronic elevation in the left side filling pressures, resulting in pulmonary hypertension. Eventual right ventricular failure leads to chamber enlargement, tricuspid annular dilation, and tricuspid regurgitation. The failing right ventricle is no longer compliant, so right side filling pressures are elevated and hepatic congestion results. Right ventricular output falls, and with it, left-sided filling. Paradoxical septal motion may further impair left ventricular compliance. LV—left ventricular; mitral valve; PA—pulmonary artery; RV—right ventricular.

SUMMARY OF TREATMENT GOALS FOR VALVULAR HEART DISEASE

Pre valve replacement	AS	HOCM	AR	MS	MR	TR
Preload	Increase	Increase	M	M	M	M
Afterload	M, Increase	M-Increase	Decrease	M	Decrease	decrease pulmonary
Contractility	M	Decrease	M	M	M, Increase	Enhance RV function
Rate	M, slow	M-slow	M-faster	Decrease	Increase	M
Rhythm	*Sinus*	*Sinus*		Usually AF		
Diastolic LV dysfunction (noncompliant)	+	+				
RV dysfunction	±	±	With MR	+++	+++	++

Post valve replacement/repair	AS	HOCM	AR	MS	MR	TR
Preload	Increase	Increase				
Afterload	M, Increase	M,Increase			Decrease	Decrease pulmonary vascular resistance
Contractility	M	M		M, Increase	M, Increase	M
Rate	M, slower	M, slower	M	M	M	M
Rhythm	*Sinus*	*Sinus*	M	Usually AF	M	M
Diastolic dysfunction	++++	++++	—	—	—	—
RV dysfunction	++	++	+	++++	++++	2° to pulmonary hypertension

M = maintain; + = presence.

Figure 5-38. Summary treatment table. When combined valvular disorders exist, treatment is usually directed to the most advanced disorder. AF—atrial fibrillation; AR—aortic regurgitation; AS— aortic stenosis; HOCM—hypertrophic obstructive cardiomyopathy; MR—mitral regurgitation; MS—mitral stenosis; RV—right ventricle; TR—tricuspid regurgitation.

REFERENCES

1. Jackson JM, Thomas SJ, Lowenstein E: Anesthetic management of patients with valvular heart disease. *Semin Anesth* 1982, 1:239–252.

2. Ross J Jr: Afterload mismatch in aortic and mitral valve disease: implications for surgical therapy. *J Am Coll Cardiol* 1985, 5:811–826.

3. Lynch C, Lake CL: Cardiovascular anatomy and physiology. In *Cardiac, Thoracic, and Vascular Anesthesia*. Edited by Youngberg J, Lake CL, Roizen M, Tinker J, Wilson R. New York: Churchill-Livingstone, in press.

4. Grossman W, Jones D, McLaurin LP: Wall stress and patterns of hypertrophy in the human left ventricle. *J Clin Invest* 1975, 56:56–64.

5. Lorell BH, Grossman W: Cardiac hypertrophy: the consequences for diastole. *J Am Coll Cardiol* 1987, 9:1189–93.

6. Wray Roth DL, Rothstein P, Thomas SJ: Anesthesia for Cardiac Surgery. In Clinical Anesthesia, edn. 3. Edited by Baresh PG, Cullen BF, Stoelting RK. Philadelphia: Lippincott-Raven; 1997:835–870.

7. Rahimtoola SH: Aortic valve disease. In *Hurst's The Heart, Arteries and Veins*, edn 9. Edited by Alexander RW, Schlant RC, Furster V. New York: McGraw-Hill; 1998:1759–1788.

8. Thomas SJ, Lowenstein E: Anesthetic management of the patient with valvular heart disease. *Int Anesthesiol Clin* 1979, 17:67–96.

9. Boudoulas H, Gravanis MB: Valvular heart disease. In *Cardiovascular Disorders: Pathogenesis and Pathophysiology*. Edited by Gravanis MB. St. Louis: CV Mosby; 1993:64.

10. Marcus ML: Effects of cardiac hypertrophy on the coronary circulation. In *The Coronary Circulation in Health and Disease*. Edited by Marcus ML. New York: McGraw-Hill; 1983.

11. Grossman W: *Cardiac Catheterization and Angiography*. Philadelphia: Lea & Febiger; 1980:129.

12. Ross J Jr, Braunwald E: Aortic stenosis. *Circulation*.1968, 38(Suppl V):61.

13. Levine RA: Echocardiographic assessment of the cardiomyopathies. In *Principles and Practice of Echocardiography*, edn 2. Edited by Weyman AE. Philadelphia: Lea & Febiger; 1994, 781–823.

14. Savage RM, Lytle BW, Mossad E, *et al.*: Hypertrophic obstructive cardiomyopathy. In *Clinical Transesophageal Echocardiography: A Problem-Oriented Approach*. Edited by Oka Y, Konstadt SN. Philadelphia: Lippincott-Raven Publishers; 1996: 199–222.

15. Maron BJ, Bonow RO, Cannon RO, *et al.*: Hypertrophic cardiomyopathy; interrelations of clinical manifestations, pathophysiology, and therapy. *N Engl J Med* 1987, 316:844–852.

16. Rackley CE, Edwards JE, Wallace RB, Katz NM: Valvular Heart Disease. In *The Heart*, edn. 6. Edited by Hurst JW. New York: McGraw-Hill; 1986:729–754.

17. Kawanishi DT, Rahimtoola SH: Mitral stenosis. In *Valvular Heart Diseases*. Edited by Rahimtoola SH. St. Louis: CV Mosby; 1996, 8.1–8.24.

18. Schlant RC: Altered Cardiovascular Function of Rheumatic Heart Disease and Other Aquired Valvular Disease. In *The Heart*, edn. 2. Edited by Hurst JW. New York: McGraw-Hill; 1970:754.

19. Rahimtoola SH, Enriquez-Sarano M, Schaff JV, Frye RL: Mitral valve disease. In *Hurst's The Heart Arteries and Veins*. Edited by Alexander RW, Schlant RC, Furster V. New York: McGraw-Hill; 1998, 1789–1820.

20. Jackson JM: Valvular heart disease. In *Manual of Cardiac Anesthesia*, edn 2. Edited by Thomas SJ, Kramer JL. New York: Churchill-Livingstone; 1993, 81–128.

21. Jackson JM, Thomas SJ: Valvular heart disease. In *Cardiac Anesthesia*, edn. 3. Edited by Kaplan JA. Philadelphia: WB Saunders; 1993:629–680.

6

Anesthetic Considerations for Lung Transplantation and Thoracic Aortic Surgery

Mark Stafford Smith and Katherine P. Grichnik

Thoracic aortic aneurysm and end-stage lung disease are conditions with high morbidity and mortality. While this consideration justifies some of the significant risk associated with thoracic aortic and lung transplantation surgeries, if risk is to be minimized, it is imperative to develop a proficient operating team to optimize patient care. Although many of the considerations for anesthesia for lung transplant and thoracic aortic surgery are similar to those for other thoracic and cardiovascular surgeries, we have focused the contents of this chapter upon what we feel are the unique clinical elements and issues for these procedures, especially since these procedures are not done frequently in everyday clinical practice.

Management of the patient for lung transplantation involves a knowledge of all aspects of the patient's history, disease process, projected surgery, and anticipated postoperative care. Firstly, a detailed knowledge of the primary disease process for which the patient is receiving a transplant is crucial to the planning and execution of the anesthetic. The pathophysiology of a disease process usually presents as a spectrum of signs and symptoms that may wax and wane or grow progressively more critical. Patients presenting for transplantation, in general, are not expected to live more than 12 to 24 months due their primary disease process. For the anesthesiologist, the time of transplantation may be when the patient is still ambulatory and functional, or it may be when the patient is in a critical care setting. Knowledge of the pathophysiology and progression of the primary disease process allows one to predict clinical care needs for patients in all stages of disease.

Once the decision to identify a patient for transplantation has been made, the anesthesiologist should become involved in the planning of the transplant process. This involves preoperative assessment of the patient, planning for the intraoperative monitoring, predicting probable intraoperative complications, and planning for cardiopulmonary bypass (CPB). The preoperative condition of the patient, the type of operation planned, (single-lung transplant [SLT], double-lung transplant [DLT], or heart-lung transplant [HLT]), determines the surgical incision and probable need for CPB. Further, the anesthesiologist should be part of the multidisciplinary team caring for the patient postoperatively and thus should be familiar with the postoperative considerations for the transplant patient. If a patient is not deemed suitable for transplantation, one should also be aware of the alternative therapies to transplantation, some of which may involve caring for the patient in the operating room.

The factors that contribute to optimal anesthetic care for thoracic aortic surgery are similar to those for lung transplantation. In addition to general considerations already mentioned, the anesthesiologist is required to be familiar with the anatomy and pathophysiology of the aortic disease (and vessel occlusion) in a particular patient, and the immediate and delayed consequences of the circulatory strategy used to gain access to the diseased aorta. Stable hemodynamic management during the post-repair phase is also essential, to minimize bleeding, avoid further injury to vessel walls, and minimize stress on new suture lines.

Strategies to combat the three most frequent major complications of aortic surgery (bleeding diathesis, neurologic deficit, and renal injury) represent important developing areas of research and clinical practice. Major advances in the reduction of bleeding have been aided through the introduction of antifibrinolytic agents, and improved techniques to maintain normothermia. In addition, advances leading to more selective blood product transfusion when required have included the availability of better rapid infusion methods, blood salvage and predonation, and improved hematocrit and coagulation monitoring. In contrast, there have been fewer significant improvements in renal and neurologic protection. Many promising approaches to monitoring for organ ischemia, maintaining organ perfusion, and assuring optimal hypothermia throughout critical periods during surgery are currently in use, but no single technique has emerged as a major advance.

Some of the most challenging and infrequent cases for the cardiothoracic anesthesiologist are lung transplant and thoracic aortic surgeries. The opportunity for preparation and consultation prior to these cases is rarely optimal, since they often occur in the middle of the night, usually with little time between initial patient assessment and surgery. In order to minimize the major morbidity and mortality associated with these procedures, the anesthesiologist must be knowledgeable and aid in the development of a clinical team capable of rapid and effective delivery of optimal patient care.

PATHOLOGY OF END-STAGE LUNG DISEASE

A. CLASSIFICATION OF PULMONARY DISEASES LEADING TO LUNG TRANSPLANTATION

Restrictive pulmonary diseases	Pulmonary vascular diseases	Obstructive pulmonary diseases
Definition: A group of diseases characterized by injury to the alveolar wall leading to diffuse scarring or fibrosis. Features include decreased compliance of the lung, generalized decreases in lung volume, impairment of diffusion, disturbance of gas exchange and possible pulmonary hypertension. Diagnosis usually involves lung biopsy.	Definition: Abnormality of lung vessels leading to high intravascular pressures within the lung tissue. Pulmonary artery mean pressure should be greater than 20 mm Hg. The abnormality of the lung vessels may be a primary event or secondary such as that due to acquired and congenital cardiac disease or chronic pulmonary emboli. Narrowed or occluded pulmonary vessels include the muscular small arteries, arterioles and muscular veins. Diagnosis is via right heart catheterization and may include lung biopsy.	Definition: A group of diseases characterized by a persistent increase in resistance to bronchial airflow. Lung volumes are increased; dilated air spaces may lose elastic recoil or may be occupied by infectious material. Diagnosis is multimodal but may often be made by chest radiograph.
Selected major disease states: idiopathic pulmonary fibrosis, sarcoidosis	Selected major disease state: primary pulmonary hypertension	Selected major disease states: emphysema, bronchiectasis
PFTs: Decreased FEV_1 and FVC, normal FEV_1/FVC ratio, decreased DLCO	PFTs: May be normal except for a decrease in diffusion capacity.	PFTs: Decreased FVC and FEV_1, decreased FEV_1/FVC ratio, decreased MMFR, air trapping (increased RV, TLC and FRC). May have decreased DLCO
Treatments: Steroids, cytotoxic agents, lung transplant. (See Fig. 6-1B.)	Treatment: Treatment of the causative problem such as mitral stenosis, anticoagulants, systemic and pulmonary vasodilators, prostacyclin, lung transplant.	Treatments: Bronchodilators, chest physiotherapy and rehabilitation, early treatment of infection, steroids, low flow oxygen, lung transplant [1].

Figure 6-1. Classification of pulmonary diseases leading to lung transplantation, **A.**
(Continued on next page)

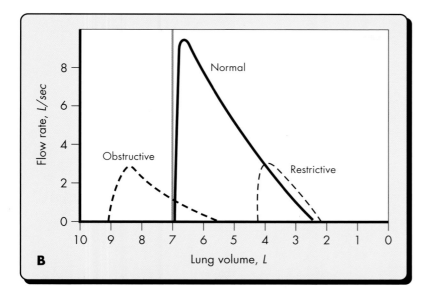

Figure 6-1. (*Continued*) **B**, Pulmonary disease patterns. DLCO—diffusion capacity for carbon monoxide; FEV_1—forced expiratory volume in 1 sec; FRC—functional reserve capacity; FVC—forced vital capacity; MMFR—maximum mid-expiratory flow. (Part B *adapted from* West [1]; with permission.)

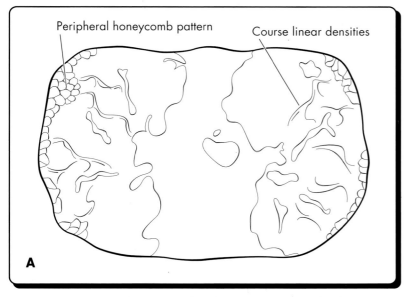

Figure 6-2. Pathophysiology of idiopathic pulmonary fibrosis. Idiopathic pulmonary fibrosis (IPF) is one of the multiple terms used to describe patients with a pulmonary inflammatory reaction of uncertain etiology leading to interstitial thickening and distortion. Other names include usual interstitial pneumonia, chronic interstitial pneumonia, and

B. PROPOSED MECHANISM FOR IPF

Unknown etiology

Parenchymal injury with alveolar inflammation (*continued etiological exposure* vs *lung defenses and individual susceptibility determine extent of injury and progression*).

Chronic alveolitis and progressive injury

Fibrin deposition and organization of fibrinous exudates

Simultaneous organization of multiple alveoli leads to patches of lung destruction

End-stage lung disease

cryptogenic fibrosing alveolitis. Depending on the extent of the fibrotic process, the lung architecture can become almost completely destroyed. The most common age of presentation is 40 to 70 years old. The disease is characterized by dyspnea, dry rales, and clubbing. The diagnosis is often made by lung biopsy to investigate a suspicious chest radiograph including "honeycomb" lung. Patients have a mean survival of 5 years after diagnosis. **A**, Schematic representation of chest computed tomography in IPF, showing coarse linear densities and a peripheral honeycomb pattern. **B**, A proposed mechanism for the pathogenesis of IPF [2].

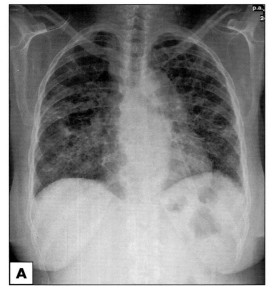

Figure 6-3. Pathophysiology of sarcoidosis. Sarcoidosis is a disorder of multiple organ systems with noncaseating granuloma formation. Although the lung and the hilar lymph nodes are the most commonly involved tissues, other systems involved may include the heart, the eyes (uveitis and inflammation), the skin (papules and erythema nodosum), the liver, and the endocrine organs. There may be multiple immunologic abnormalities, including delayed hypersensitivity characterized by depression of the cellular immune system and hyperactivity of the humoral immune system characterized by hyperglobulinemia. Symptoms include progressive dyspnea and clubbing. The chest radiograph may demonstrate enlarged lymph nodes (especially hilar) and interstitial lung disease. Lung, skin, or salivary gland biopsy may demonstrate noncaseating granulomas. The natural history of the disease is variable with some patients enjoying resolution of their symptoms and others progressing to end-stage lung disease. Therapy usually involves steroid administration. **A**, Chest radiograph of sarcoidosis.

(*Continued on next page*)

Figure 6-3. (*Continued*) B, Classification of sarcoidosis [3,4].

B. CLASSIFICATION OF SARCOIDOSIS

Early
  Bilateral hilar lymph node enlargement
    Miliary nodules
    Early interstitial lung disease
Intermediate
  Nodules
  Reticular pattern on radiograph
Late
  Extensive fibrosis with bullae and/or
  Superimposed infection
  Alveolar granulomas

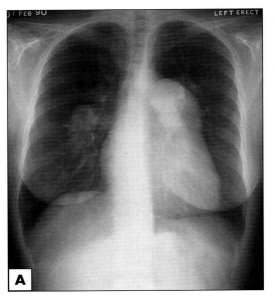

Figure 6-4. Pathophysiology of pulmonary hypertension. Pulmonary hypertension can be primary or secondary to congenital heart

B. SAMPLE RIGHT HEART CATHETERIZATION PRESSURES

Systemic arterial blood pressure: 110/70
Right atrial pressure: 45/10
Right ventricular pressure: 80/10
Pulmonary artery pressure: 80/40
Pulmonary capillary wedge pressure: 10
Severe tricuspid regurgitation noted

disease or severe lung disease. Primary pulmonary hypertension (PPH) is defined as idiopathic pulmonary arterial hypertension. Pulmonary arteries in PPH are characterized by vasoconstriction, medial thickening, cellular proliferation, and the deposition of plexiform lesions and dilatation [5,6]. Females are affected 2:1 *vs* males. Clinical symptoms include dyspnea, fatigue, syncope, and rarely hemoptysis. A suspicious chest radiograph may show right ventricular enlargement, dilated central pulmonary vessels, and decreased peripheral vascular markings. The diagnosis is made with a right heart catheterization. Patients with PPH have a mean survival of about three years after diagnosis. Associated problems may include collagen-vascular diseases or immunologic diseases. **A,** Radiograph demonstrating PPH. **B,** Sample right heart catheterization data from a patient with PPH [5].

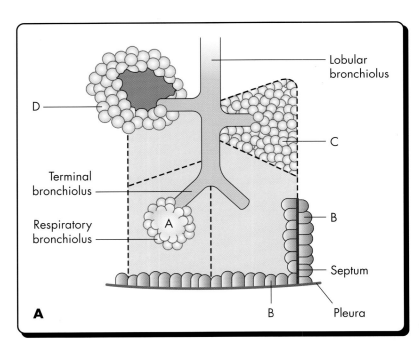

A

Figure 6-5. Pathophysiology of emphysema. The definition of emphysema is "a condition of the lung characterized by abnormal, permanent enlargement of air spaces distal to the terminal bronchiole, accompanied by the destruction of their walls, and without obvious fibrosis." Emphysema occurs distal to the terminal bronchiole and thus is limited to the gas-exchanging alveolated elements of the lung or acinus. There are five recognized types of emphysema. For example, alpha-1 antitrypsin deficiency leads to a severe, early-onset panacinar emphysema. All types of emphysema are associated with tobacco use. On chest radiography, the emphysematous lung is characterized by hyperinflation. Associated changes include flattening of the diaphragm, increased anterior-posterior diameter of the chest cavity, and the appearance of a small vertical heart on chest radiograph. Post-bronchodilator forced expiratory volume in 1 sec (FEV_1) and mean pulmonary artery pressures are the major predictors of prognosis in patients with chronic obstructive lung disease. **A,** Diagram of bronchioles in emphysema.

(*Continued on next page*)

B. CLASSIFICATION OF EMPHYSEMA

A. Centriacinar
B. Periacinar
C. Panacinar
D. Irregular (scar)
E. Bullous

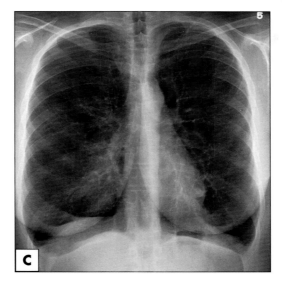

Figure 6-5. (*Continued*) **B,** Classification of emphysema [7–9] (*A–D* correspond to letters in *panel A; E* not shown). **C,** Radiograph of a patient with alpha-1-anti-trypsin deficiency. (Part A *from* Reid [7]; with permission.)

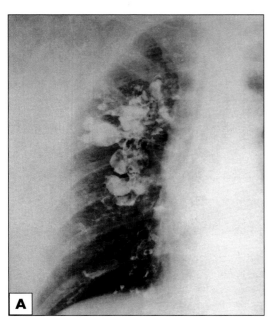

Figure 6-6. Pathophysiology of bronchiectasis. **A,** Bronchogram of patient with saccu-

B. PATHOGENESIS OF BRONCHIECTASIS

1. Infection (or airway collapse due to bronchial obstruction from noninfectious etiology) in patient with normally branching bronchial tree.
2. Inflammatory injury leading to airway distortion and scar. Marked dilation of proximal airways.
3. Peripheral airways not patent with obliteration of the normal branched bronchial tree.
4. Dilated airways often filled with secretions, which may be purulent.
5. Bronchial arteries may enlarge and cause hemoptysis.

lar bronchiectasis. Bronchiectasis is a permanent abnormal dilatation of the bronchi, as a generalized or localized process. The pathogenesis is described in **B.** It is characterized by shortness of breath, chronic cough, and sputum production; it is not necessarily due to smoking. Significant airway obstruction occurs. Bronchiectasis is subcategorized as cylindrical, varicose, or saccular, depending on the amount of bronchial dilatation and degree of terminal bronchiole obstruction by purulent secretions. Alternatively, it may be classified as "wet" vs "dry." Wet bronchiectasis refers to the massive production of sputum, and dry bronchiectasis is characterized by hemoptysis due to bronchiole arteriole dilatation. Therapy for bronchiectasis includes antibiotics, intensive chest physiotherapy, selected pulmonary resection, and lung transplantation [8–11]. (Part A *from* Weinberger [12]; with permission.)

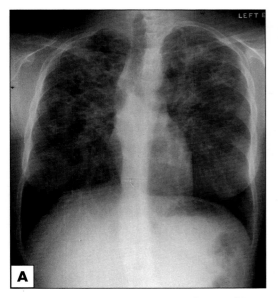

Figure 6-7. Pathophysiology of cystic fibrosis (CF). CF is the most common lethal inher-

B. CF FACTS

Defects: Abnormal, thick immobile secretions of exocrine glands and within the lungs.
Diagnosis: Elevated sweat chloride concentration.
Problems: Recurrent lung infections, pancreatic insufficiency, malnutrition, end stage lung disease.
Complications: Pneumothorax, massive hemoptysis, respiratory failure, cor pulmonale.

ited disorder of caucasians. The mean survival of patients with CF is approximately 30 years of age. It is inherited in an autosomal recessive manner with an incidence of 1 in 2500. It is primarily a disease of the secretions of exocrine glands with the production of thick, tenacious mucus that blocks the ducts of the secreting gland. Patients with CF have apparently normal lungs at birth but are abnormally sensitive to infection. This, combined with hypertrophy of the mucous glands in the lungs leads to airway plugging and tissue destruction, resulting in the characteristic bronchiectasis-like picture of CF. The clinical presentation includes severe obstructive lung disease, pancreatic insufficiency, and serum electrolyte abnormalities. Therapy includes chest physiotherapy, antibiotics, bronchodilators, oral pancreatic enzyme therapy, and lung transplantation. **A,** Radiograph of a patient with CF. **B,** Facts about CF [8].

CRITERIA FOR LUNG TRANSPLANTATION

End stage lung disease (life expectancy 12–24 mo)

No other major organ dysfunction

Not immunosuppressed, steroid use < 15 mg prednisone/d

Age less than 65 for SLT, age less than 55 for BLT

Compliance with medical regimens

Stable psychological profile with good social support

Adequate nutrition and ambulatory (oxygen use acceptable)

Disease suitable for transplantation:
  Chronic obstructive lung disease (SLT > BLT, or SLT with contralateral lung volume reduction surgery)
    Emphysema, alpha-1 antitrypsin
  Bronchiectasis (BLT)
  Cystic fibrosis (BLT)
  Pulmonary hypertension (primary BLT > SLT, secondary *eg* Eisenmenger's syndrome HLT)
  Idiopathic pulmonary fibrosis (SLT/BLT)
  Sarcoidosis (SLT/BLT)
  Miscellaneous (SLT/BLT)
    Extrinsic allergic alveolitis, eosinophilic granuloma, drug-induced lung disease, lymphangiomyomatosis

Figure 6-8. Criteria for lung transplantation. The criteria for lung transplantation are in a continuous process of evolution, dramatically changed from prior criteria. Single lung transplantation (SLT) is advocated for disease processes in which the remaining lung would not adversely impact the functioning of the transplanted lung. Examples include chronic obstructive lung disease and idiopathic pulmonary fibrosis. Bilateral lung transplantation (BLT) is performed for diseases in which the transplanted lung could become soiled by infection, impaired by abnormal gas flow or receive abnormal amounts of vascular flow due to the primary lung disease in the native remaining lung. Examples include chronic obstructive lung disease, bronchiectasis, cystic fibrosis, and primary pulmonary hypertension. Heart-lung transplant is reserved for pulmonary disease with cardiac dysfunction not expected to resolve after transplantation. An example is Eisenmenger's syndrome [10,13,14]. HLT—heart-lung transplantation.

PREOPERATIVE ASSESSMENT FOR LUNG TRANSPLANTATION

History and physical
  Type of lung disease, length of disease, status of disease, comorbidities

Radiology: chest radiograph and chest computed tomography
  Can determine which side to operate on first, rule out concurrent neoplasm

Laboratory investigation
  Serologies, blood group, histocompatibility antigens, panel reactive antibodies, blood chemistry, complete blood count, clotting parameters

Pulmonary workup
  Pulmonary function tests, bronchoscopy as indicated, differential lung ventilation and perfusion scan

Cardiac workup
  Transthoracic echocardiogram: assess heart function, patent foramen ovale
  Right and left heart catheterization
  Intracardiac pressures can predict need for CPB or nitric oxide, determine right vs left ventricular ejection fraction, rule out concurrent coronary artery disease
  24-hour ECG monitor

Allergies
  Cystic fibrosis and bronchiectasis patients are likely to be resistant or allergic to antibiotics; they may need desensitization

Psychosocial profile

Figure 6-9. Preoperative assessment for lung transplantation. The preoperative workup should focus on the abnormalities that can be altered or improved prior to surgery. Further, the preoperative workup can identify the possible need for cardiopulmonary bypass (such as pulmonary arterial pressures greater than two thirds of systemic pressures). Intraoperative complications may be anticipated and appropriate preparations can be made (such as the need for a cell saver in a patient with a history of prior thoracic surgery). The full preoperative workup should be available to the anesthesia team for review so that interventions pertinent to the anesthetic care can be made prior to transplantation (such as optimization of treatment for systemic hypertension). Further, the preoperative work up should be accessible 24 hours a day for review, because surgery often occurs on an emergent basis outside of regular working hours. CPB—cardiopulmonary bypass.

ADDITIONAL MONITORING FOR LUNG TRANSPLANTATION

Radial arterial line

Femoral arterial line
   Radial arterial line may dampen or become dysfunctional with positioning or during surgery

Oximetric pulmonary artery catheter
   Will need to pull back with pulmonary artery anastomosis

Transesophageal echocardiogram
   Assess for right and left heart function, intraoperatively assess for shunts
   Assess flow in pulmonary veins after transplant

Urinary catheter

Fiberoptic bronchoscope
   To assure accurate endotracheal tube (ET) placement and lung isolation (double lumen [DLET] or single lumen [SLET] with endobronchial blocker)

Accurate ventilator measurements
   Peak and mean airway pressures, lung volumes, amounts of positive end expiratory pressure and pressure support
   Nitric oxide concentration measurement

Figure 6-10. Additional monitoring for lung transplantation. In addition to the usual American Society of Anesthesiology monitors, one needs to consider additional monitoring for the transplant patient, as shown in this table. These monitors enable the anesthesiologist to quickly diagnose and effectively treat the expected hemodynamic and respiratory compromise that occurs intraoperatively. Patients also need large bore IV access that does not kink with positioning (antecubital lines are prone to this) to treat intravascular volume losses as they occur [13,14].

INTRAOPERATIVE ANESTHETIC MANAGEMENT FOR LUNG TRANSPLANTATION

Asepsis with line placement

Assure immunosuppresive agents and antibiotics given prior to surgery

Assure ability to maintain normothermia

Assure blood products available and in operating room

Position carefully, check pressure points

Assure accurate DLET or SLET with a bronchial blocker placement

Limit fluids as is possible

Assure proper ventilator availability
   Need ventilator able to deliver pressure-limited ventilation
   Reassess tidal volume, inspiratory pressures and minute ventilation frequently anticipate sudden changes
   Beware of potential for dynamic hyperinflation

Have vasopressors ready: significant cardiopulmonary dysfunction can occur
   Dopamine, epinephrine, milrinone and dobutamine useful
   Consider cardiopulmonary bypass early when vasopressor therapy is not effective

Expect and attempt to prevent pulmonary edema
   Occurs often between the first and second lung transplant in a bilateral sequential transplant

May need to tolerate significant hypercapnea

May need to change DLET to SLET prior to transport to the intensive care unit

Figure 6-11. Intraoperative anesthetic management for lung transplantation. The intraoperative management of the patient for lung transplantation is among the most challenging tasks one can undertake. Preoperatively patients are critically ill with severe cardiopulmonary disease. The nature of the operation induces further dysfunction with one-lung ventilation, surgical manipulation, intravascular volume loss, sudden and unexpected changes in ventilatory function, severe acid-base abnormalities, and difficulties with oxygenation. Some of the considerations for intraoperative management are listed in this table. However, one must be aware of the significant potential for unexpected problems and be ready to react quickly to treat sudden changes in multiple physiological functions [13,14]. DLET—double-lumen endotracheal tube; SLET—single-lumen endotracheal tube.

CRITERIA FOR CONSIDERATION FOR THE USE OF CPB DURING LUNG TRANSPLANTATION

Significant preexisting pulmonary hypertension and/or
  hypoxemia during one-lung ventilation
  Pulmonary artery pressures two thirds or greater than systemic
    arterial pressures
Deterioration of native lung function during one lung ventilation
Acute pulmonary edema unresponsive to therapy in first trans-
  planted lung during the implantation of the second lung of a
  double lung transplant
Acute cardiac decompensation
Vasodilatation leading to refractory hypotension
  May see sepsis-like syndrome with cystic fibrosis patients
Living-related lobar lung transplant
  Transplanted lobes may decompensate with one lung ventila-
    tion and perfusion of the patient's full cardiac output
Combined lung and heart transplant

Figure 6-12. Criteria for consideration for the use of cardiopulmonary bypass (CPB) during lung transplantation. The decision to undertake CPB for lung transplant surgery is not to be taken lightly. Bleeding complications secondary to anticoagulation and fibrinolysis can be profound. Further, oxygenation postoperatively may be depressed. These patients are already prone to disseminated intravascular coagulation postoperatively (intraoperative stressors include low cardiac output states, hypothermia, prolonged operative procedures, large areas of raw bleeding surfaces, sepsis due to prior infections, and preoperative coagulation abnormalities), which can be aggravated by exposure to cardiopulmonary bypass. Conversely, one should not postpone CPB in the face of profound cardiopulmonary compromise—a reversible situation can quickly become difficult to manage and may result in irreversible organ dysfunction [13,14].

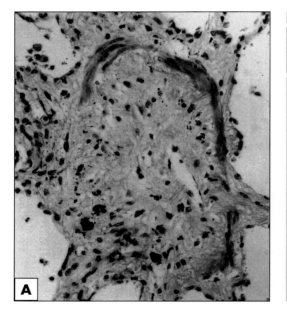

B. POSTOPERATIVE CARE FOR LUNG TRANSPLANT PATIENTS

Determinants of severity of illness postoperatively
  Severity of pulmonary disease, prior infection, SLT *vs* DLT *vs* HLT, type of incision,
    need for CPB
Multidisciplinary team effort essential
  Surgeon, pulmonologist, anesthesiologist, respiratory therapist, physical therapist,
    nutritionist, transplant coordinator, social worker
Selected postoperative procedures
  Perfusion scan to assess vascular anastomoses, aggressive prevention and treatment of
    noncardiogenic pulmonary edema, thoracic epidural placement for pain management,
    exquisite attention to parameters of ventilation, surveillance bronchoscopy, infection
    prophylaxis, immunosuppression
Selected complications after lung transplantation
  Infection (bacterial, fungal, viral), severe perfusion to ventilation mismatch, bronchial and
    vascular constriction or thromboses, gastroparesis, rejection, bronchiolitis obliterans

Figure 6-13. Postoperative considerations for lung transplantation. The postoperative care of the lung transplant patient is challenging at best and may involve multiple procedures in the intensive care unit. Optimization of management is best achieved by a multidisciplinary team effort with one person leading the team. Patients vary in severity of illness, the postoperative procedures needed, and the complications that may occur. All of the usual considerations for a critically ill patient may be complicated by the risks of immunosuppression, the risks of infection, and the risk of an ischemic-reperfusion injury (characterized by noncardiogenic pulmonary edema). Once a patient has survived the immediate postoperative period, bronchiolitis obliterans is a feared consequence of transplantation and may occur in up to 50% of patients after transplant [10,15]. (Part A *from* Yousem [16]; with permission.)

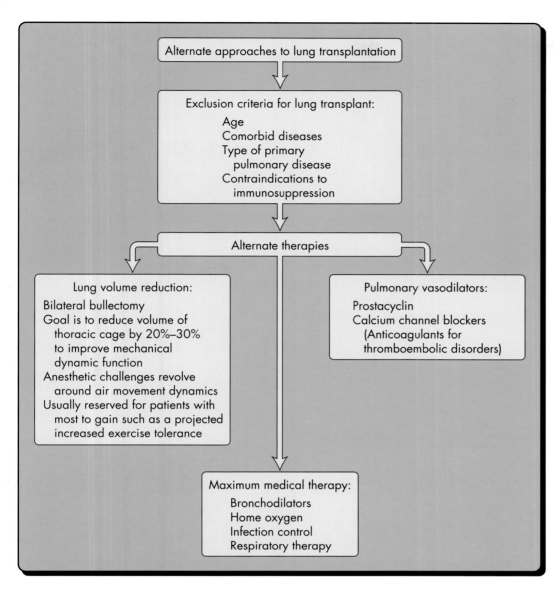

Alternate approaches to lung transplantation

↓

Exclusion criteria for lung transplant:

Age
Comorbid diseases
Type of primary
   pulmonary disease
Contraindications to
   immunosuppression

↓

Alternate therapies

Lung volume reduction:

Bilateral bullectomy
Goal is to reduce volume of
   thoracic cage by 20%–30%
   to improve mechanical
   dynamic function
Anesthetic challenges revolve
   around air movement dynamics
Usually reserved for patients with
   most to gain such as a projected
   increased exercise tolerance

Pulmonary vasodilators:

Prostacyclin
Calcium channel blockers
   (Anticoagulants for
   thromboembolic disorders)

Maximum medical therapy:

Bronchodilators
Home oxygen
Infection control
Respiratory therapy

Figure 6-14. Alternate approaches to lung transplantation. Patients who are unable to have lung transplant surgery may still present to the operating room for procedures to treat their pulmonary diseases. Alternative therapies to lung transplantation involve both surgical and medical approaches. Should a patient present for lung reduction surgery, one must consider the patient to be as frail as a patient (*eg*, lung reduction) presenting for transplantation. Further, the patient undergoes a surgical procedure with frequent intraoperative problems that may not result in improved lung function for a period of time postoperatively [17].

AORTIC DISEASE

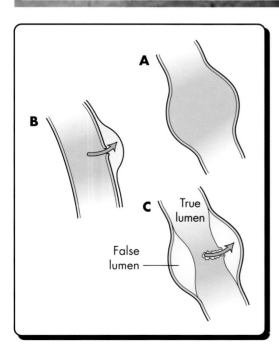

Figure 6-15. Types of aortic aneurysmal dilatation. **A,** A true aneurysm involves all layers of the aorta. The expanded lumen is the result of stretched and thinned tissues, which are vulnerable to subsequent rupture or dissection. The aneurysm may contain a laminated thrombus. **B,** Aortic pseudoaneurysm represents a contained rupture of the intima and media of the vessel wall. The resulting hemorrhage is contained within the adventitia or periaortic tissues and may thrombose or progress to free rupture over time. **C,** A dissecting aortic aneurysm develops as blood separates medial layers following an intimal tear of the vessel wall. The resulting false lumen causes vessel wall expansion with compression of the true vessel lumen. Aortic dissection may lead to obstruction or rupture of the aorta and branch vessels. Atherosclerotic plaque may limit the propagation of aortic dissection.

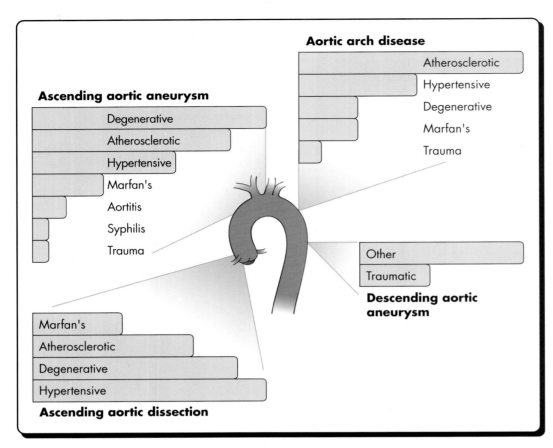

Figure 6-16. Pathophysiology and relative frequency of aortic disease. Thoracic aortic aneurysm is a rare disease, with an incidence of 6 per 100,000 person-years [18]. The disease is generally seen after the third decade, occurring approximately equally among men and women. Location in the ascending (51%) and descending (38%) aorta is more common than in the aortic arch (11%) [19]. Causes of thoracic aortic aneurysmal dilatation vary by location [19]. The relative frequency of different etiologic factors contributing to thoracic aortic disease is depicted, by location, in this figure [18,19]. Approximately, 40% to 50% of patients will present with either aortic dissection or traumatic disruption [18,19].

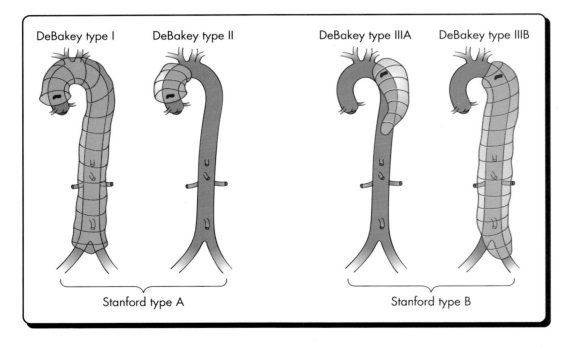

Figure 6-17. Classification of aortic dissection. The location of the intimal tear and extent of dissection are key to the DeBakey classification (I, II, IIIA, IIIB) of aortic dissection [20]. In contrast, the Stanford classification [21] identifies only the presence (type A) or absence (type B) of ascending aortic involvement in the dissection. While type B aortic dissections are best treated with medical therapy in the absence of further complications (*eg*, rupture, organ ischemia), mortality without surgery is extremely high for type A dissections [22]. (*Adapted from* DeBakey and coworkers [20].)

Figure 6-18. Anesthetic considerations for thoracic aortic surgery.

ANESTHETIC CONSIDERATIONS FOR THORACIC AORTIC SURGERY

Aortic pathology
  Location, extent of aneurysm (*vs* placement of aortic crossclamps)
  Type of aneurysm, *eg* dissection, traumatic
  Symptomatic (leaking *vs* ruptured)
  Requirements for resuscitation or blood pressure control prior to surgery
  Presence of end organ ischemia (*eg*, kidney)
  Associated cardiac problems (aortic insufficiency/pericardial tamponade/coronary
      artery occlusion)
  Risk of aortic rupture during patient transfer and anesthetic procedures (*eg* central line,
      endotracheal tube or transesophageal echo probe placement)
  Presence of vessel occlusion vs arterial line placement
Surgical Approach
  Ascending aorta and aortic arch - supine, median sternotomy
  Descending aorta - left side up with femoral artery/vein access, left thoracotomy
Ventilation/Perfusion Considerations
  Ascending aorta
    Left radial arterial line placement
  Descending aorta
    Right radial arterial line placement
    Lung isolation strategy (right lung ventilation during repair)
    Lower body perfusion strategy
      Unassisted: post-repair reversal of low dose heparin +/- treatment of reperfusion
        acidosis
      Assisted: attention to upper vs lower body perfusion; post-repair reversal of high
        dose heparin
    Vasopressor drug and fluid management (especially during 'unclamping')
  Aortic arch (if deep hypothermic circulatory arrest planned)
    Early placement of ice around head
    If retrograde cerebral perfusion planned, consider monitoring superior vena
        cava pressure
Hemostatic considerations
  Minimize drug-related hemostatic impairments
  Optimize homeostasis (*eg*, avoid hypothermia, hemodilution)
  Consider antifibrinolytic/antiinflammatory agents
  Frequent hemostatic assessment to guide blood product usage

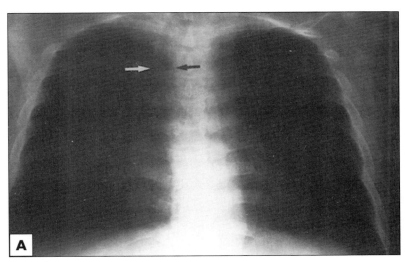

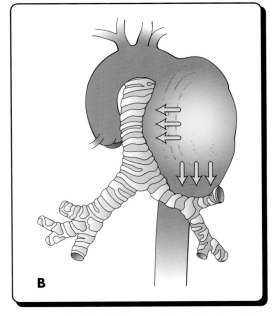

Figure 6-19. Special considerations for lung isolation with thoracic aortic surgery. **A,** Thoracic aortic aneurysms (*arrows* identify deviated trachea) may compress and distort mediastinal structures including the airway [23]. **B,** The trachea and left mainstem bronchus can be narrowed and deviated by an aneurysm, and the angle of the left mainstem bronchus with the trachea altered significantly. One-lung anesthesia is desirable for surgical repair of descending thoracic aortic aneurysms; however, lung isolation may be technically challenging. Placement of a single lumen endotracheal tube and left mainstem bronchus blocker (or Univent tube [Fuji Systems, Japan]) using fiberoptic bronchoscopy may be simpler than double-lumen tube intubation and also avoids the necessity for reintubation after surgery. Vigorous intubation attempts should be avoided, since this may risk rupture of the aneurysm. (Part A *from* Hunt and Schwab [23]; with permission.)

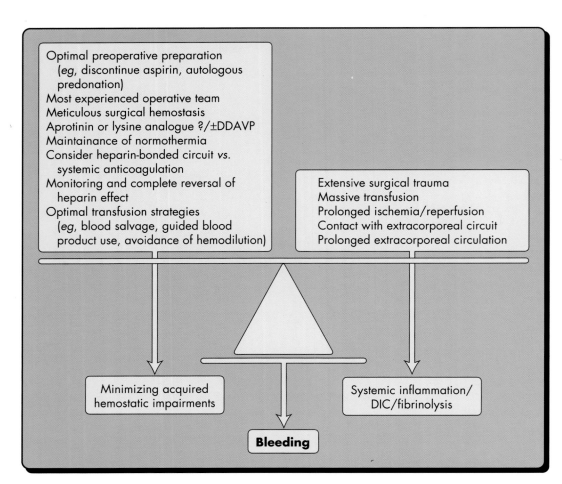

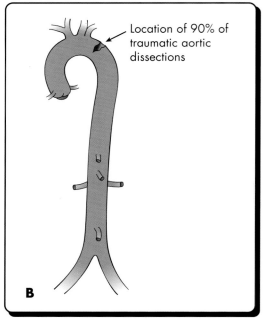

Figure 6-20. Factors influencing hemostasis during thoracic aortic surgery. Bleeding associated with thoracic aortic surgery is a major cause of perioperative morbidity and mortality. Many factors contribute to impaired hemostasis during thoracic aortic surgery. A common pathway for some of them is disseminated intravascular coagulation (DIC) and fibrinolysis. It is imperative therefore that careful attention is paid to those perioperative factors that can be influenced by the anesthesiologist to minimize additional acquired hemostatic impairments [24].

SURGERY OF THE DESCENDING THORACIC AORTA

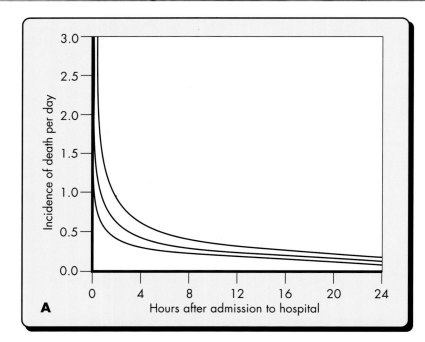

Figure 6-21. Traumatic aortic dissection. Since the risk of rupture following traumatic aortic dissection is significant (**A**), the highest priority is placed upon immediate surgery when this is diagnosed. Traumatic aortic dissection usually occurs related to a blunt trauma involving rapid deceleration; horizontal impacts displace the heart and aortic arch anteriorly, causing injury at the isthmus of the descending aorta (**B**) where the descending aorta is 'fixed' to the chest wall (about 90% of all cases). In contrast, aortic injuries involving vertical deceleration (*eg*, falls) usually injure the ascending aorta or aortic arch.

(Continued on next page)

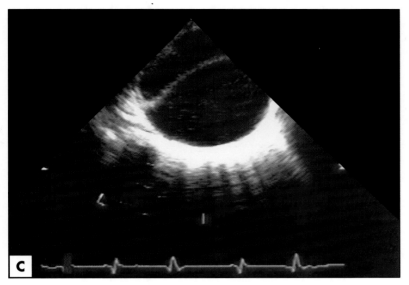

Figure 6-21. (*Continued*) Typical chest radiographic findings include widened mediastinum, obscured aortic knob, presence of nearby high impact injuries (*eg*, second rib fracture), and right tracheal displacement [25,26]. Definitive diagnosis can be made by aortography, computed tomography, magnetic resonance imaging or transesophageal echocardiography (**C**) [27]. Major comorbidities associated with traumatic aortic dissection, such as closed head and unstable neck injuries and myocardial and pulmonary contusions, should always be suspected. Other life-threatening injuries may require surgery prior to, or at the same time as, traumatic aortic aneurysm repair. (Part A *from* Kirklin and Barratt-Boyes [28]; with permission.)

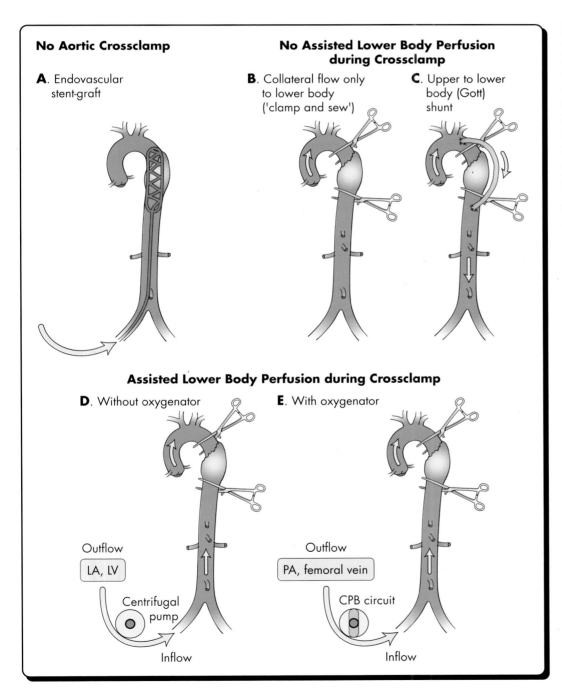

No Aortic Crossclamp

A. Endovascular stent-graft

No Assisted Lower Body Perfusion during Crossclamp

B. Collateral flow only to lower body ('clamp and sew')

C. Upper to lower body (Gott) shunt

Assisted Lower Body Perfusion during Crossclamp

D. Without oxygenator

Outflow
LA, LV
Centrifugal pump
Inflow

E. With oxygenator

Outflow
PA, femoral vein
CPB circuit
Inflow

Figure 6-22. Circulatory strategies for descending thoracic aortic aneurysm repair. For thoracoabdominal aneurysm surgery, the standard left thoracotomy incision must be extended to a midline abdominal incision for access to the abdominal aorta. Different lower body perfusion strategies (**A–E**) have significant implications for anesthetic technique and problems that can be expected: After separation from assisted lower-body perfusion techniques, reversal of full systemic anticoagulation is required, while significant metabolic acidosis may result from lower-body reperfusion using the 'clamp and sew' method. In contrast, controlled hypotension is necessary during endovascular stent-graft deployment, a procedure that may be complicated by profound reflex bradycardia [29]. Common to all circulatory strategies is the importance of hemodynamic stability throughout the procedure, which requires cooperation of the surgeon and the anesthesiologist, especially during the period of aortic crossclamp placement and removal. No technique has proven to be superior regarding mortality or the occurrence of major complications, including paraplegia or renal failure.

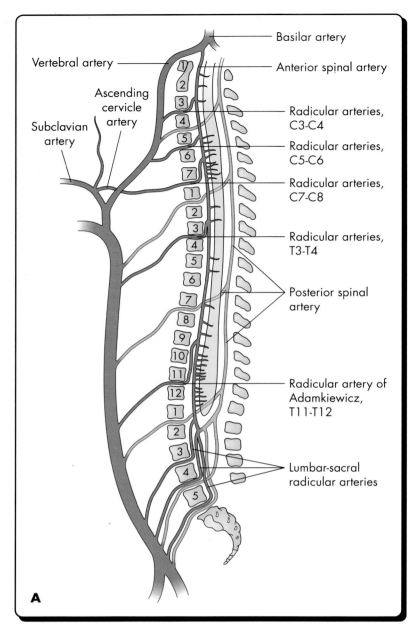

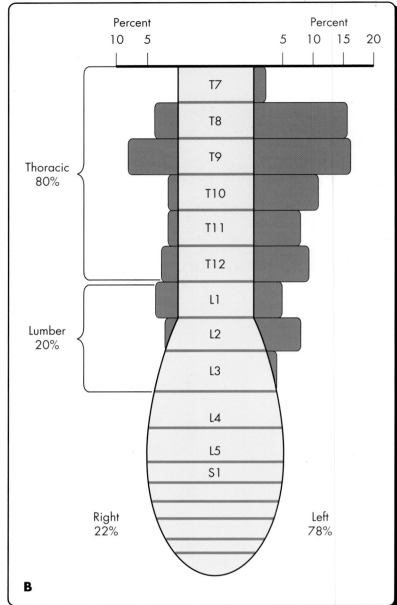

Figure 6-23. Arterial blood supply of the spinal cord. Knowledge of the spinal cord blood supply is particularly important during surgery of the descending thoracic aorta, since paraplegia due to spinal cord ischemia is a catastrophic and distressingly common (5% to 20%) complication of this surgery. The vulnerability of the spinal cord during manipulation of the descending thoracic aorta is due to the reliance of up to 50% of spinal cord perfusion, including that of the spinal lumbosacral enlargement, upon the integrity of the artery of Adamkiewicz (**A**), a major vessel that is supplied from this region of the aorta [30]. While other spinal cord supply vessels enter the spinal canal, they are usually small, and represent a poor anastamotic network. The origin of the artery of Adamkiewicz is variable (**B**); the vessel usually enters the spinal canal between T8 and L3 (78% in thoracic region), most commonly on the left side (80%) [31]. (Part A *adapted from* Simpson [32]; with permission; part B *adapted from* Djindjian [30]; with permission.)

SPINAL CORD PROTECTION FOR DESCENDING THORACIC AORTIC SURGERY

Strategies to preserve spinal cord perfusion
 Avoidance of aortic crossclamping
  Endovascular stent-graft placement [33]
 Maintenance of spinal perfusion pressure (PPsc = BPsc - CSFpress) during aortic cross-clamp
  Maintenance of BPsc
   Maintenance of systemic, supra-clamp blood pressure [34]
   Monitoring of lower body perfusion pressure: femoral arterial line
   Lower body perfusion during crossclamping
    Gott shunt [35], axillofemoral bypass [36]
    mechanically assisted (CPB with oxygenator, centrifugal pump) [37]
  Decrease CSF pressure
   lumbar drain [38], hyperventilation, thiopental
 Focus on the integrity of critical spinal vessels
  Identification of vessels for preservation (*eg* artery of Adamkiewicz)
   preoperative angiography [39]
   intraoperative: selective vessel injection and spinal tracer sensing [40]
  SSEP changes with vessel clamping [41]
  Reimplantation of intercostal arteries [42]
  Guidance with on line spinal ischemia monitoring (*eg* SSEP, MEP) [43]
 Alternate spinal oxygen delivery strategies
  Intrathecal oxygenated perflurocarbon emulsion [44]
General neuroprotective techniques
 Shortest possible period of potential spinal cord ischemia
 Hypothermia
  Total body (± circulatory arrest, ± retrograde cerebral perfusion) [45]
  Epidural cooling [46]
 Pharmaceutical therapy
  Barbiturates, isoflurane
  Calcium channel blockers, naloxone
 Glucose management

Figure 6-24. Spinal cord protection for descending thoracic aortic surgery. As survival has improved, paraplegia following descending thoracic aortic surgery has emerged as a major morbidity of this procedure. Numerous strategies have been devised in attempts to reduce the incidence of this tragic complication. There is currently no consensus in the literature regarding the best way to protect the spinal cord from injury. In general, the risk of paraplegia is related to the extent and the type of aortic pathology. BP_{sc}— spinal cord arterial pressure; CSFpress—cerebral spinal fluid pressure; MEP—motor evoked potential; PP_{sc}— spinal cord perfusion pressure; SSEP—somatosensory evoked potential.

SURGERY OF THE AORTIC ARCH AND ASCENDING AORTA

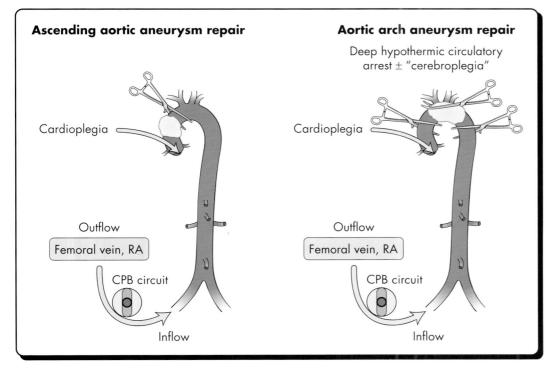

Ascending aortic aneurysm repair

Cardioplegia

Outflow
Femoral vein, RA

CPB circuit

Inflow

Aortic arch aneurysm repair

Deep hypothermic circulatory arrest ± "cerebroplegia"

Cardioplegia

Outflow
Femoral vein, RA

CPB circuit

Inflow

Figure 6-25. Circulatory strategies for ascending and arch aortic aneurysm repair. Femoral arterial cannulation for standard cardiopulmonary bypass is used during ascending aortic aneurysm repair. Deep hypothermia prior to circulatory arrest for aortic arch repair is achieved by packing the head in ice and prolonged cooling with cardiopulmonary bypass, and may be maintained by continued cerebral perfusion ('cerebroplegia') during arrest. Ventricular distension in the presence of aortic valve insufficiency may be necessitate aortic crossclamping prior to the achievement of deep hypothermia.

NEUROPROTECTIVE STRATEGIES FOR DEEP HYPOTHERMIC CIRCULATORY ARREST (14–19°C) FOR AORTIC ARCH SURGERY

Cerebral hypothermia (methods to achieve and maintain)
   Packing the head in ice [47]
   Extended (> 20 min) CPB cooling prior to circulatory arrest [48]
      Nasopharyngeal temperature may underestimate brain temperature by 4–5°C [49]. It is suggested to maintain cooling 5–8 min after achievement of target temperature.
Enhanced hypothermia plus other possible benefits
   Arterial blood gas management:
      pH Stat improved outcomes vs alpha Stat in some data [50].
      (Proposed mechanism: enhanced cooling [51] and decreased energy consumption with intracellular acidosis, or possible interaction of CO_2 effect with mechanism of cerebral ischemic injury)
   Additional cold cerebral perfusion during circulatory arrest ('cerebroplegia') [52]
      Continuous vs intermittent, retrograde vs antegrade
      (Proposed mechanism in addition to enhanced cooling: preservation of intracellular pH and energy state) [53]
      Transcranial doppler monitoring may aid in determining optimal low-flow rate [54]
Modified Ultrafiltration
   May reduce inflammatory mediators [55]
   (eg, TNF, complement, proinflammatory interleukins)
General Neuroprotective Techniques
   Shortest possible period of circulatory arrest [56]
   Pharmaceutical therapy
      Barbiturates, isoflurane
      Calcium channel blockers, naloxone
   Glucose management

Figure 6-26. Neuroprotective strategies for deep hypothermic circulatory arrest (14°–19°C) for aortic arch surgery. Deep hypothermic circulatory arrest is frequently employed as a neuroprotective strategy during aortic arch surgery. However, even in patients whose surgery includes a "safe" period of circulatory arrest, up to 30% of patients develop postoperative neurologic complications. While research into alternate approaches to reduce these complications continues, achieving and maintaining brain temperatures between 14 and 19°C remains the most effective method of neuroprotection. Several ways to ensure accurate and effective initial brain cooling, and subsequent maintenance of hypothermia are shown in this table. The ideal approach to "cerebroplegia" (cerebral perfusion during deep hypothermic circulatory arrest to maintain hypothermia) has not been defined; effective methods include intermittent versus continuous and antegrade versus retrograde. The mechanism by which ultrafiltration contributes to neuroprotection (in an animal model) is yet to be defined but may hold promise as a future strategy, complementary to hypothermia. CPB—cardiopulmonary bypass; TNF—tumor necrosis factor.

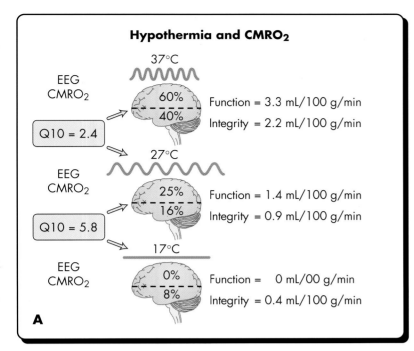

Hypothermia and CMRO₂

37°C

EEG
CMRO₂

60%
40%

Function = 3.3 mL/100 g/min
Integrity = 2.2 mL/100 g/min

Q10 = 2.4

27°C

EEG
CMRO₂

25%
16%

Function = 1.4 mL/100 g/min
Integrity = 0.9 mL/100 g/min

Q10 = 5.8

17°C

EEG
CMRO₂

0%
8%

Function = 0 mL/00 g/min
Integrity = 0.4 mL/100 g/min

A

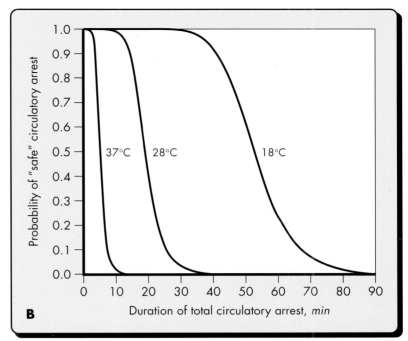

B

Figure 6-27. Estimation of "safe" circulatory arrest duration. A period of circulatory arrest is often necessary during aortic arch surgery. The brain is generally agreed to be the organ most vulnerable to the damaging effects of a period of circulatory arrest. The "safe" duration of cerebral circulatory arrest may be extended from 5–10 min with normothermia by using hypothermia to slow brain activity and metabolism. Hypothermia has a predictable effect on brain metabolism that may be described in terms of changes in the global consumption of oxygen by the brain ($CMRO_2$) (**A**) [57]. Reduced temperature predictably affects the oxygen requirements of the brain by lowering energy requirements for both maintenance of basic cellular integrity and other brain activity (*ie*, electroencephalographic activity, EEG). Michenfelder *et al* [57] proposed a theoretical relationship among temperature, brain function (EEG), and $CMRO_2$, described by the ratio of metabolic rates at two temperatures separated by 10°C (Q10). While experimental evidence suggests that for a broad range of temperatures the Q10 for human brain is approximately 2.4, a striking increase in Q10 (decrease in $CMRO_2$) is observed when extreme hypothermia is employed, suggesting that a step decrease in brain metabolism occurs with abolition of brain function (*ie*, isoelectric EEG) at temperatures below 18°–21°C. Theoretical calculations of the "safe" arrest period proposed by Michenfelder, using the Q10 temperature coefficient, may be compared with brain viability estimates following circulatory arrest derived from histologic and operative outcome data compiled by Kirklin and Barratt-Boyes [58] (**B**). (Part A *from* Michenfelder [57]; with permission; part B *from* Kirklin and Barratt-Boyes [58]; with permission.)

REFERENCES

1. West J: *Respiratory Physiology: The Essentials*. Baltimore: Williams and Wilkins; 1979:143–169.

2. Spencer H: Pulmonary Diseases of Uncertain Aetiology. In *Pathology of the Lung* (Excluding Pulmonary Tuberculosis). Oxford: Permagon Press Ltd; 1977:697–772.

3. Groskin S: Chronic Interstitial Lung Disease. In *Heitzman's The Lung: Radiologic-Pathologic Correlations*. St. Louis: Mosby; 1993:235–359.

4. Weinberger S: Interstitial Lung Diseases of Unknown Etiology, In *Principals of Pulmonary Medicine*. Edited by Weinberger S. Philadelphia: WB Saunders; 1992:146–158.

5. Burke A, Farb A, Virmani R: The pathology of primary pulmonary hypertension. *Mod Path* 1991, 4:269–282.

6. Burke A, Virmani R, Farb A: Primary Pulmonary Hypertension and Venoocclusive Disease. In *Pathology of Pulmonary Disease*. Edited by Saldana M. Philadelphia: JB Lippincott; 1994:235–246.

7. Reid L: Chronic Obstructive Pulmonary Diseases. In *Pulmonary Diseases and Disorders*. Edited by Fishman A. New York: McGraw-Hill; 1988:1247–1272.

8. Groskin S: Chronic Obstructive Pulmonary Disease. In *Heitzman's The Lung: Radiologic-Pathologic Correlations*. St. Louis: Mosby; 1993:429–466.

9. Sobonya R: Emphysema, In *Pathology of Pulmonary Disease*. Edited by Saldana M. Philadelphia: JB Lippincott; 1994:275–286.

10. Tapson V, Baz M: Lung Transplantation. In *Textbook of Pulmonary Diseases*. Edited by Baum G, Crapo J, Celli B, Karlinsky J. Philadelphia: Lippincott-Raven; 1998:1007–1017.

11. deMello D, Reid L: Bronchiectasis. In *Pathology of Pulmonary Disease*. Edited by Saldana M. Philadelphia: JB Lippincott; 1994:295–308.

12. Weinberger S: Bronchiectasis. In *Principals of Pulmonary Medicine*. Edited by Weinberger S. Philadelphia: WB Saunders; 1992:106–117.

13. Myles P, Weeks A, Buckland M, *et al.*: Anesthesia for bilateral sequential lung transplantation: experience of 64 cases. *J Cardiothorac Vasc Anesth* 1997, 11:177–183.

14. Bracken C, Gurkowski M, Naples J: Lung transplantation: historical perspective, current concepts, and anesthetic considerations. *J Cardiothorac Vasc Anesth* 1997, 11:220–241.

15. Keller CA, Cagle PT, Brown RW, *et al.*: Bronchiolitis obliterans in recipients of single, double, and heart-lung transplantation. *Chest* 1995, 107(4):973–80.

16. Yousem S: Transplantation Pathology. In *Pathology of Pulmonary Disease*. Edited by Saldana M. Philadelphia: JB Lippincott; 1994:819–826.

17. Sciurba F: Improvement in pulmonary function and elastic recoil after lung-reduction surgery for diffuse emphysema. *N Engl J Med* 1996, 334:1095–1099.

18. Bickerstaff L, Pairolero P, Hollier L, *et al.*: Thoracic aortic aneurysms: a population-based study. *Surgery* 1982, 92:1103–1108.

19. Ikonomidis JS, Weisel RD, Mouradian MS, *et al.*: Thoracic aortic surgery. *Circulation* 1991, 84(5 Suppl):III1–6.

20. DeBakey M, McCollum C, Crawford E, *et al.*: Dissection and dissecting aneurysms of the aorta: Twenty-year follow-up of five hundred twenty-seven patients treated surgically. *Surgery* 1982, 92:1118–1134.

21. Miller D, Stinson E, Oyer P, *et al.*: Operative treatment of aortic dissections. Experience with 125 patients over a sixteen-year period. *J Thorac Cardiovasc Surg* 1979, 78:365–382.

22. Wheat MW, Jr: Acute dissecting aneurysms of the aorta: diagnosis and treatment—1979. *Am Heart J* 1980, 99(3):373–387.

23. Hunt D, Schwab F: Chest trauma. *In Diagnostic Radiology in Emergency Medicine*. Edited by Rosen P, Doris P, Barkin R, *et al*. St. Louis: Mosby-Year Book; 1992:77–100.

24. de Figueiredo LF, Coselli JS: Individual strategies of hemostasis for thoracic aortic surgery. *J Card Surg* 1997, 12(2 Suppl):222–228.

25. Creasy JD, Chiles C, Routh WD, Dyer RB: Overview of traumatic injury of the thoracic aorta. *Radiographics* 1997, 17(1):27–45.

26. Oh J, Seward J, Tajik A: Diseases of the aorta. In *The Echo Manual: From the Mayo Clinic*. Boston: Little, Brown; 1994:195–203.

27. von Segesser LK, Fischer A, Vogt P, Turina M: Diagnosis and management of blunt great vessel trauma. *J Card Surg* 1997, 12(2 Suppl):181–192.

28. Kirklin J, Barratt-Boyes B: Acute traumatic aortic dissection. In *Cardiac Surgery*: Morphology, Diagnostic Criteria, Natural History, Techniques, Results, and Indications. New York: Churchill Livingstone; 1986:1451–1470.

29. Schoenwald P, Sprung J, Sullivan T: Anesthetic considerations for treatment of abdominal aortic aneurysm with an endovascular graft. *Anesth Analg* 1998, 86:S99.

30. Djindjian R: Arteriography of the spinal cord. *Am J Roentgenol Radium Ther Nucl Med* 1969, 107(3):461–78.

31. Usubiaga JE: Neurological complications following epidural anesthesia. *Int Anesthesiol Clin* 1975, 13(2):1–153.

32. Simpson J: Anesthesia for descending thoracic aortic surgery. In *Anesthesia for Aortic Surgery*. Boston: Butterworth-Heinemann; 1997:175–198.

33. Mitchell RS: Endovascular stent graft repair of thoracic aortic aneurysms. *Semin Thorac Cardiovasc Surg* 1997, 9(3):257–268.

34. Cernaianu AC, Olah A, Cilley JH, Jr, *et al.*: Effect of sodium nitroprusside on paraplegia during cross-clamping of the thoracic aorta [see comments]. *Ann Thorac Surg* 1993, 56(5):1035–1038.

35. Verdant A, Cossette R, Page A, *et al.*: Aneurysms of the descending thoracic aorta: three hundred sixty-six consecutive cases resected without paraplegia. *J Vasc Surg* 1995, 21(3):385–391.

36. Comerota AJ, White JV: Reducing morbidity of thoracoabdominal aneurysm repair by preliminary axillofemoral bypass. *Am J Surg* 1995, 170(2):218–222.

37. Bonatti J, Watzka S, Antretter H, *et al.*: Spinal cord protection in descending and thoracoabdominal aortic surgery—the role of distal perfusion. *Thorac Cardiovasc Surg* 1996, 44(3):136–139.

38. Murray MJ, Bower TC, Oliver WC, Jr, *et al.*: Effects of cerebrospinal fluid drainage in patients undergoing thoracic and thoracoabdominal aortic surgery. *J Cardiothorac Vasc Anesth* 1993, 7(3):266–272.

39. Illuminati G, Koskas F, Bertagni A, *et al.*: Variations in the origin of the artery of Adamkiewicz. *Riv Eur Sci Med Farmacol* 1996, 18(2):61–66.

40. Svensson LG: Intraoperative identification of spinal cord blood supply during repairs of descending aorta and thoracoabdominal aorta. *J Thorac Cardiovasc Surg* 1996, 112(6):1455–1461.

41. Griepp RB, Ergin MA, Galla JD, *et al.*: Looking for the artery of Adamkiewicz: a quest to minimize paraplegia after operations for aneurysms of the descending thoracic and thoracoabdominal aorta. *J Thorac Cardiovasc Surg* 1996, 112(5):1202–1215.

42. Svensson LG, Hess KR, Coselli JS, Safi HJ: Influence of segmental arteries, extent, and atriofemoral bypass on postoperative paraplegia after thoracoabdominal aortic operations. *J Vasc Surg* 1994, 20(2):255–262.

43. Grabitz K, Sandmann W, Stuhmeier K, *et al.*: The risk of ischemic spinal cord injury in patients undergoing graft replacement for thoracoabdominal aortic aneurysms. *J Vasc Surg* 1996, 23(2):230–240.

44. Maughan RE, Mohan C, Nathan IM, *et al.*: Intrathecal perfusion of an oxygenated perfluorocarbon prevents paraplegia after aortic occlusion. *Ann Thorac Surg* 1992, 54(5):818–825.

45. Okita Y, Takamoto S, Ando M, *et al.*: Repair for aneurysms of the entire descending thoracic aorta or thoracoabdominal aorta using a deep hypothermia. *Eur J Cardiothorac Surg* 1997, 12(1):120–126.

46. Cambria RP, Davison JK, Zannetti S, *et al.*: Clinical experience with epidural cooling for spinal cord protection during thoracic and thoracoabdominal aneurysm repair. *J Vasc Surg* 1997, 25(2):234–243.

47. Mault JR, Ohtake S, Klingensmith ME, *et al.*: Cerebral metabolism and circulatory arrest: effects of duration and strategies for protection. *Ann Thorac Surg* 1993, 55(1):57–64.

48. Kern FH, Jonas RA, Mayer JE, Jr, *et al.*: Temperature monitoring during CPB in infants: does it predict efficient brain cooling? *Ann Thorac Surg* 1992, 54(4):749–754.

49. Cook DJ, Oliver WC, Jr, Orszulak TA, Daly RC: A prospective, randomized comparison of cerebral venous oxygen saturation during normothermic and hypothermic cardiopulmonary bypass. *J Thorac Cardiovasc Surg* 1994, 107(4):1020–1029.

50. Jonas RA, Bellinger DC, Rappaport LA, *et al.*: Relation of pH strategy and developmental outcome after hypothermic circulatory arrest. *J Thorac Cardiovasc Surg* 1993, 106(2):362–368.

51. Watanabe T, Miura M, Inui K, *et al.*: Blood and brain tissue gaseous strategy for profoundly hypothermic total circulatory arrest. *J Thorac Cardiovasc Surg* 1991, 102(4):497–504.

52. Pagano D, Carey JA, Patel RL, *et al.*: Retrograde cerebral perfusion: clinical experience in emergency and elective aortic operations (published erratum appears in *Ann Thorac Surg* 1995, 60(1):228). *Ann Thorac Surg* 1995, 59(2):393–397.

53. Skaryak LA, Chai PJ, Kern FH, *et al.*: Blood gas management and degree of cooling: effects on cerebral metabolism before and after circulatory arrest. *J Thorac Cardiovasc Surg* 1995, 110(6):1649–1657.

54. Astudillo R, van der Linden J, Ekroth R, *et al.*: Absent diastolic cerebral blood flow velocity after circulatory arrest but not after low flow in infants. *Ann Thorac Surg* 1993, 56(3):515–519.

55. Skaryak LA, Kirshbom PM, DiBernardo LR, *et al.*: Modified ultrafiltration improves cerebral metabolic recovery after circulatory arrest. *J Thorac Cardiovasc Surg* 1995, 109(4):744–752.

56. Ergin MA, Galla JD, Lansman L, *et al.*: Hypothermic circulatory arrest in operations on the thoracic aorta. Determinants of operative mortality and neurologic outcome. *J Thorac Cardiovasc Surg* 1994, 107(3):788–799.

57. Michenfelder J: The hypothermic brain. In *Anesthesia and the brain*. New York: Churchill Livingstone; 1988:23–34.

58. Kirklin J, Barratt-Boyes B: Hypothermia, circulatory arrest, and cardiopulmonary bypass. In *Cardiac Surgery: Morphology, Diagnostic Criteria, Natural History, Techniques, Results, and Indications*. New York: Churchill Livingstone; 1986:29–83.

End-Stage Heart Failure and Cardiac Transplantation

Christopher J. O'Connor and Kenneth J. Tuman

Congestive heart failure is a relatively common disorder, affecting more than 2 million persons in the United States [1]. Despite recent advances in diagnosis and treatment, however, the incidence has remained relatively unchanged and increases considerably with advancing age. Heart failure is defined as myocardial dysfunction resulting in inability of the heart to generate sufficient flow to satisfy metabolic requirements of body tissues, or generation of adequate flow only with elevated intracardiac filling pressures [1]. It is a complex clinical syndrome that involves a variety of pathophysiologic derangements that produce decreased effort tolerance from low cardiac output, dyspnea from vascular and pulmonary congestion, and ultimately, a markedly diminished survival rate [1].

The treatment of heart failure encompasses pharmacologic and mechanical interventions to improve myocardial function, reduce cardiac filling pressures, attenuate abnormal physiologic changes associated with low cardiac output, improve quality of life, and reduce mortality. When conventional medical therapy fails, patients with end-stage heart failure may be candidates for ventricular assist devices and eventual cardiac transplantation.

The limited data on perioperative outcome in patients with end-stage heart failure suggest increased risk for perioperative cardiac complications in patients with active heart failure undergoing major noncardiac surgery [2]. The perioperative outcome of patients with well-compensated and stable heart failure is less well defined, although perioperative management of these patients should minimize further depression of ventricular function and excessive increases in either preload or afterload that may precipitate an acute exacerbation of heart failure. Perioperative management may necessitate invasive hemodynamic monitoring (*ie,* systemic and pulmonary artery catheterization) of patients with severe heart failure undergoing major abdominal or thoracic surgery. In addition, avoidance of large doses of cardiodepressant intravenous induction agents or high concentrations of volatile anesthetics is advisable. Lower concentrations of inhaled anesthetics are commonly combined with modest doses of opioids in such patients. Major conduction blockade with epidural or spinal anesthesia is appealing because reduction in systemic vascular resistance may favorably influence left ventricular (LV) function, provided that systemic and coronary perfusion pressures are maintained [3,4].

Perioperative management of patients undergoing placement of implantable left ventricular assist devices is similar to that for patients with severe LV dysfunction undergoing conventional cardiac surgery, although there is frequent need for pharmacologic support of the right ventricle (especially drugs with inotropic or vasodilating properties, including inhaled nitric oxide) before separation from cardiopul-

monary bypass (CPB). Similarly, although anesthetic and monitoring concerns during cardiac transplantation are comparable to conventional cardiac surgical procedures, other aspects of management are unique. These include proper timing of administration of antibiotics and immunosuppressive agents, recognition of the potential for significant blood loss in individuals with preexisting assist devices, and the recognition and treatment of systemic vasodilation and right ventricular dysfunction of the donor allograft before separation from CPB.

To optimize management of these high-risk patients, it is essential to understand the basic pathophysiology of end-stage heart failure, including anatomic and functional classifications of myocardial dysfunction, the fundamental physiologic derangements that accompany ventricular failure, and the current therapeutic modalities available for treatment. Familiarity with these important scientific and clinical aspects of heart failure is prerequisite to achieving a successful perioperative outcome after cardiac as well as noncardiac surgical procedures.

CLASSIFICATION OF HEART FAILURE

NEW YORK HEART ASSOCIATION FUNCTIONAL CLASSIFICATION OF HEART FAILURE

Class I	No limitation of daily physical activity.
Class II	Slight limitation of activity. Comfortable at rest but ordinary physical activity produces fatigue and dyspnea.
Class III	Marked limitation of physical activity. Fatigue and dyspnea results from minimal physical activity.
Class IV	Severe physical limitation. Dyspnea at rest and unable to carry on physical activity without severe symptoms.

Figure 7-1. New York Heart Association classification of heart failure. The functional classification of patients with congestive heart failure developed by the New York Heart Association [5] is based on the amount of activity tolerated by patients before the onset of symptoms. Despite the limitations of this subjective classification, it is a useful descriptive system and remains the standard by which patients with heart failure are compared.

CLASSIFICATION AND ETIOLOGY OF HEART FAILURE

Systolic dysfunction	Diastolic dysfunction
Dilated cardiomyopathy	Hypertrophic cardiomyopathy
Ischemic	thy
Hypertensive	Hypertrophic obstructive
Primary myopathy	cardiomyopathy
Infectious (*eg*, viral, parasitic)	Hypertension
Toxic (*eg*, alcohol, drugs)	Ischemia
Idiopathic	Restrictive cardiomyopathy
Familial	Sarcoidosis
Valvular disease	Amyloidosis
Congenital heart disease	Subendocardial fibrosis
High-output failure	
Anemia	
Thyrotoxicosis	
Beriberi disease	
Systemic arteriovenous fistulas/shunts	
Paget's disease	
Multiple myeloma	

Figure 7-2. Classification of heart failure. Heart failure may be classified according to anatomic or physiologic abnormalities or by etiologic mechanisms. In this table, heart failure is primarily distinguished by pathophysiologic changes in systolic or diastolic function, and is then further subdivided according to anatomic changes such as dilation or restriction of cardiac chambers. Specific etiologies tend to be subgrouped according to the primary anatomic or physiologic abnormalities present.

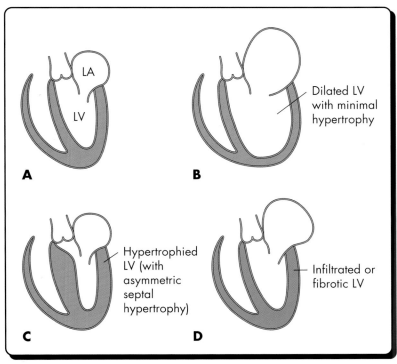

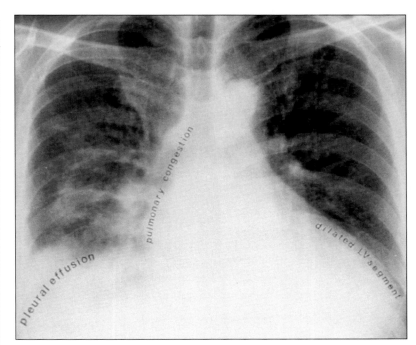

Figure 7-3. An anatomic classification of heart failure is depicted in this figure. Normal heart (**A**). The ventricular cavities are dilated with minimal compensatory hypertrophy in dilated cardiomyopathy (**B**), whereas hypertrophy of the ventricular wall and septum are characteristic of hypertrophic cardiomyopathy (**C**). Asymmetric hypertrophy of the ventricular septum out of proportion to the other ventricular walls is present in most patients with hypertrophic cardiomyopathy. Although obstruction of the left ventricular (**LV**) outflow tract may be present, the principal abnormality is impaired ventricular compliance due to inappropriate myocardial hypertrophy. Restrictive cardiomyopathy (**D**) is characterized by smaller ventricular cavities and thicker walls than normal, although the degree of wall thickness is less than that seen with hypertrophic cardiomyopathy. The primary myocardial defect of this disease is impaired diastolic relaxation and restricted ventricular filling. LA—left atrium. (*From* Fang and coworkers [6]; with permission.)

Figure 7-4. Radiographic appearance of acute pulmonary edema. This upright chest radiograph demonstrates several of the characteristic features of acute pulmonary edema in a patient with dilated cardiomyopathy, including cardiac dilatation, pulmonary congestion with interstitial edema, and vascular redistribution to the upper lobe vessels, as well as pleural effusions. LV—left ventricle. (*From* Wada [7]; with permission).

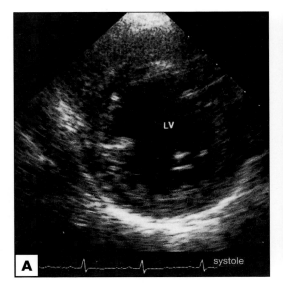

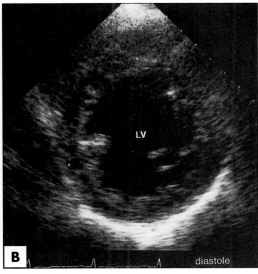

Figure 7-5. Transthoracic echocardiograms from a patient with dilated cardiomyopathy. These parasternal short-axis echocardiographic images of the left ventricle (LV) (**A** and **B**) demonstrate the increased end-diastolic and end-systolic volumes characteristic of dilated cardiomyopathies. The similar end-systolic and end-diastolic areas and the relative lack of myocardial wall thickening during systole also reflect the markedly reduced ejection fraction. (*From* Wada [7]; with permission.)

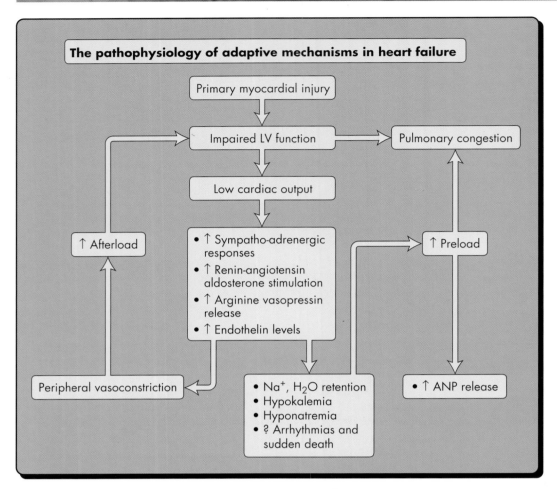

The pathophysiology of adaptive mechanisms in heart failure

Figure 7-6. The pathophysiology of adaptive mechanisms in heart failure. A complex series of neurohormonal changes take place in the presence of heart failure that are directly related to low cardiac output and elevated intracardiac filling pressures. These events, which include increased adrenergic activity, activation of the renin-angiotensin-aldosterone system, and the augmented release of vasopressin (antidiuretic hormone) and endothelin (a potent endogenous vaso-constrictor), are adaptive responses that increase cardiac contractility and expand the circulating blood volume, thus maintaining arterial blood pressure and vital organ perfusion. As heart failure becomes chronic, however, many of these compensatory responses cause undesirable consequences such as increased preload, afterload, and potentially fatal arrhythmias that are deleterious and ultimately limit survival in patients with chronic congestive heart failure. This series of events creates the "vicious circle" of heart failure. The increased release of atrial natriuretic peptide (ANP) opposes these adverse responses by increasing salt and water excretion and reducing vascular tone [8]. LV—left ventricular.

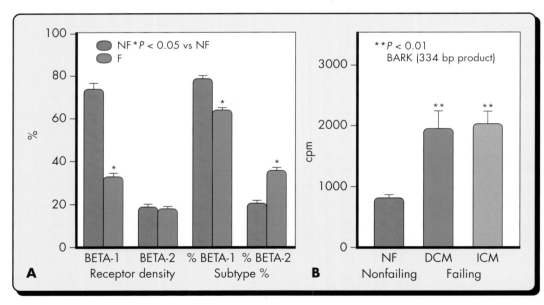

Figure 7-7. Alterations in β-adrenergic receptors in patients with chronic heart failure (**A**). Myocardium from patients with heart failure shows a marked reduction in β-adrenergic receptor density that is postulated to be mediated by increased circulating levels of norepinephrine. This down-regulation of β-receptors is proportional to the severity of heart failure and involves primarily β_1-, but not β_2-receptors. **B,** In addition, an increase in β-adrenergic receptor kinase (BARK), an enzyme that produces uncoupling of β_1-receptors, is also observed in heart failure and contributes further to the unresponsiveness of the β_1-receptor. BP—base pair; CPM—counts per minute; DCM—dilated cardiomyopathy; F—failing; ICM—idiopathic cardiomyopathy; NF—nonfailing. (*Part A from* Bristow [9]; part B *from* Ungerer and coworkers [10]; with permission.)

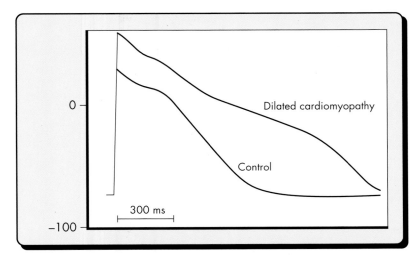

Figure 7-8. Abnormal action potentials in failing myocardium. The action potential of an isolated myocyte from a dilated failing ventricle is markedly prolonged and may contribute to lethal arrhythmias, which are felt to be one of the major causes of sudden death in patients with heart failure. (*From* Beuckelmann and coworkers [11]; with permission).

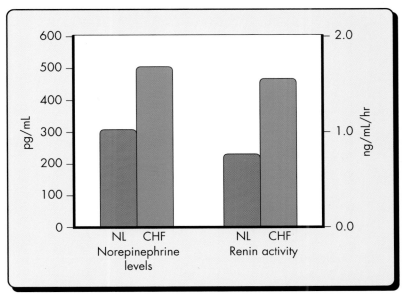

Figure 7-9. Plasma norepinephrine levels and renin activity in patients with and without heart failure. Activation of neurohormonal systems in patients with heart failure is evidenced by increases in plasma norepinephrine levels and plasma renin activity. The extent of elevation of norepinephrine levels correlates with both the severity of heart failure and with cardiac mortality, although it is unclear whether elevated norepinephrine levels are directly responsible for sudden death via arrhythmogenic or vasoconstrictor effects, or are merely a manifestation of severe end-stage heart failure [12]. CHF—congestive heart failure; NL—normal. (*From* Francis and coworkers [13]; with permission.)

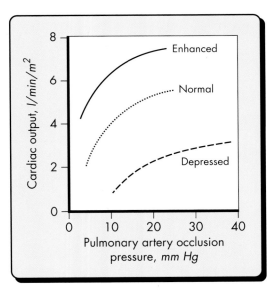

Figure 7-10. Frank-Starling ventricular function curves in normal and exercising individuals and in patients with heart failure. An increase in preload in normal individuals, as reflected by an increased pulmonary artery occlusion pressure, augments myocardial contractility and thus cardiac output (CO). During exercise, enhanced ventricular function is observed due to the effects of circulating catecholamines and sympathetic nervous system activation. In contrast, CO is reduced in heart failure and is maintained only by increased end-diastolic fiber length as reflected by increased ventricular filling volumes. Unfortunately, in heart failure there is impaired augmentation of CO with these increased filling pressures and pulmonary vascular congestion results which, if untreated, may progress to frank hypotension. (*From* Little and Braunwald [14]; with permission).

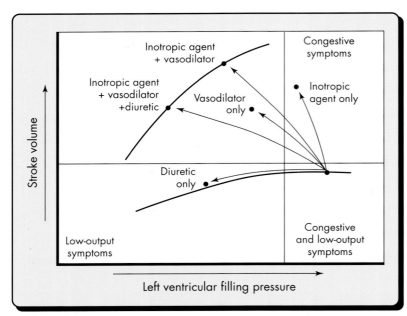

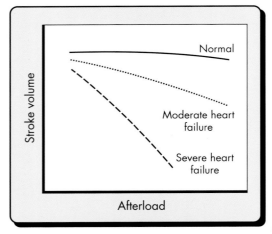

Figure 7-11. Hemodynamic effects of pharmacologic interventions for heart failure. Preload reduction with diuretics and vasodilators (*eg*, nitrates) reduces left ventricular (LV) filling pressures and pulmonary congestion yet has minimal impact on stroke volume and low-output symptoms. In contrast, inotropic agents such as dobutamine or milrinone improve contractility and low-output symptoms and shift the ventricular function curve upward. Arterial vasodilators such as nitroprusside or captopril may also improve ventricular function and reduce filling pressures. A combination of these agents achieves the most dramatic improvement in cardiac output and congestive symptoms. (*From* Smith and Kelly [15]; with permission.)

Figure 7-12. The effect of changes in afterload on ventricular function in heart failure. Although an increase in outflow resistance (afterload) results in arterial hypertension with minimal change in stroke volume in normal hearts, increasing resistance produces a dramatic decline in stroke volume in the presence of moderate or severe heart failure. Consequently, vasodilators that reduce afterload dramatically improve ventricular function in patients with heart failure but have minimal impact on the function of normal ventricles [16]. (*From* Bozjnak [17].)

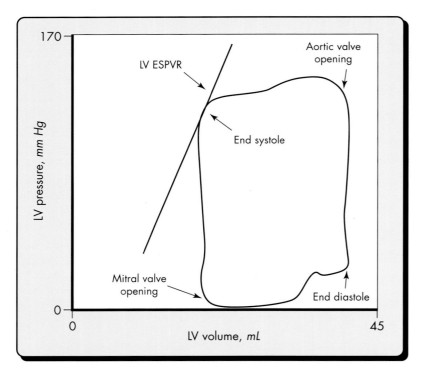

Figure 7-13. Left ventricular pressure-volume loop. Left ventricular pressure-volume loops represent the changes in left ventricular pressure and volume during the cardiac cycle and can be used to demonstrate the responses of the left ventricle (LV) to changes in preload, afterload, and contractility. The slope of the LV end-systolic pressure-volume relation (LV ESPVR) is a measure of contractility that is relatively load-independent. Decreased contractility, as seen with heart failure, shifts the slope of the LV ESPVR line downward and to the right. Conversely, increased contractility shifts the LV ESPVR line upward and to the left. (*From* Little and Braunwald [14]; with permission.)

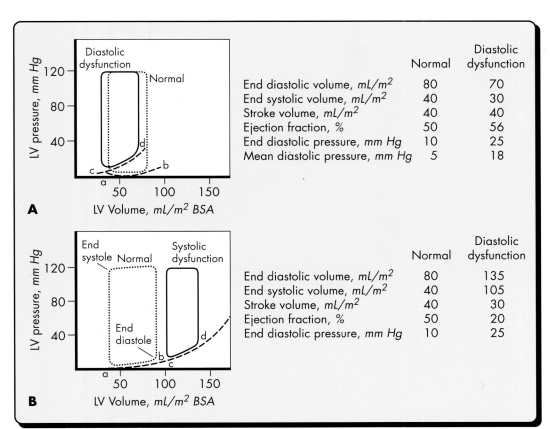

	Normal	Diastolic dysfunction
End diastolic volume, mL/m²	80	70
End systolic volume, mL/m²	40	30
Stroke volume, mL/m²	40	40
Ejection fraction, %	50	56
End diastolic pressure, mm Hg	10	25
Mean diastolic pressure, mm Hg	5	18

	Normal	Diastolic dysfunction
End diastolic volume, mL/m²	80	135
End systolic volume, mL/m²	40	105
Stroke volume, mL/m²	40	30
Ejection fraction, %	50	20
End diastolic pressure, mm Hg	10	25

Figure 7-14. The effect of systolic and diastolic dysfunction on pressure-volume loops. In the presence of isolated diastolic dysfunction (**A**), the pressure-volume loop is shifted to the left (*curve a-b* shifted to *curve c-d*) and left ventricular (LV) end-diastolic pressures increase while stroke volume and ejection fraction are unchanged or increased. Systolic dysfunction (**B**) is demonstrated by an increase in both end-systolic and end-diastolic volumes while stroke volume and ejection fraction decrease. LV end-diastolic pressures increase due to increased end-diastolic volumes that accompany compensatory ventricular dilation. The *dashed lines* highlight the diastolic pressure-volume relations with reduced ventricular compliance (δV/δP) and increased elastance (δP/δV) in heart failure compared with normal. BSA—body surface area. (*From* Zile [18]; with permission.)

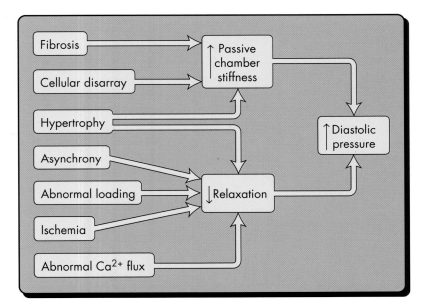

Figure 7-15. The etiology and consequences of ventricular diastolic dysfunction. Approximately 30% of patients with congestive heart failure have primarily diastolic heart failure characterized by abnormalities in ventricular filling that lead to reduced ventricular compliance and increased end-diastolic pressures. Typically, systolic function is normal or near normal in these patients. The primary manifestation of diastolic failure is pulmonary and systemic venous congestion secondary to high ventricular filling pressures. An example is hypertrophic cardiomyopathy in which ventricular hypertrophy leads to increased chamber stiffness and reduced chamber relaxation. Myocardial ischemia may also lead to acute changes in ventricular compliance that are relieved with anti-ischemic therapy such as nitrates or β-adrenergic receptor blockade [19]. (*From* Gaasch and Izzi [20]; with permission.)

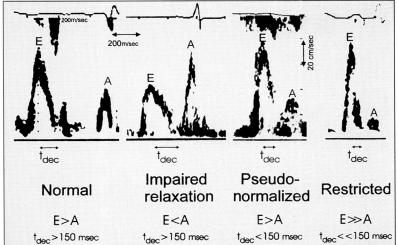

Figure 7-16. Abnormal Doppler mitral inflow velocities with diastolic dysfunction. Various patterns of abnormal diastolic dysfunction can be described echocardiographically by the absolute values and ratio of the mitral inflow velocities during early diastolic filling (E wave) and late diastole during atrial contraction (A wave). Normally the E/A ratio is > 1 and the time required for deceleration of the early diastolic inflow (t_{dec}) is > 150 msec. With impaired relaxation, as might be seen with left ventricular hypertrophy or arterial hypertension, the E/A ratio is reversed (< 1). In patients with more severe impairment of diastolic function, the E/A ratio is > 1, but the t_{dec} is faster (< 150 msec) than normal, reflecting the increased left atrial pressure compensation for the slowed rate of ventricular relaxation. With more severe abnormalities of diastolic function, as with severe pulmonary congestion or restrictive cardiomyopathies, early diastolic filling greatly exceeds that during atrial contraction and the E/A ratio is > 2 with a very short t_{dec}. (*From* Little and Braunwald [14]; with permission.)

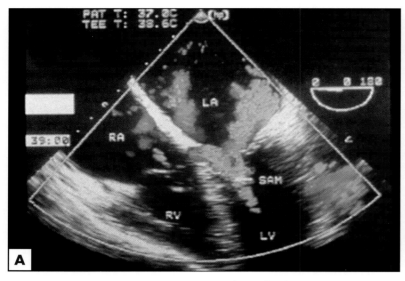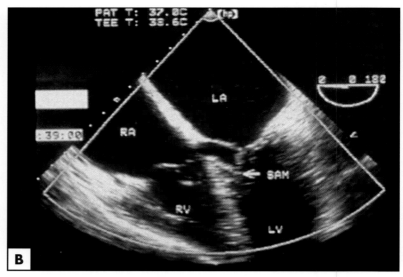

Figure 7-17. Intraoperative transesophageal echocardiogram of a patient with idiopathic hypertrophic subaortic stenosis, a form of hypertrophic cardiomyopathy. This basal short-axis view demonstrates several characteristic pathologic features of IHSS including asymmetric septal hypertrophy, systolic anterior motion of the mitral valve (SAM), turbulent flow in the left ventricular (LV) outflow tract due to the SAM-septal contact, and mitral regurgitation. LA—left atrium; RA—right atrium; RV—right ventricle. (*From* Savage and coworkers [21]; with permission.)

TREATMENT

CHARACTERISTICS OF THE β-ADRENORECEPTOR IN THE HUMAN HEART

Newly described receptor that *inhibits* cardiac contractility

Resistance to chronic catecholamine-induced β-adrenergic receptor down-regulation

May be responsible for the unexplained negative inotropic effects of catecholamines and may thus be involved in pathophysiologic mechanisms leading to chronic heart failure

May explain the therapeutic benefits of β-adrenergic receptor antagonists in the treatment of heart failure.

Figure 7-18. In 1996, Gauthier and colleagues first described a new β-adrenergic receptor, the β$_3$-receptor, whose primary function is inhibitory [22]. Although still incompletely defined, the implications of this fascinating new discovery for the treatment of heart failure are provocative and far-reaching [23].

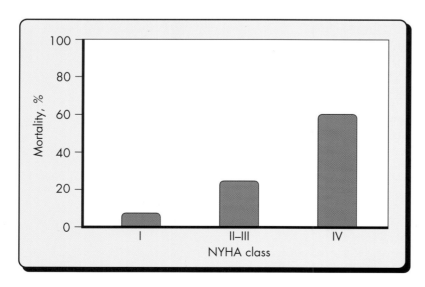

Figure 7-19. One-year mortality in patients with heart failure. Based on data from several clinical trials employing placebo-treated groups, 1-year mortality is approximately 60% in untreated New York Heart Association (NYHA) Class IV patients. This high mortality emphasizes the importance of establishing early therapy with agents such as angiotensin-converting enzyme inhibitors, which limit the progression of heart failure and improve survival [24].

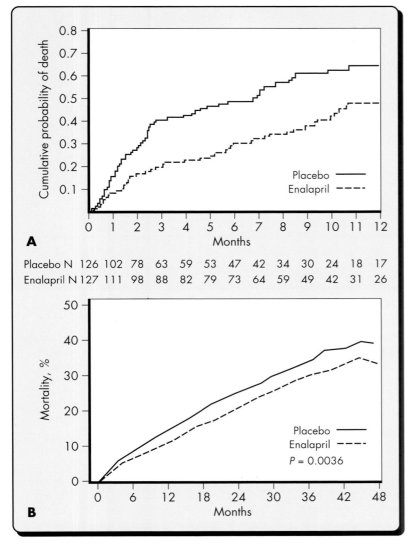

Placebo N 126 102 78 63 59 53 47 42 34 30 24 18 17
Enalapril N 127 111 98 88 82 79 73 64 59 49 42 31 26

Figure 7-20. Impact of angiotensin-converting enzyme (ACE) inhibitors on mortality. Data from the CONSENSUS (Cooperative Northern Scandinavian Enalapril Survival Study (**A**) and SOLVD (Studies On Left Ventricular Dysfunction) (**B**) trials have convincingly demonstrated that ACE inhibitor therapy improves survival in patients with heart failure and reduces or delays the onset of congestive heart failure when used early in the course of the disease. (Panel A *from* The Consensus Trial Study Group [25]; with permission; and panel B *from* The SOLVD Investigators [26]; with permission.)

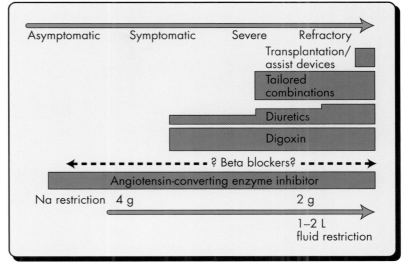

Figure 7-21. Treatment protocol for patients with heart failure. Treatment of patients with heart failure follows a stepwise process beginning with salt restriction and angiotensin-converting enzyme (ACE) inhibitor therapy for asymptomatic patients, followed by the addition of digoxin and diuretics for progressive symptoms. Tailored combinations refer to the use of additional inotropic agents or vasodilators (usually in combination with an ACE inhibitor), in conjunction with invasive hemodynamic monitoring for more severely symptomatic individuals. Eventually, refractory heart failure may require circulatory assist devices and cardiac transplantation. Although seemingly contradictory in the treatment of heart failure due to their potential cardiodepressant properties, current data suggest that β-adrenergic antagonists in low doses may improve symptoms and possibly reduce mortality in patients with symptomatic heart failure. However, large-scale, prospective randomized trials are necessary to confirm and more precisely quantify the benefits of β-adrenergic receptor blockade in the treatment of heart failure suggested by earlier studies [27]. (*From* Smith and coworkers [28]; with permission.)

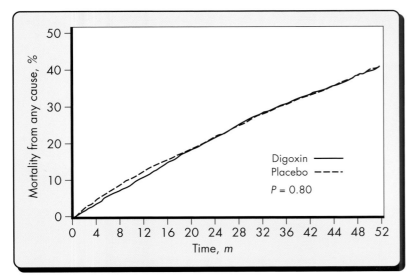

Figure 7-22. The effect of digoxin on mortality in patients with heart failure. The impact of digoxin therapy on morbidity and mortality was investigated in this landmark study of 7000 patients with heart failure treated with digoxin or placebo, in addition to diuretics and an angiotensin-converting enzyme (ACE) inhibitor. Although the risk of hospitalization was reduced by the use of digoxin, mortality was unaffected. The inability of digoxin to reduce mortality limits its use to patients with persistent symptoms despite the use of other agents such as ACE inhibitors, diuretics, or β-adrenergic antagonists [29]. (*From* The Digitalis Investigation Group [30]; with permission.)

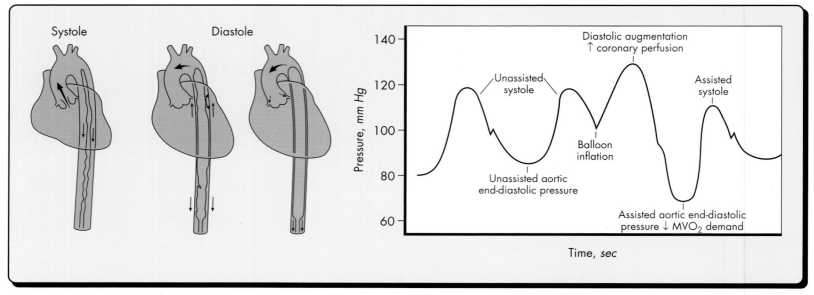

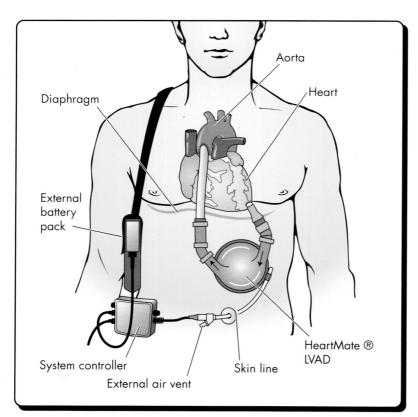

Figure 7-23. Intra-aortic balloon counterpulsation device. The intra-aortic balloon counterpulsation device (IABP) is most commonly used for the treatment of severe left ventricular failure in patients unable to be separated from cardiopulmonary bypass. It is positioned in the descending thoracic aorta with the tip below the left subclavian artery. The balloon is inflated during diastole and forces blood from the aorta proximally into the coronary arteries and distally into the peripheral circulation, thus augmenting coronary blood flow and myocardial oxygen supply and, to a lesser extent, systemic perfusion (less than 0.5 L/min). The balloon is rapidly deflated during the isovolumetric phase of ventricular systole just prior to opening of the aortic valve. This produces an effective reduction in afterload and a decrease in myocardial oxygen consumption ($M\dot{V}O_2$). The net effect of reduced myocardial work and improved coronary perfusion is a favorable shift in the myocardial oxygen supply-demand ratio and an increase in cardiac output and systemic perfusion [31]. (*From* High and coworkers [32]; with permission; and *from* Galla and coworkers [33]; with permission.)

Figure 7-24. HeartMate® left ventricular assist device. The HeartMate® is one of the more commonly used implantable left ventricular assist devices that provide mechanical circulatory support to patients with end-stage heart failure awaiting cardiac transplantation. During placement, the left ventricular apex is cannulated for removal of oxygenated blood that will pass through the assist device into the proximal ascending aorta. The pump is placed preperitoneally in the abdominal wall and is connected to either an external air power supply or, as depicted here, is electrically powered by a portable battery pack. Blood flow is pulsatile and minimal anticoagulation is required. The average waiting time until transplantation typically varies from several months to as long as 1 to 2 years. (Redrawn with permission from Thermo Cardiosystems, Inc., Woburn, MA)

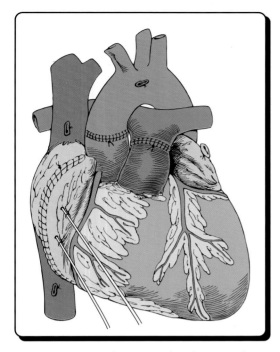

Figure 7-25. The surgical technique of cardiac transplantation. The donor left atrium is anastomosed first to the recipient left-atrial remnant along the posterolateral atrial wall, followed by the right atrial anastomosis, which is usually begun at the level of the coronary sinus using the recipient right atrial cuff. Once the atrial anastomoses are completed, the pulmonary artery anastomosis is then performed, followed finally by the aortic anastomosis. The implantation typically requires from 45 to 60 minutes. After successful de-airing of the heart, the pulmonary artery catheter can be readvanced into the pulmonary artery and the patient weaned from cardiopulmonary bypass (CPB). A period of time ranging from 30 to 60 minutes is usually required for the heart to recover from the effects of ischemic injury prior to separation from CPB [34]. (*From* Laks and coworkers [35]; with permission.)

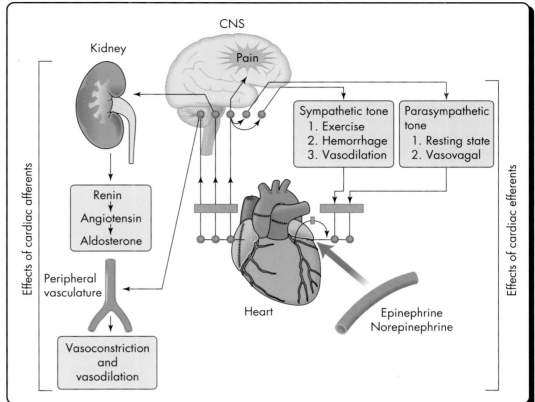

Figure 7-26. The effects of cardiac denervation after heart transplantation. The loss of afferent cardiac innervation may interfere with several reflex cardiac mechanisms including salt and water regulation via the renin-angiotensin-aldosterone system, reflex control of the peripheral vasculature, and the sensation of cardiac pain. In contrast, loss of efferent vagal tone to the sinus node results in a 30% higher resting heart rate than the normally innervated heart. Reflex increases in heart rate and contractility normally brought about by exercise, hemorrhage, or vasodilation are also attenuated by the loss of efferent sympathetic impulses. Finally, denervation may produce hypersensitivity to catecholamines due to a lack of adrenergic neuronal uptake. Because of these changes in cardiac innervation, heart transplant recipients rely primarily on a rapid increase in stroke volume via the Starling mechanism to maintain cardiac output in the face of exercise, rather than on increases in heart rate (which are more gradual and secondary to increased circulating catecholamines). Cardiac output after transplantation is therefore highly preload dependent and adequate intravascular volume must be maintained during subsequent surgical procedures, especially if spinal or epidural anesthesia is employed. In addition, the heart rate response to indirect acting pharmacologic agents such as atropine, glycopyrrolate, pancuronium, digoxin, phenylephrine, and anticholinesterases will be absent or markedly attenuated [36,37]. (*From* Hosenpud and Greenberg [36]; with permission.)

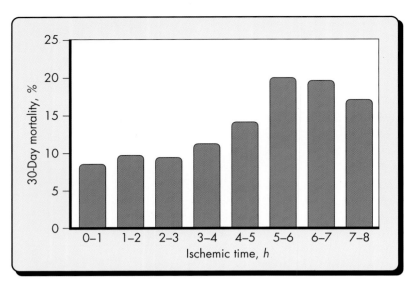

Figure 7-27. The effect of donor ischemic time on early survival after cardiac transplantation. Early survival after transplantation is related to the ischemic time of the donor (defined as the time from donor aortic cross-clamping to aortic cross-clamp release in the recipient) and therefore ischemic time is limited to 4 to 6 hours, with average ischemic times ranging between 3 to 4 hours [38]. Despite limited ischemic times and standard myocardial preservation, however, some ischemic damage occurs to the cardiac allograft. As a result, most centers routinely employ inotropic and chronotropic support with isoproterenol or dobutamine when separating from cardiopulmonary bypass after cardiac transplantation [36,38]. (*From* Hosenpud and Greenberg [36]; with permission.)

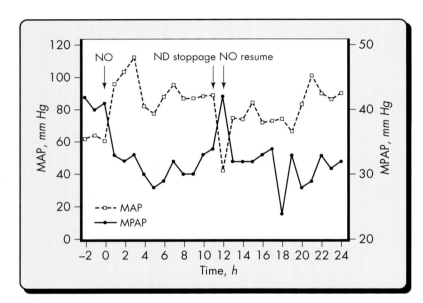

Figure 7-28. Right ventricular dysfunction secondary to pulmonary hypertension after cardiac transplantation. Right ventricular failure is a common cause of early mortality after cardiac transplantation and is frequently due to pulmonary hypertension in the recipient, donor allograft ischemic injury, size mismatch between donor and recipient, and the denervated state of the donor heart. In this figure, right ventricular dysfunction developed 4 days after transplantation and is illustrated in this figure as pulmonary hypertension accompanied by systemic hypotension refractory to dobutamine, dopamine, epinephrine, isoproterenol, milrinone, and nitroprusside. The latter two agents were not tolerated due to hypotension. A trial of nitric oxide (NO), a selective pulmonary artery vasodilator with minimal effect on systemic blood pressure, produced a prompt reduction in mean pulmonary artery pressures (MPAP) and an increase in mean arterial pressure (MAP). When NO was temporarily discontinued, the MPAP increased while the MAP dropped precipitously. These changes reversed promptly with the reinstitution of NO. This demonstrates one of the more common and serious intraoperative problems that may develop immediately after transplantation and before separation from cardiopulmonary bypass. In some instances, a right ventricular assist device may be required for temporary support of the right ventricle. (*From* Girard and coworkers [39]; with permission.)

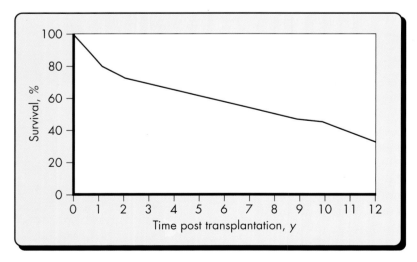

Figure 7-29. Survival statistics after cardiac transplantation. Survival at 1 year after cardiac transplantation is over 80% at most centers and may exceed 90% in some instances. Factors that may adversely influence survival include recipient age less than 5 years and greater than 65 years, older donor age, non-O blood type, longer donor ischemic time, and recipient ventilator dependence at the time of transplantation [40]. (*From* Hosenpud and coworkers [41].)

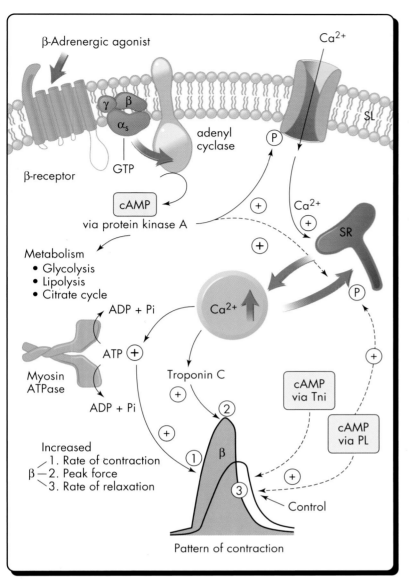

Figure 7-30. Mechanism of increased myocardial contractility by β-adrenergic stimulation. β-Receptor stimulation by β-adrenergic agonists such as epinephrine or isoproterenol initiates a complex series of cellular interactions that ultimately result in increased intracellular calcium (Ca^{2+}) concentrations. Initial stimulation of the β-receptor produces stimulation of G proteins, also known as guanine nucleotide regulatory proteins, to activate adenylate cyclase. Adenylate cyclase increases cyclic adenosine monophosphate (cAMP) production which mediates increased metabolism (*left*) and protein kinase phosphorylation of the Ca^{2+} channel protein (P). This leads to opening of the calcium channel and increased influx of calcium through the sarcolemma (SL) of the myocyte. These Ca^{2+} ions then cause release of more calcium from the sarcoplasmic reticulum (SR) which increases cytosolic calcium. The combination of calcium's interaction with troponin C and enhanced myosin adenosinetriphosphatase (ATPase) activity produces an increase in the rate and peak force of contraction (enhanced inotropy). Inhibition of phosphodiesterases (by drugs such as amrinone and milrinone), leads to increased cAMP and intracellular Ca^{2+} levels and, consequently, enhanced contractility. An increased lusitropic (relaxant) effect of β-receptor stimulation is produced by cAMP activation of the protein phospholamban (PL). ADP—adenosine phosphate; ATP—adenosine triphosphate; GTP—guanosine triphosphate; P_i—inorganic phosphate; Tni—troponin-I. (*From* Opie [42]; with permission.)

A. PHARMACOLOGIC THERAPY FOR END-STAGE HEART FAILURE

Drug	Indication	Dose	Mechanism	Therapeutic Benefit	Adverse effects
Renin-angiotensin system antagonists	First-line therapy for CHF		Vasodilation	Improved survival	Renal dysfunction
			Blunting of sympathetic stimulation	Reduce disease progression	Hypotension
			Inhibit neuroendocrine responses	Favorable effects on myocardial remodelling	Hyperkalemia
			↓ Preload		
Captopril		6.25–50 mg po q8h			
Enalapril		2.5–10 mg po q12h			
Enalaprilat		0.5–2 mg IV q12h			
Lisinopril		2.5–20 mg po q12–24h			
Ramipril		1.25–5 mg po qd			
Losartan		25–50 mg q 12h	Angiotensin II receptor blockade	Similar to ACEI, less cough	

Figure 7-31. Pharmacologic therapy for end-stage heart failure (**A–D**). ACEI—angiotensin-converting enzyme inhibitor; cAMP—cyclic adenosine monophosphate; CHF—congestive heart failure; IV—intravenous; NO—nitric oxide; PDE—phosphodiesterase enzyme; PVR—pulmonary vascular resistance; SVR—systemic vascular resistanc.

(Continued on next page)

B. PHARMACOLOGIC THERAPY FOR END-STAGE HEART FAILURE

Drug	Indication	Dose	Mechanism	Therapeutic Benefit	Adverse effects
Vasodilators					
Nitroglycerin	Acute chronic therapy	10–200 µg/min IV 10–60 mg po qid	NO donor	Preload > afterload reduction Coronary vasodilation	Hypotension Tolerance
Nitroprusside	Acute therapy	10–200 µg/min	NO donor	Preload reduction ↓ PVR Improved ventricular-arterial coupling	Cyanide, thiocyanate toxicity Hypotension $\dot{V}/\dot{Q}$ mismatching → hypoxemia
Hydralazine	Chronic therapy, ACEI intolerance	10–100 mg po q6h	Unclear	Direct arterial vasodilation	Hypotension Tachycardia Tolerance
Ibopamine	Chronic therapy; not in current use		Dopaminergic and β-receptor stimulation producing primarily vasodilation	Afterload reduction Mild inotropic effect	Enhanced mortality in recent studies

C. PHARMACOLOGIC THERAPY FOR END-STAGE HEART FAILURE

Drug	Indication	Dose	Mechanism	Therapeutic Benefit	Adverse effects
Phosphodiesterase inhibitors	Acute therapy		PDE III inhibition → ↑ cAMP	Vasodilation Positive inotropic activity	Enhanced mortality with chronic therapy; for short-term IV use **only**
Milrinone		50 µg/kg load IV, then 0.25–1.0 µg/kg/min			Hypotension
Amrinone		0.5 mg/kg IV load, then 2–20 µg/kg/min			Thrombocytopenia limits use
Vesnarinone	Only orally active, PDE inhibitor	60 mg qd	Multiple mechanisms	Awaits further study	Enhanced mortality at higher doses

Figure 7-31. (*Continued*)

D. PHARMACOLOGIC THERAPY FOR END-STAGE HEART FAILURE

Drug	Indication	Dose	Mechanism	Therapeutic Benefit	Adverse effects
β-Adrenergic agonists	Acute therapy only				Enhanced mortality
Dobutamine		2–20 µg/kg/min	β-Receptor stimulation	Inotropic effect Vasodilation ↓ PVR	Tachycardia, tachy-arrhythmias
Dopamine		2–20 µg/kg/min	Dopaminergic, α, β-receptor stimulation Enhanced norepineph-rine release	Selective renal vasodilation at low dose Inotropic and vasoconstictor effects at higher doses	Tachycardia, arrhythmias Increased SVR Less effective in heart failure patients than dobutamine
Epinephrine	Acute therapy accompanied by hypotension	1–20 µg/min	α,β-Receptor stimulation	Inotropic and vasoconstrictor effects	Tachycardia, arrhythmias, vasoconstric-tion
Dopexamine		0.25–5.0 µg/kg/min	$β_2$, dopaminergic stimulation	Inotropic, vasodila-tor effects Intermediate between dobutamine and dopamine	Significant tachycardia
Norepinephrine	Acute therapy accompanied by hypotension	1–20 µg/min	α, β-Receptor stimulation	Potent vasoconstrictor	Vasoconstriction
Digoxin	Chronic therapy	0.125–0.25 mg qd	Inhibition of the Na^+, K^+-ATPase sodium pump → ↑ intracel-lular Ca^{2+} ↓ central sympathetic tone	Weak positive inotropic effect Inhibits compen-satory neurohu-moral effects	Arrhythmias Conduction disturbances

Figure 7-31. (*Continued*)

REFERENCES

1. Braunwald E, Colucci WS, Grossman W: Clinical aspects of heart failure: high output heart failure; pulmonary edema. In *Heart Disease. A Textbook of Cardiovascular Medicine*, edn 5, Vol 1. Edited by Braunwald E. Philadelphia: WB Saunders;1997:445–470.

2. Goldman C, Caldera D, Nussbaum S, *et al.*: Multifactoral index of cardiac risk in noncardiac surgical procedures. *N Engl J Med* 1977, 297:846–850.

3. Sharrock NE, Bading B, Mineo R, *et al.*: Deliberate hypotensive epidural anesthesia for patients with normal and low cardiac output. *Anesth Analg* 1994, 79:899–904.

4. Rooke GA, Freund PR, Jacobson AF: Hemodynamic response and change in organ blood volume during spinal anesthesia in elderly men with cardiac disease. *Anesth Analg* 1997, 85:99–105.

5. The Criteria Committee, New York Heart Association, Inc. Diseases of the Heart and Blood Vessels, Nomenclature and Criteria for Diagnosis, edn 6. Boston: Little, Brown, 1964: 114.

6. Fang K, Dec A, Lilly LS: The Cardiomyopathies. In *Pathophysiology of Heart Disease*. Edited by Lilly LS. Philadelphia: Lea & Febiger; 1993:167–168.

7. Wada T: *Basic and Advanced Visual Cardiology. Illustrated Case Report Multi-Media Approach*. Philadelphia: Lea & Febiger; 1991:165–167.

8. Colucci WS, Braunwald E: Pathophysiology of heart failure. In *Heart Disease: A Textbook of Cardiovascular Medicine*, edn 5, Vol 1. Edited by Braunwald E. Philadelphia; WB Saunders; 1997:394–420.

9. Bristow MR: Changes in myocardial and vascular receptors in heart failure. *J Am Coll Cardiol* 1993, 22:61A–71A.

10. Ungerer M, Böhm M, Elce JS, *et al.*: Altered expression of β-adrenergic receptor kinase and $β_1$-adrenergic receptors in the failing human heart. *Circulation* 1993, 87:454–463.

11. Beuckelmann DJ, Näbauer M, Erdmann E: Intracellular calcium han-dling in isolated ventricular myocytes from patients with terminal heart failure. *Circulation* 1992, 85:1046–1055.

12. Colucci W, Braunwald E: Pathophysiology of heart failure. In *Heart Disease. A Textbook of Cardiovascular Medicine*, end 5, Vol 1. Edited by Braunwald E. Philadelphia: WB Saunders; 1997:394–420.

13. Francis GS, Benedict C, Johnstone DE, *et al.*: Comparison of neuroen-docrine activation in patients with left ventricular dysfunction with and without congestive heart failure: a substudy of the studies of left ven-tricular dysfunction (SOLVD). *Circulation* 1990, 82:1724–1729.

14. Little WC, Braunwald E: Assessment of cardiac function. In *Heart Disease: A Textbook of Cardiovascular Medicine*, edn 5, Vol 1. Edited by Braunwald E. Philadelphia: WB Saunders; 1997:421–444.

15. Smith TW, Kelly RA: Therapeutic strategies for CHF in the 1990's. *Hospital Practice* 1991, 26:127–150.

16. Smith TW, Kelly RA, Stevenson LW, *et al.*: Management of heart failure. In *Heart Disease. A Textbook of Cardiovascular Medicine*, edn 5, Vol 1. Edited by Braunwald E. Philadelphia: WB Saunders; 1997:492–514.

17. Bozjnak Z, Kampine JP: Physiology of the heart. In *Cardiac Anesthesia: Principles and Clinical Practice*. Edited by Estafanous FG, Barash PG, Reves JG. Philadelphia: JB Lippincott; 1994:3–17.

18. Zile MR: Diastolic dysfunction: detection, consequencees, and treatment. *Mod Concepts Cardiovasc Dis* 1990, 59:1.

19. Colucci WS, Braunwald E: Pathophysiology of heart failure. In *Heart Disease: A Textbook of Cardiovascular Medicine*, edn 5, Vol 1. Edited by Braunwald E. Philadelphia: WB Saunders; 1997:394–404.

20. Gaasch WH, Izzi G: Clinical diagnosis and management of left ventricular diastolic dysfunction. In *Cardiac Mechanics and Function in the Normal and Diseased Heart*. Edited by Hori M, Suga H, Baan J, Yellen EL. New York: Springer-Verlag; 1989:296

21. Savage RM, Lytle BW, Mossad E, *et al.*: Hypertrophic obstructive cardiomyopathy. In *Clinical Transesophageal Echocardiography: A Problem-Oriented Approach*. Edited by Oka Y, Konstadt SN. Philadelphia: Lippincott-Raven Publishers; 1996:199–222.

22. Gauthier C, Tavernier G, Charpentier F, *et al.*: Functional β_3-adrenoceptor in the human heart. *J Clin Invest* 1996, 98:556–562.

23. Bond RA, Lefkowitz RJ: Editorial. The third beta is not the charm. *J Clin Invest* 1996, 98:241.

24. Braunwald E, Colucci WS, Grossman W: Clinical aspects of heart failure: high output heart failure; pulmonary edema. In *Heart Disease. A Textbook of Cardiovascular Medicine*, edn 5, Vol 1. Edited by Braunwald E. Philadelphia: WB Saunders; 1997:445–470.

25. The Consensus Trial Study Group: Effects of enalapril on mortality in severe congestive heart failure. Results of the Cooperative North Scandinavian Enalapril Survival Study (CONSENSUS). *N Engl J Med* 1987, 316:1429–1435.

26. The SOLVD Investigators: Effect of enalapril on survival in patients with reduced left ventricular ejection fractions and congestive heart failure. *N Engl J Med* 1991, 325:293–302.

27. Doughty RN, Rodgers A, Sharpe N, *et al.*: Effects of beta-blocker therapy on mortality in patients with heart failure: a systematic overview of randomized controlled trials. *Eur Heart J* 1997, 18:560–565.

28. Smith TW, Kelly RA, Stevenson LW, Braunwald E: Management of heart failure. In *Heart Disease: A Textbook of Cardiovascular Medicine*, edn 5, Vol 1. Edited by Braunwald E. Philadelphia: WB Saunders; 1997:492–514.

29. Packer M: End of the oldest controversy in medicine—are we ready to conclude the debate on digitalis? *N Engl J Med* 1997, 336:575–576.

30. The Digitalis Investigation Group: The effect of digoxin on mortality and morbidity in patients with heart failure. *N Engl J Med* 1997, 336:525–533.

31. Richenbacher WE, Pierce WS: Assisted Circulation and the Mechanical Heart. In *Heart Disease. A Textbook of Cardiovascular Medicine*, edn 5, Vol 1. Edited by Braunwald E. Philadelphia: WB Saunders; 1997:534–547.

32. High KM, Pierce WS, Skeehan TM: Circulatory assist devices. In *The Practice of Cardiac Anesthesia*. Edited by Hensley FA Jr, Martin DE. Boston: Little, Brown & Co; 1990:642–661.

33. Galla JD, Silvay G, Griepp RB, *et al.*: Circulatory assist devices. In *Cardiac Anesthesia*, edn 3. Edited by Kaplan JA. Philadelphia: WB Saunders; 1993:1122–1148.

34. Frazier OH, Radovancevic B: The HeartMate™ left ventricular assist device. In *Atlas of Heart-Lung Transplantation*. New York: McGraw-Hill; 1994:17–24.

35. Laks H, Martin SM, Grant PW: Heart transplantation: Part III. In *Atlas of Heart-Lung Transplantation*. New York: McGraw-Hill; 1994:51–74.

36. Hosenpud JD, Greenberg BH: *Congestive Heart Failure. Pathophysiology, Diagnosis, and Comprehensive Approach to Management*. New York: Springer-Verlag; 1993:717–740.

37. Cheng DCH, Ong DD: Anesthesia for non-cardiac surgery in heart-transplanted patients. *Can J Anaesth* 1993, 40:981–988.

38. Perlroth MG, Reitz BA: Heart and heart-lung transplantation. In *Heart Disease: A Textbook of Cardiovascular Medicine*, end 5, Vol 1. Edited by Braunwald E. Philadelphia: WB Saunders; 1997:515–533.

39. Girard C, Durand PG, Vedrinne C, *et al.*: Inhaled nitric oxide for right ventricular failure after heart transplantation. *J Cardiothoracic Vasc Anesth* 1993, 7:481–485.

40. Bourge RC, Naftel DC, Costanzo-Nordin MR, *et al.*: Pretransplantation risk factors for death after heart transplantation: a multi-institutional study. The transplant cardiologists research database group. *J Heart Lung Transplant* 1993, 12:549–562.

41. Hosenpud JD, Novick RJ, Breen TJ, Daily OP: The registry of the International Society for Heart and Lung Transplantation: Eleventh Official Report. *J Heart Lung Transplant* 1994, 13:561–570.

42. Opie LH: Normal and abnormal circulatory function: Part II. In *Heart Disease: A Textbook of Cardiovascular Medicine*, edn 5, Vol 1. Edited by Braunwald E. Philadelphia: WB Saunders; 1997:360–393.

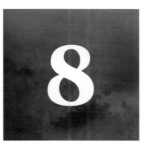

Electrocardiography and Monitoring of the Cardiothoracic Patient

Jacqueline M. Leung and Joseph L. Romson

Since its development nearly 100 years ago, electrocardiography has evolved into a primary monitoring modality in the perioperative care of the cardiothoracic patient. Continuous electrocardiographic monitoring is unsurpassed in providing an inexpensive and noninvasive means of detecting cardiac rhythm disturbances and myocardial ischemia.

Early clinical electrocardiographic equipment required the subject to place both arms and the left leg in buckets of conducting solution. As early as 1856, Kolliker and Muller demonstrated that action currents were associated with each cardiac cycle in a beating frog heart preparation. It was not until 1902, however, when the father of electrocardiography, Willem Einthoven [1], first employed the string galvanometer to register an accurate, quantitative representation of the electrical currents produced by the beating human heart.

More recently introduced, transesophageal echocardiography has rapidly assumed an important role in monitoring the cardiothoracic patient. Although initial acquisition costs are high, echocardiography provides information about the cardiac status of critically ill patients that may be unattainable by any other means. Specifically, the detection of regional wall motion abnormalities, the evaluation of valvular disorders, and the assessment of ventricular loading conditions can readily be accomplished in the operating room with transesophageal echocardiography. An advantage of transesophageal echocardiography is its portability. Because it is unobtrusive, imaging can continue while surgery is going on. Furthermore, high quality images of cardiac structures can be obtained without radiation exposure to patients or health care providers. Because it is minimally invasive, the complication rate resulting from the use of transesophageal echocardiography in appropriately selected patients is acceptably low.

At the most basic level, intraoperative transesophageal echocardiography is useful as a sensitive means of detecting myocardial ischemia (manifest as regional wall motion abnormalities) and as a means of assessing volume status (left ventricular end diastolic area). Skill in evaluating valvular function, more sophisticated means of assessing ventricular loading conditions, and examination of the aorta can be developed with additional training.

With nearly a century separating the clinical introduction of these two techniques, the current state of monitoring of the cardiothoracic patient relies heavily on the often complementary information yielded by electrocardiography and transesophageal echocardiography. This chapter highlights the important aspects of these two monitoring techniques.

ELECTROCARDIOGRAPHY

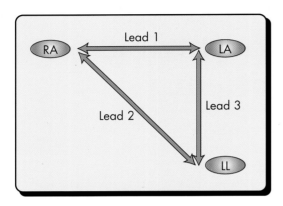

Figure 8-1. Limb leads. Three standard limb leads have been in use for 90 years. Lead 1 connects the patient's right and left arms, lead 2 connects the right arm with the left leg; and lead 3 connects the left arm with the left leg. Each lead records the potential between the two connected limbs. All three standard limb leads are in the frontal plane of the body. LA—left arm; LL—left leg; RA—right arm.

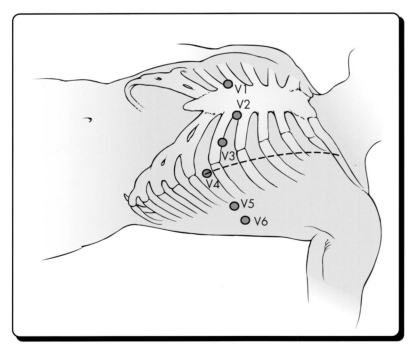

Figure 8-2. Precordial leads. Additional chest leads (precordial leads) may be applied to obtain different views of the heart. When one electrode is placed on the limb and the other at a precordial position, the limb lead is called the "indifferent" electrode and the precordial lead is called the "exploring" electrode. The standard limb leads are *bipolar*, because they represent the potential between two points. The precordial leads are *unipolar* because they are more influential than the limb leads, which are more distally located. Unipolar limb leads are created by reversing the standard electrode positions, placing the exploring electrode on the limb and the indifferent electrode on the chest. Depending on the limb to which the exploring electrode is connected, the leads are labeled VR (right arm), VL (left arm), and VF (left leg). Because the amplitude in these leads is small, the potential is augmented by a device, as indicated by the prefix "a," giving rise to leads aVR, aVL, and aVF. (*Adapted from* Thys [1a].)

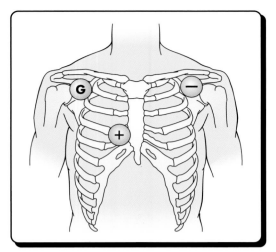

Figure 8-3. Modified chest lead (MCL_1). The MCL_1 lead was introduced in 1968 primarily for use in the intensive care unit. The positive electrode is placed in the V_1 position and the negative electrode is placed at the left shoulder. The ground may be placed anywhere. The advantages of this lead configuration are that because it imitates a V_1 lead, right bundle branch block (RBBB) and left bundle branch block (LBBB) can be differentiated, left versus right ventricular ectopy can be distinguished, and one may be able to distinguish left ventricular ectopy from RBBB aberration. P wave morphology in the MCL_1 lead may not be as informative as in lead II, especially when ectopic or retrograde conduction of the P wave results in a biphasic morphology. G—ground. (*Adapted from* Marriott [2]; with permission).

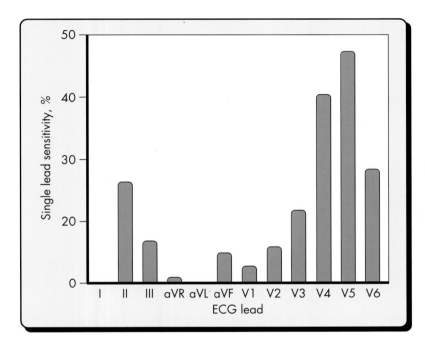

Figure 8-4. Lead sensitivity in detecting myocardial ischemia. To determine which leads best detect ischemia in the perioperative setting, London *et al.* [3] studied 105 patients with or at risk for coronary artery disease (CAD) undergoing noncardiac surgery. Using microprocessor-assisted continuous 12-lead electrocardiography (ECG), they found 51 episodes of ischemia. Forty-five manifested as ST segment depression and six as concurrent ST elevation in some leads and ST depression in others. Lead V_5 demonstrated the highest single-lead sensitivity (75%). Lead II alone had very low sensitivity (33%), but, when combined with lead V_5 (the most widely used two-lead system intraoperatively), sensitivity increased to 80%. The use of leads II, V_4, and V_5 permitted detection of 96% of intraoperative ischemic episodes. These data indicate that it is important to monitor several carefully chosen and precisely placed leads to enhance the ability of intraoperative ECG in detecting ischemia. (*Adapted from* London and coworkers [3]; with permission.)

Figure 8-5. Nonischemic causes of T-wave and ST-segment changes. ST-T wave changes may also occur in settings where there is no active ischemia.

NONISCHEMIC CAUSES OF T WAVE AND ST SEGMENT CHANGES

Ventricular hypertrophy
Changes in body temperature
Serum electrolytes (especially potassium)
Ventilatory changes
Administration of drugs such as quinidine and digitalis
Electrical stimulation of the right stellate ganglion
Left sympathetic stimulation

INCIDENCE OF ARRHYTHMIAS

Study	Year	Number	Subjects	Arrhythmias (%)
Sabotka [4]	1981	50	Women 22–28 years old without heart disease	54 (ventricular)
				64 (atrial premature)
Brodsky [5]	1977	50	Male medical students	56 (atrial premature)
				50 (ventricular)
Vanik [6]	1968	5013	Surgical patients	17.9
Kuner [7]	1967	154	Surgical patients	61.7
Bertrand [8]	1971	100	Surgical patients	84
Angelini [9]	1974	128	Cardiac surgery	50
O'Kelly [10]	1992	230	Noncardiac surgical patients with risk factors for or documented coronary artery disease	21 (ventricular)

Figure 8-6. Incidence of arrhythmias. The incidence of arrhythmias in the normal population as compared with those undergoing surgery and anesthesia is shown here. Certain subgroups have been shown to be at increased risk of developing intraoperative arrhythmias. For example, Bertrand *et al.* [8] reported a 60% incidence of ventricular arrhythmias in patients with known cardiac disease, as compared with an incidence of 37% in patients without known heart disease. The studies differ regarding the prognostic significance of intraoperative arrhythmias, however. One study by Angelini *et al.* [9] reported that in patients undergoing valve and coronary artery bypass graft surgery, postoperative arrhythmias were associated with surgical mortality in 80% of the cases. Two other studies, however, one in noncardiac [10] and one in cardiac [10a] surgery, suggest that perioperative arrhythmias are not associated with an increased risk of postoperative cardiac complications.

CAUSES OF PERIOPERATIVE ARRHYTHMIAS

Electrolyte disturbances (hypokalemia, hypocalcemia, hypomagnesemia)

Hypothermia

Medications such as digitalis, theophylline, anesthetic agents

Metabolic alkalosis

Presence of indwelling central venous or pulmonary artery catheters

Sympathetic stimulation (hypoxia, hypercarbia, endotracheal intubation, surgical incision, pain)

Parasympathetic stimulation (pain, distention of bladder or bowel)

Figure 8-7. Causes of perioperative arrhythmias. Perioperatively, a number of conditions can give rise to the development of arrhythmias. These conditions are outlined in the accompanying figure.

COMMON ARTIFACTS ASSOCIATED WITH PERIOPERATIVE ECG MONITORING

Electrical signals generated from the skin

Electromyographic signals

Baseline wander resulting from the epidermal layer of the skin being stretched as during respiration in which voltages of several mV are generated

Improper electrode contact

Loss of integrity of lead wires or cables

60 Hz electrical noise from other power source

Figure 8-8. Common artifacts associated with perioperative ECG monitoring. Inadequate preparation of the skin can greatly reduce the clinical utility of ECG monitoring [11].

RECOMMENDATIONS FOR PERIOPERATIVE TRANSESOPHAGEAL ECHOCARDIOGRAPHY

Category I indications	Category II indications	Category III indications
Supported by strongest evidence. Transesophageal echocardiography (TEE) is frequently useful in improving clinical outcomes and is often indicated.	*Supported by weaker evidence. TEE may be useful in improving clinical outcomes, but appropriate indications are less certain.*	*Little current scientific support. TEE is infrequently useful in improving clinical outcomes. Appropriate indications are uncertain.*
Evaluation of acute, persistent hemodynamic disturbances	Patients with increased risk of myocardial ischemia or infarction	Evaluation of myocardial perfusion or coronary artery anatomy
All types of valve surgery	Patients with increased risk of hemodynamic disturbances	Evaluation of repair of other cardiomyopathies (see Category I)
Congenital heart surgery	Assessment of repair of cardiac aneurysms	Monitoring for emboli during orthopedic procedures
Repair of hypertrophic obstructive cardiomyopathy	Evaluation of removal of cardiac masses	Evaluation of pleuropulmonary diseases
More detailed examination for suspected endocarditis	Detection of cardiac foreign bodies	Placement of intra-aortic balloon or pulmonary artery catheter
Suspected thoracic aortic aneurysms, dissection, or disruption	Detection of air emboli during cardiac or neurosurgical procedures	Monitoring cardioplegia administration
Evaluation of pericardial window procedures	Evaluation of intracardiac thrombectomy	
	Monitoring during pulmonary embolectomy procedures	
	Evaluation of suspected cardiac trauma	
	Detection of aortic atheromatous disease or other sources of emboli	
	Evaluation of anastomotic sites in heart or lung transplantation	
	Monitoring of placement of assist devices	

Figure 8-9. Indications for perioperative use of transesophageal echocardiography. The American Society of Anesthesiologists and the Society of Cardiovascular Anesthesiologists performed a systematic review of outcome data relating to the use of intraoperative echocardiography. These groups then developed the practice guidelines for the use of intraoperative transesophageal echocardiography outlined here [12]. The perioperative use of transesophageal echocardiography is limited by a few factors, one of which is the expense of acquisition of the equipment. Initial costs would typically be $150,000 to $200,000 to purchase a multiplane echocardiographic probe and monitor and its associated hardware. Second, developing skill in image acquisition and interpretation requires time and dedication. Basic skills for ischemia monitoring and assessing left ventricular volume can be learned relatively quickly, however, when combined with training in the recognition of cardiac tomography.

Figure 8-10. Contraindications to intraoperative transesophageal echocardiography.

CONTRAINDICATIONS TO PERIOPERATIVE TRANSESOPHAGEAL ECHOCARDIOGRAPHY

Esophageal strictures
Esophagitis
Esophageal varices
Previous esophageal surgery
Other serious esophageal disease (tumors, etc.)

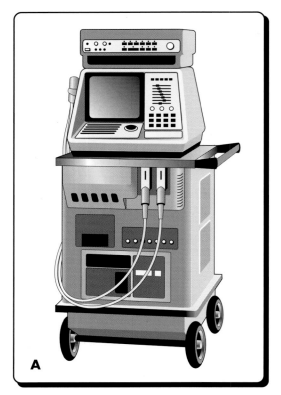

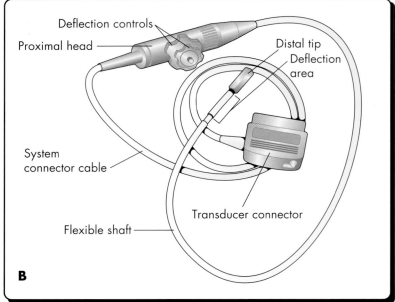

Figure 8-11. Transesophageal echocardiography equipment. The basic equipment package for transesophageal echocardiography is shown in these two figures. The ultrasound unit (**A**) is typically placed on a cart with wheels to aid in mobility. Accompanying the recording unit is a videorecorder and often a video printer. The transesophageal echocardiography probe (**B**) is a gastroscope mounted with a multiplane transducer at the distal end. Control wheels (deflection controls) at the proximal end of the probe guide the probe tip in the anterior/posterior and left/right directions. The scan sector of a multiplane probe is manipulated by a control located near the control wheels (not shown). (*Courtesy of* Hewlett Packard Company, Andover, MA.)

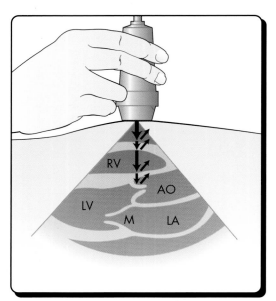

Figure 8-12. Ultrasound wave propagation and acoustic impedance. Cardiac imaging by ultrasonography relies on the propagation of high-frequency sound waves, in the range of 2 to 7 megahertz (MHz or millions of cycles per second) through biologic tissues. The sound waves travel straight through a homogenous medium until either being gradually absorbed (attenuated) or impacting on an interface of differing tissue density (or, loosely stated, differing acoustic impedance). The ultrasound beam is then either reflected, refracted (bent), or further absorbed. It is the reflected ultrasound energy, which returns to the transducer, that is electronically processed to generate the image. This figure shows a schematic of a transducer placed on the patient's chest. The ultrasonic beam produced by the transducer encounters multiple changes in acoustic impedance as it penetrates the heart.

Ultrasonic waves travel poorly through air and are nearly entirely reflected by dense tissues such as bone, calcium deposits, or metal. This near total reflection severely limits ultrasound beam penetration so that objects beyond the reflecting boundary will not be imaged, also referred to as "echo shadowing."

The resolution of objects by ultrasound imaging can be enhanced by utilizing higher frequency sound waves. Higher-frequency beams undergo relatively greater degrees of absorption and scattering, however, thus, the depth of tissue penetration by the beam is less. Ultimately, the choice of interrogating frequency is a tradeoff between deeper penetration/lower resolution (lower frequency) and higher resolution/less penetration (higher frequency). Ao—aorta; LA—left atrium; LV—left ventricle; M—mitral valve; RV—right ventricle. (*From* Hamer [13].)

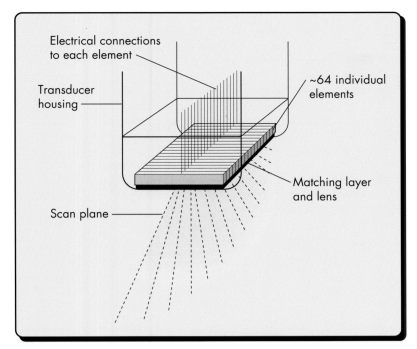

Electrical connections to each element

Transducer housing

Scan plane

~64 individual elements

Matching layer and lens

Figure 8-13. Production of the ultrasound beam. The core of the ultrasound transducer is the piezoelectric ("pressure-electric") material, which has the property of undergoing shape changes when an electric current is applied to the crystal. As the crystal expands and contracts, ultrasonic waves are produced, with the wavelength being a function of the thickness of the crystal. When sonic energy hits piezoelectric materials, as in an echo returning to the transducer, a shape change occurs in the crystal, which generates an electric current. This current forms the basis of creating the ultrasound image.

Modern transducers use a series of individual crystals that are electronically linked to perform as one larger crystal. This phased array system has advantages with regard to producing, focusing and steering the ultrasound beam, which is described in Figure 8-14. (*From* Monoghan [14]; with permission.)

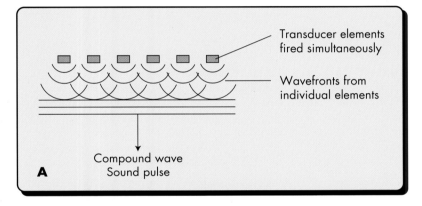

Transducer elements fired simultaneously

Wavefronts from individual elements

Compound wave Sound pulse

A

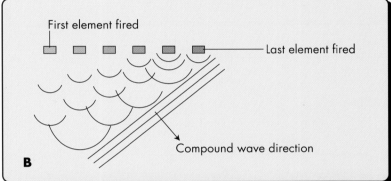

First element fired

Last element fired

Compound wave direction

B

Figure 8-14. Modification of the ultrasound beam. When electrically stimulated, each crystal of the phased array independently emits an ultrasonic impulse. Depending on the timing and firing sequence of each crystal in the array, summation of the individual waves produces a compound wave, which can be "driven" in different directions. If each crystal is fired simultaneously, the compound wave travels in a direction perpendicular to the transducer face (**A**). If the firing sequence is altered, the compound wave direction of travel will change (**B**). The same technique makes it possible to alter the shape of the compound wave to focus the beam at various depths of tissue penetration (**C**). (*From* Monaghan [14] and Feigenbaum [15]; with permission.)

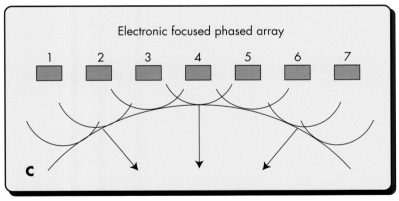

Electronic focused phased array

1 2 3 4 5 6 7

C

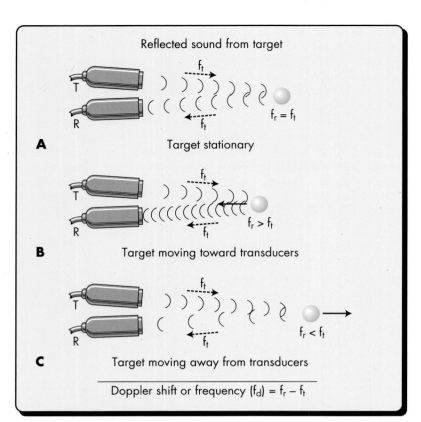

Figure 8-15. Doppler effect. Determination of the relative velocity and direction of blood flow relies on the Doppler effect, described by Christian Johann Doppler in 1842. Doppler noted that the change in frequency of a sound-emitting object is a function of the velocity and direction of travel of the object relative to the listener. It is possible to evaluate erythrocyte direction and velocity of travel with one transducer (T) emitting the ultrasound and the receiving transducer (R) evaluating the returning echo from the erythrocyte. If the target is stationary (**A**), then the transmitted frequency (Ft) is equal to the reflected frequency (Fr). The Fr is greater than the Ft if the red cell is moving toward the transducer (**B**), and the converse is true if the erythrocyte is moving away (**C**). The magnitude of the change in frequency (Ft versus Fr), known as the Doppler shift, is proportional to the velocity of the moving target. (*From* Feigenbaum [15]; with permission.)

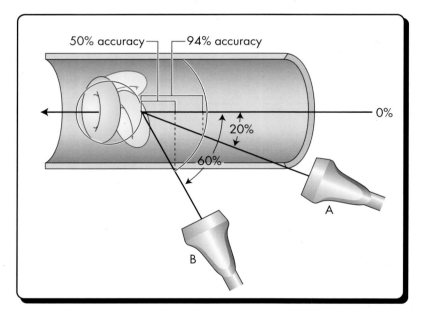

Figure 8-16. Angle of interrogation and Doppler accuracy. Accurate measurement of blood flow velocity utilizing the Doppler effect requires careful alignment of the interrogating beam **parallel** to the direction of blood flow. The velocity of the moving target and the Doppler shift are related by the cosine of the incident angle of the ultrasound beam relative to the direction of travel of the target. Incident angles of 20° or less do not markedly affect the accuracy of determining the target velocity. (*From* Obeid [16]; with permission.)

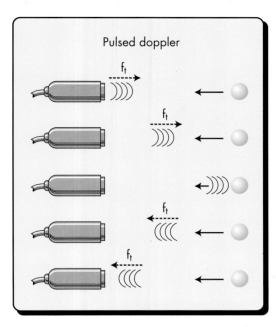

Pulsed doppler

Figure 8-17. Continuous versus pulsed wave Doppler. Figure 8-15 demonstrates a system in which the transmitting transducer delivers the interrogating beam on a continuous basis. The transmitting transducer is operating continuously; thus, all moving targets in the beams' path will return echoes to the receiver. A drawback to this system is that no "range" information (*ie*, the distance from the target to the transducer) is available. Because the echocardiographer is frequently interested in measuring blood flow velocities at specific places in the heart, pulsed wave Doppler was developed. Here, the interrogating beam (Ft) is emitted in short bursts, and the returning echoes (Fr) are received by the same transducer. Because the speed of sound in tissue is nearly constant, the area of interest (sample volume) can be selected by time gating the returning signals—only accepting echo information that required the "correct" amount of time to return from the target. The main drawback to pulsed wave Doppler is that greater Doppler shifts (*ie*, greater changes in frequency between Ft and Fr) representing higher blood flow velocities cannot be accurately measured, because the transducer alternates between send and receive modes. Thus, to measure accurately high peak-blood-flow velocities through a valvular lesion like aortic stenosis, continuous-wave Doppler must be used. (*From* Feigenbaum [15]; with permission.)

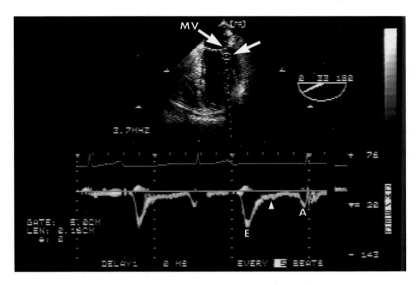

Figure 8-18. Mitral valve flow assessed by pulsed-wave Doppler. With the sample volume (*arrow*) placed at the tips of the mitral valve (MV) during diastole, the velocity of blood flowing from the left atrium to the left ventricle can be measured. Shown is an example of a normal pulsed-wave Doppler profile. Early in diastole (E), blood flow transiting the mitral valve increases in velocity. A period of decreased left ventricular filling occurs (diastasis period, *arrowhead*). Atrial contraction then causes a transient increase in blood flow velocity (A) through the mitral valve.

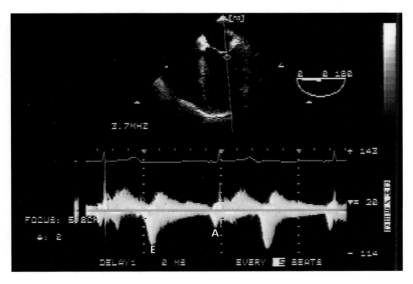

Figure 8-19. Mitral valve flow assessed by continuous-wave Doppler. For comparison purposes, blood flow velocities through the mitral valve in the same patient as in Fig. 8-18 were measured with continuous-wave Doppler. Unlike in the case of the pulsed-wave Doppler measurement, blood flow velocity information is being obtained all along the cursor line (*eg*, left atrium through the mitral valve into the left ventricle). It is preferable to use pulsed-wave Doppler to measure the relatively low blood flow velocities occurring through the mitral valve. A—atrial contraction; E—early diastolic filling.

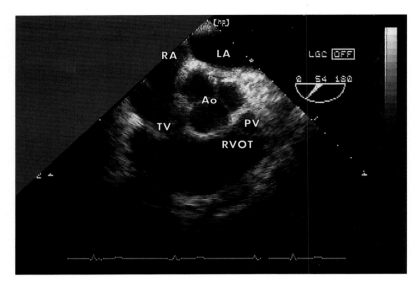

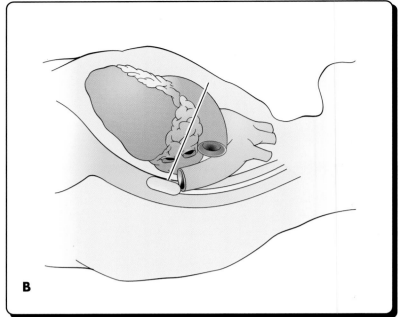

Figure 8-20. Cardiac structures at base of the heart. By introducing the echo probe to a depth of 30 cm from the incisors, a transverse view of the aortic valve is obtained (**A**). The position of the transducer is shown in **B**. A true cross-section of the aortic valve (*AO*) annulus is achieved by using the adjustable scan angulation feature of the multiplane probe to an indicated angle of 15° to 45°. (In this example, it was necessary to scroll the sector scan to 54° to obtain the desired cross-section of the aortic valve annulus.) Other identifiable structures in this view are the left atrium (*LA*) and right atrium (*RA*), separated by the interatrial septum, tricuspid valve (*TV*); and right ventricular outflow track (*RVOT*) with portions of the pulmonic valve (*PV*). In this view, color flow mapping across the pulmonic valve can detect pulmonic insufficiency. Often, the best view of the pulmonic valve can be obtained with the scan angulation at 90°. (*Part B from* Labovitz and Pearson [17]; with permission.)

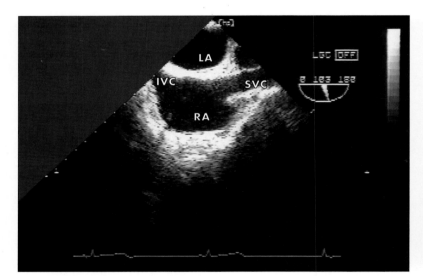

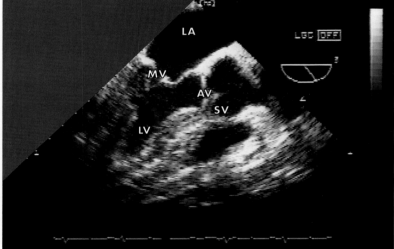

Figure 8-21. Bicaval view. With the probe at a depth of 30 cm from the incisors and the scan angulation set at 90°, rotating the probe to the left (around the long axis of the probe) shows the right atrium (*RA*) flanked by the superior vena cava (*SVC*) and the inferior vena cava (*IVC*). This view is useful for examining the interatrial septum. LA—left atrium.

Figure 8-22. View at base of heart (120°). With the probe remaining at a depth of 30 cm from the incisors, this view is obtained by rotating the scan angulation to 120°. The aortic root can be examined from the sinus of Valsalva (*SV*) to the proximal aortic arch. Color flow mapping across the aortic valve (*AV*) or mitral valve (*MV*) can be used in this view to detect valvular stenosis or insufficiency. LA—left atrium; LV—left ventricle.

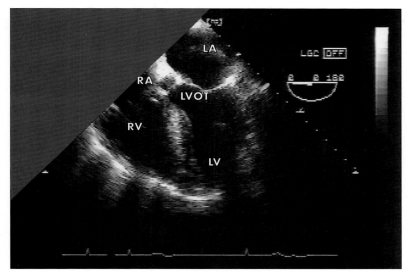

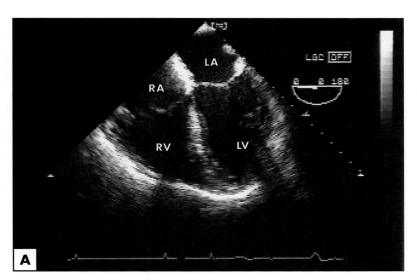

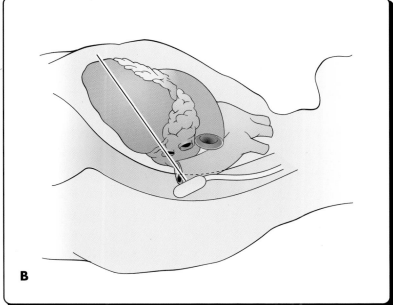

Figure 8-23. Five chamber view. By advancing the probe approximately 0.5 to 1 cm (midway between upper esophageal and midesophageal levels) and retroflexing the probe 10° to 30°, the sonographer obtains a "five-chamber view," consisting of the left (*LA*) and right atria (*RA*), left (*LV*) and right ventricles (*RV*), and the left ventricular outflow tract (*LVOT*). Detection of aortic insufficiency, mitral stenosis, and mitral insufficiency is accomplished with two-dimensional (2D) imaging and color flow Doppler. Multiple cross-sectional views of the mitral valve with 2D and color Doppler imaging may be obtained by decreasing the probe retroflexion back to neutral and then advancing and withdrawing the probe in millimeter increments. This technique minimizes the potential for missing significant, but localized disease of the mitral valve.

Figure 8-24. Four-chamber view. Advancing another 1 to 2 cm and retroflexing the probe 10° to 30° reveals the "four-chamber" view (**A**). The position of the transducer is shown in **B**. Here, the relative size and function of the right (*RA*) and left atria (*LA*) and left (*LV*) and right ventricles (*RV*) can be appreciated. This view is unique because it provides a simultaneous image of the function of all four cardiac chambers. Atrial disease such as arrhythmias, atrial dilation, and thrombi may be detected. Regional wall motion abnormalities of both the right and the left ventricle are easily visualized. Further evaluation of mitral and tricuspid valve function can easily be accomplished. (*From* Labovitz and Pearson [17]; with permission.)

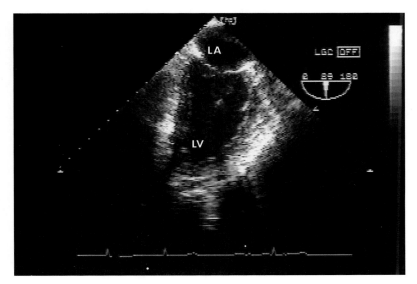

Figure 8-25. Two-chamber-long axis view. With the left atrium and left ventricle centered on the screen, switching to the longitudinal axis yields the "two-chamber long axis" view. Here, the anterior wall of the left ventricle (*LV*) is on the right, and the inferior wall is on the left. This view may provide the best image of the left ventricular apex. The left atrium (*LA*) and, occasionally, the left atrial appendage (not seen in this example) are visualized.

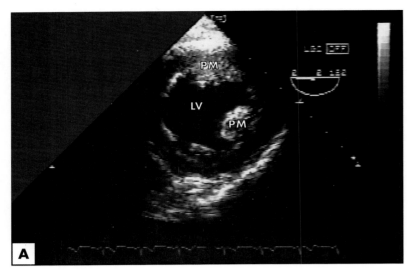

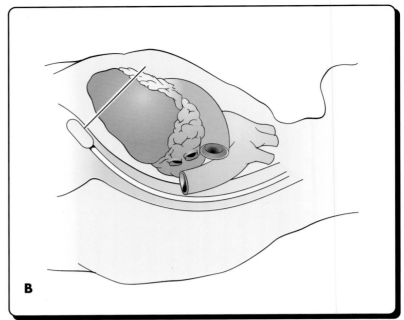

Figure 8-26. Transgastric, midpapillary short axis view. At an approximate depth of 40 cm and with anteroflexion of the probe, the "short axis midpapillary" view is obtained (**A**). The position of the transducer is shown in **B**. This view is often regarded as the best single view for monitoring regional left ventricular (*LV*) wall motion, global ventricular function, and left ventricular filling. The true transverse cross-section of the left ventricle is obtained with the middle portion of both papillary muscles (*PM*) visualized. Detection of regional wall motion abnormalities can be subtle, requiring training and experience for accurate interpretation [18,19]. Artifactual regional myocardial dysfunction can occur when an oblique section instead of a true transverse section of the left ventricle is obtained. (*From* Labovitz and Pearson [17]; with permission.)

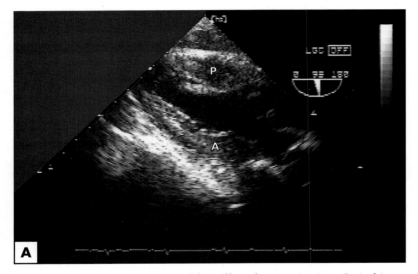

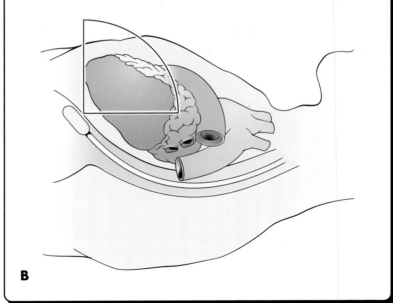

Figure 8-27. Transgastric, midpapillary long-axis view. Switching to the midpapillary longitudinal view (by scrolling the scan sector to 90°) provides additional cross-sectional views for evaluation of regional myocardial function. In this cross-section, the posterior wall (*P*) is closest to the transducer (nearest the apex of the 2-D scan sector) and the anterior wall (*A*) farthest away (**A**). The position of the transducer is shown in **B**. Each wall can be further divided into basal, mid-, and apical segments (*eg,* posterobasal, midanterior) and independently assigned a regional wall motion score (*eg,* normal, hypokinetic, and so forth) (See Figure 8-28). Unfortunately, in this cross-sectional view the left ventricular apex is not always visible. (*From* Labovitz and Pearson [17]; with permission.)

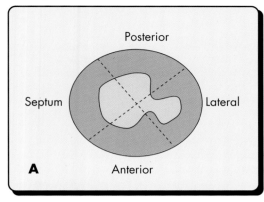

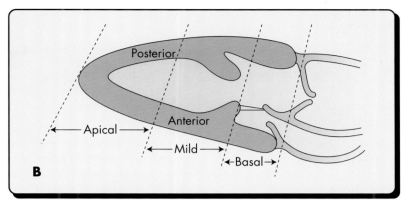

Figure 8-28. Regional division of echocardiographic images of the left ventricle. The circumferential view (**A**) of the left ventricle is traditionally [20] divided into four segments, encompassing the anterior wall, inferior wall, lateral free wall, and interventricular septum. The longitudinal view (**B**) is divided into anterior and posterior walls, which are further subdivided into apical, mid, and basal segments. Assessment of regional myocardial function is based on evaluation of coordinated inward motion of the left ventricle and uniform wall thickening during systole. Each wall segment can be independently graded as being unable to score, hyperkinetic, normal, hypokinetic, akinetic, or dyskinetic (0–5, respectively).

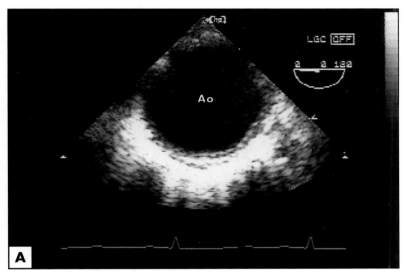

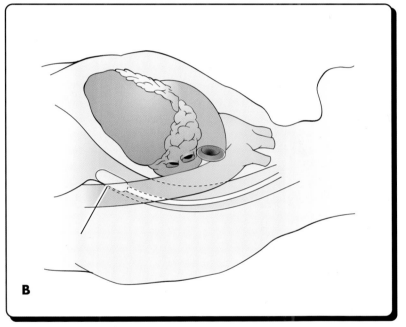

Figure 8-29. Descending aorta. Withdrawing the probe to the level of the aortic valve (30 cm) and rotating the probe 180° around the long axis of the probe permit the examination of the descending aorta (**A**). The position of the transducer is shown in **B**. Setting the depth selector to 40 mm will enlarge the pulsating aorta. Assess-ment of the extent of atherosclerotic disease can be accomplished by gradually advancing and withdrawing the probe with the scan sector set at 0° (transverse view) or 90° (longitudinal view). (*From* Labovitz and Pearson [17]; with permission.)

REFERENCES

1. Einthoven W: Un nouveau galvanometre. *Arch N Sc Ex Nat* 1901, 6:625–630.

1a. Thys D: The normal ECG. In *The ECG in Anesthesia and Critical Care.* Edited by Thys D, Kaplan J. New York: Churchill Livingstone; 1987.

2. Marriott HJL: *Practical Electrocardiography*, edn 8. Baltimore: Williams & Wilkins; 1984:1–8.

3. London M, Hollenberg M, Wong M, *et al.*: Intraoperative myocardial ischemia: localization by continuous 12-lead electrocardiography. *Anesthesiology* 1988, 69:232–241.

4. Sabotka P, Mayer J, Bauernfeind R, *et al.*: Arrhythmias documented by 24-hour continuous ambulatory electrocardiographic monitoring in young women without apparent heart disease. *Am Heart J* 1981, 101:753–759.

5. Brodsky M, Wu D, Denes P, *et al.*: Arrhythmias documented by 24-hour continuous ambulatory monitoring in 50 male medical students without apparent heart disease. *Am J Cardiol* 1977, 39:390–395.

6. Vanik P, Davis H: Cardiac arrhythmias during halothane anesthesia. *Anesth Analg* 1968, 47:299–307.

7. Kuner J, Enescu V, Utsu F, *et al.*: Cardiac arrhythmias during anesthesia. *Dis Chest* 1967, 52:580–587.

8. Bertrand C, Steiner N, Jameson A, Lopez M: Disturbances of cardiac rhythm during anesthesia and surgery. *JAMA* 1971, 216:1615–1617.

9. Angelini L, Feldman M, Lufschonowski R, Leachman R: Cardiac arrhythmias during and after heart surgery: diagnosis and management. *Prog Cardiovasc Dis* 1974, 16:469–495.

10. O'Kelly B, Browner W, Massie B, *et al.*: Ventricular arrhythmias in patients undergoing noncardiac surgery. *JAMA* 1992, 268:217–221.

10a. Smith R, Leung J, Keith F, *et al.*: SPI Research Group: Ventricular dysrhythmia in patients undergoing coronary artery bypass surgery: incidence, characteristics, and prognostic importance. *Am Heart J* 1992, 123:73–81.

11. Mirvis D, Berson A, Goldberger A: Instrumentation and practice standards for electrocardiographic monitoring in special care units: a report for health professionals by a task force of the council on clinical cardiology, American Heart Association. *Circulation* 1989, 79:464–471.

12. ASA/SCA Task Force on Perioperative TEE: Guidelines for perioperative transesophageal echocardiography. *Anesthesiology* 1996, 84:986–1006.

13. Hamer JPM: *Echocardiography 1*. Netherlands: Boehringer Ingelheim; 1987.

14. Managhan MJ: *Practical Echocardiography and Doppler*. New York: John Wiley & Sons; 1990.

15. Feigenbaum H: *Echocardiography*, edn 5. Philadelphia: Lea & Febiger; 1994.

16. Obeid AI: *Echocardiography in Clinical Practice*. Philadelphia: J.B. Lippincott; 1992.

17. Labovitz AJ, Pearson AC: *Transesophageal Echocardiography: Basic Principles and Clinical Applications*. Philadelphia: Lea & Febinger; 1993:23–31.

18. Bergquist B, Leung JM, Bellows WH: Transesophageal echocardiography in myocardial revascularization: I. Accuracy of intraoperative real-time interpretation. *Anesth Analg* 1996, 82:1132–1138.

19. Bergquist B, Bellows WH, Leung JM: Transesophageal echocardiography in myocardial revascularization II. Influence on intraoperative decision making. *Anesth Analg* 1996, 82:1139–1145.

20. American Society of Echocardiography Committee on Standards, Subcommittee on Quantitation of Two-Dimensional Echocardiograms: recommendations for quantitation of the left ventricle by two-dimensional echocardiography. *J Am Soc Echocardiogr* 1989, 2:358–367.

Cardiopulmonary Bypass

Randall M. Schell, Richard L. Applegate, and J.G. Reves

Extracorporeal circulation was successfully used for the first time in 1953 to facilitate cardiac surgery. An atrial septal defect was closed in a young woman while her blood was oxygenated and pumped by a machine and modern cardiac surgery was born. Since that time the use of cardiopulmonary bypass (CPB) has become routine, practiced an estimated 2000 times each day worldwide [1]. Current uses of CPB include cardiac surgery, thoracic aortic aneurysm surgery, resection of renal cell carcinoma, neurosurgery (neurobasilar aneurysms), resuscitation, trauma, support for angioplasty, liver transplantation, and pulmonary transplantation.

The primary function of CPB is to provide optimal conditions for surgery by pumping oxygenated blood from the venous system to the arterial system bypassing the left and right heart. Secondary functions include control of systemic temperature, myocardial preservation by delivery of cardioplegia solutions into the aorta or the coronary sinus, and removal of blood from the operative field by pump cardiotomy suctions and vents with return to the patient. Specialized functions may include delivery of anesthetic agents and removal of excess water by ultrafiltration.

The study of CPB and extracorporeal flow [2–5] can be divided into two general areas: the mechanical devices used and the pathophysiologic response to this nonphysiologic mode of oxygenating and perfusing the body. However, debate continues on which mechanical devices should be used (ie, roller or centrifugal pump, bubble or membrane oxygenator), what physiologic perfusion parameters are optimal (ie, perfusion pressure, flow rate, temperature, mode of perfusion [pulsatile, nonpulsatile], blood gas management) and methods to prevent organ injury (ie, brain, heart) and reduce the systemic inflammatory response that occurs during CPB. Although the majority of CPB is performed with membrane oxygenators, centrifugal pumps, the use of arterial line microfilters, crystalloid priming solutions, alpha-stat arterial blood gas pH management, and intraoperative cell salvaging procedures [6], no uniformly accepted standard method for CPB has been defined. The mechanical equipment and physiologic perfusion parameters used during CPB are often based on institutional preferences.

It is the role of the perfusionist to maintain and operate the CPB equipment and each institution achieves its own balance with regard to perfusionist responsibility to the cardiac surgeon and cardiac anesthesiologist. When accidents during extracorporeal perfusion occur, it is usually due to human error [7–9]. Vigilance in monitoring; communication between the cardiac surgeon, cardiac anesthesiologist, and perfusionist during CPB; and familiarity with CPB equipment and perfusion techniques are necessary for those applying this nonphysiologic process (extracorporeal circulation), which has been called by some a "state of controlled shock" [10]. This chapter reviews the equipment, techniques, physiology, and complications of CPB.

EQUIPMENT AND TECHNIQUES

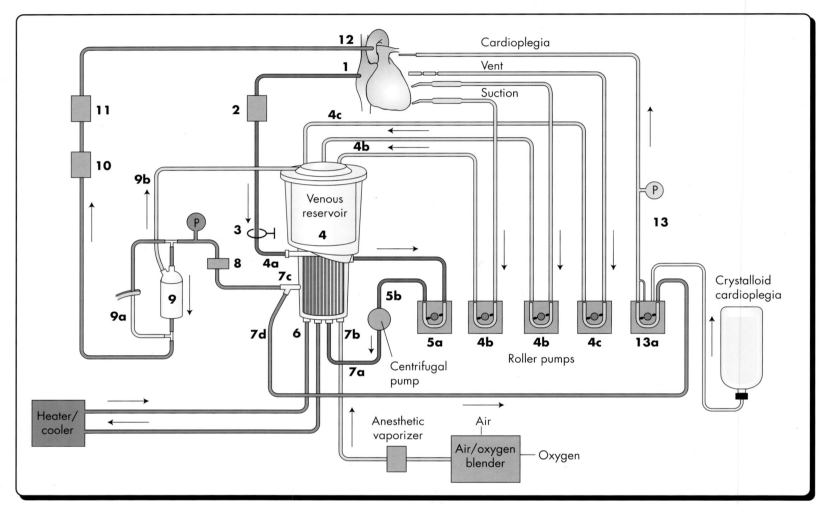

Figure 9-1. The anatomy of a "modern" cardiopulmonary bypass (CPB) circuit. Deoxygenated, venous blood exits the right atrium and vena cava through a venous cannula (1) and drains by gravity through a large polyvinyl chloride tubing toward the venous reservoir (4). An in-line blood gas monitor (2) may be used to continuously measure venous blood gases. A venous inflow regulating clamp (3) is used to adjust "hold" or resistance to gravity drainage of venous blood and thus filling of the heart. A single integrated, disposable unit containing the venous reservoir, heat exchanger, and oxygenator is demonstrated. The venous reservoir (4) serves as a receiving chamber for venous return (4a), suction catheters from the surgical field (4b), and vents (4c). It may be a collapsible-bag "closed" system or hardshell-reservoir "open" system and is a buffer for fluctuations and imbalances between venous return from the patient and arterial flow back to the patient. It is a trap for air, a site for adding blood, fluids, or drugs to the circuit, a source of blood for the pump, and provides a safety factor against pumping air to the patient if there is a sudden decrease in venous return. The cardiotomy suction roller pump(s) (4b) removes blood from the operative field via suction catheters and returns it to the venous reservoir. Whenever the left ventricle (LV) is unable to handle the amount of blood returning to it, an LV vent (4c) and roller pump may be used to prevent LV distention. Blood from the venous reservoir is moved through the CPB circuit by a roller (5a) or centrifugal pump (5b). The heat exchanger (6) is used to warm or cool the blood passing by it and to the patient and is usually located just proximal to the oxygenator (7). Blood is pumped from the heat exchanger into the membrane oxygenator (7a). A blended mixture of oxygen and air with or without anesthetic vapor is delivered to the oxygenator (7b). Oxygenated blood is delivered into the arterial line (7c). A fraction of the blood may be diverted to the cardioplegia delivery system (7d) to provide a blood-crystalloid cardioplegia solution. An arterial flowmeter (8) and arterial line pressure monitor (P) are present. Oxygenated blood passes through an arterial filter (9) and bubble trap or in the unlikely case of arterial filter occlusion through the filter bypass (9a). An arterial filter purge line (9b) with a unidirectional valve creates an escape route for any entrained air. A bubble detector (10) and an in-line blood gas monitor (11) may be present. Oxygenated blood is returned to the patient via the arterial cannula (12) which is usually in the ascending aorta. Cardioplegia delivery (13) and ultrafiltration (not shown) are specialized functions of the CPB circuit. A mixture of blood-crystalloid or crystalloid warm or cold cardioplegia is delivered via a roller pump (13a) past a line pressure monitor (P) to the aorta with antegrade flow down the coronary arteries or retrograde flow via the coronary sinus.

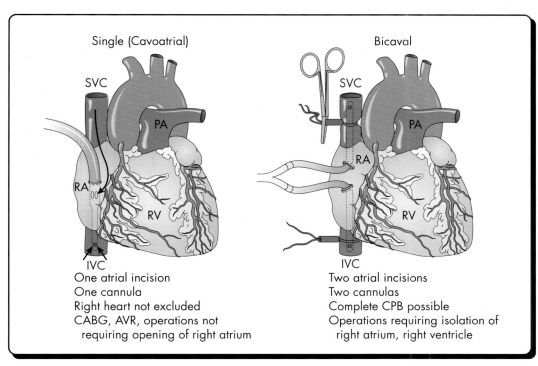

Single (Cavoatrial)

SVC

PA

RA

RV

IVC

One atrial incision
One cannula
Right heart not excluded
CABG, AVR, operations not
    requiring opening of right atrium

Bicaval

SVC

PA

RA

RV

IVC

Two atrial incisions
Two cannulas
Complete CPB possible
Operations requiring isolation of
    right atrium, right ventricle

Figure 9-2. Venous cannulation techniques. Venous blood returning to the right heart is drained by gravity to the venous reservoir or when a bubble oxygenator is used to the oxygenator itself through a venous cannula made of polyvinyl chloride (PVC) with either soft PVC tips or hard tips made of stainless steel. The majority of cardiac procedures (coronary artery bypass graft [CABG], aortic valve replacement [AVR]) using CPB are performed with venous cannulation through the right atrium, with a single "two-stage" cannula. The wider proximal section

has holes in the cannula that lie within the right atrium (RA) and a narrower distal extension is positioned in the inferior vena cava (IVC) and has end holes and side holes. "Single-stage" cannulas may be placed in the IVC and the superior vena cava (SVC) (bicaval) with heavy ligatures around the cannula and the vena cava, which may be constricted thereby diverting all blood return to the venous reservoir creating a bloodless surgical field and no ejection from the left ventricle ("total bypass"). Bicaval cannulation with caval occlusion is required whenever the right heart is going to be entered. When a two-stage cannula or bicaval cannulation without caval occlusion is used, some blood may pass into the right atrium, pulmonary circulation, and to the left ventricle resulting in left ventricular ejection and arterial pulsation or "partial bypass." Optimal venous return is dependent on drainage through a nonobstructed, adequately sized venous cannula through tubing that is not kinked or obstructed by an air lock, past venous clamps that should be open, to a venous reservoir that is positioned below the level of the patient to provide an adequate hydrostatic pressure head for gravity drainage. The technical characteristics of the different venous cannulation techniques have been reviewed [11]. PA—pulmonary artery.

Extracorporeal circuit tubing

Desirable characteristics

Low resistance to flow	Flexible	Biocompatible
Low priming volume	Kink-resistant	Low spallation rate
Transparent	Crack-rupture proof	Tolerance for heat
Resilient	Nontoxic	sterilization

Silicone   Heparin-bonded   PVC

Covalently linked heparin

Spacer molecule

Blood contact surface

Covalent

Ionically linked heparin

Blood contact surface

Ionic

Figure 9-3. Extracorporeal circuit tubing. Extracorporeal circuit tubing provides a conduit for transporting blood from the venous cannula to the reservoir, as the pumping chamber in the arterial roller pump and suction pumps, and throughout the CPB circuit. Desirable characteristics of CPB circuit tubing are listed. Keeping the tubing short and wide reduces resistance to flow

but increasing the width requires an increased priming volume. Transparent tubing allows inspection of the circuit for air and the color of the blood passing through it. It should be resilient (reexpands after compression) if it is to be repeatedly compressed in the roller pump, flexible, and kink-resistant. If cracks in the tubing occurred air might be entrained (venous side), pieces break off into the circuit (spallation), or blood leak out of the tubing. The manufacturing technique should result in nontoxic tubing that is biocompatible, minimizing the body's inflammatory response to this foreign surface exposure. The release of pieces of tubing material (spallation) resulting from trauma to the tubing from pumps and shear stress of blood passing through it should be minimal. Medical grade polyvinyl chloride (PVC) tubing meets most of these characteristics and is the most common type of tubing in CPB circuits. Silicone tubing is sometimes used in arterial roller pump heads because it is softer than PVC resulting in a truer stroke volume when compressed but is very susceptible to wear and has an increased rate of spallation. In an attempt to improve biocompatibility and thromboresistance, techniques have been developed to coat the inner surfaces of the CPB equipment that come in contact with blood. Ionic or covalent bonding of heparin [12,13] to the circuit allows it to interact with circulating unbound antithrombin III and thrombin potentially reducing the level of systemic anticoagulation required. (*Adapted from Gravlee [12]; with permission.*)

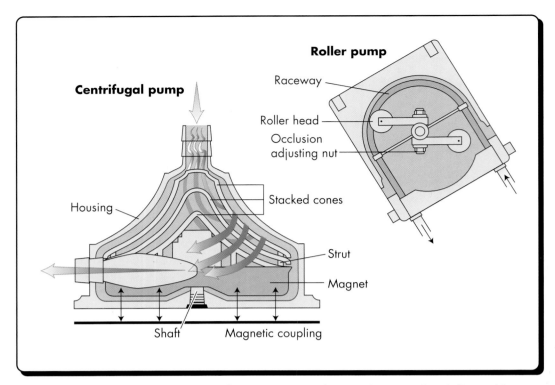

Roller pump

Raceway

Roller head

Occlusion
adjusting nut

Centrifugal pump

Housing

Stacked cones

Strut

Magnet

Shaft　　Magnetic coupling

Figure 9-4. CPB pumps. Many modern CPB circuits have an integrated and disposable venous reservoir, heat exchanger, and membrane oxygenator. If this configuration is used, blood passes from the venous reservoir to the centrifugal or roller pump and then to the heat exchanger and membrane oxygenator and back into the systemic arterial system. The pump flow is ≈ 2 to 2.5 L/min/m^2 (about 50 to 60 mL/kg/min with flow requirements related to core body temperature and metabolic rate). Flow is commonly nonpulsatile [6] although pulsatile flow may be provided in an attempt to mimic physiologic perfusion. When bubble oxygenators are used, the pump is usually placed after the oxygenator.

Centrifugal pumps consist of vane impellers or a nest of plastic cones in a plastic housing magnetically coupled with an electric motor in the permanent drive console that when spinning, causes a magnet in the base of the disposable pump head to spin at an equal rate. The spinning cones or impellers form a vortex constrained by the outside plastic housing which generates pressure to move the blood out of the pump. The pump is totally nonocclusive.

Therefore, flow may go backward exsanguinating the patient if the pump is stopped and the arterial line unclamped. It will not generate excessive pressure with possible rupture of circuit tubing if the arterial line is occluded while pumping. Flow is not determined by rotational rate of the pump alone but is pressure-sensitive. An increase in downstream resistance or a decrease in preload reduces pump flow. Therefore, a flowmeter or sensor must be incorporated into the arterial outflow to quantify pump output. The centrifugal pump is not as effective in generating pulsatile perfusion as a roller pump and it cannot pump large quantities of air to the patient if it is accidentally introduced into the circuit and fills the pump because it relies on centrifugal force to generate pressure.

Most roller pumps have two rollers driven by an electrical motor (or hand cranked in the event of electrical failure) that trap a portion of fluid and blood in the tubing between it and the pump housing and propel it forward. The pump output depends on the revolutions of the pump and volume displaced with each revolution (tubing diameter, pump occlusion). "Pump occlusion" refers to how occluded the tubing is as the roller presses it against the housing ("raceway") and is usually set in the "just occlusive" position in attempts to minimize blood trauma and hemolysis. Unlike centrifugal pumps, roller pumps have a constant stroke volume with each pump cycle, are capable of pulsatile flow, can pump large quantities of air, and are afterload-independent with the possibility of overpressurizing lines causing them to burst.

Figure 9-5. The centrifugal pump is compared and contrasted with the roller pump. Although centrifugal pumps are more expensive than roller pumps, the increased safety and less trauma to formed blood elements (especially with prolonged pumping) may justify their use despite the lack of clinical studies definitively documenting a superior outcome for routine extracorporeal circulation [14,15]. Centrifugal pumps are frequently used for temporary ventricular assistance, emergency CPB circuits, and venovenous bypass for liver transplantation.

CENTRIFUGAL PUMP VS ROLLER PUMP

Factors Compared	Centrifugal Pump	Roller Pump
Afterload	Dependent	Independent
Occlusive	No	Yes
Risk of air embolism	↓	↑
Expense	$$	$
Priming volume	Greater	Less
Generate pulsatile flow	Poor	Better
Excessive arterial line pressure	Not Possible	Possible
Reverse flow possible	Yes	No
Can hand crank	No	Yes
Trauma to bypass tubing	Less	Greater
Trauma to blood	Less	Greater
Superior outcome	?	?

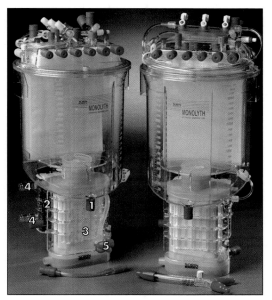

Figure 9-6. The modern membrane oxygenator [16,17], as opposed to a bubble oxygenator, is utilized in greater than 90% of adult [6] and pediatric [18] cardiac procedures utilizing CPB and is frequently supplied as an integral unit also incorporating the venous reservoir and the heat exchanger. This oxygenator imitates the natural pulmonary anatomy by interposing a thin membrane between the gas and the blood and is usually positioned after the roller or centrifugal pump similar to the right ventricle pumping blood to the lung.

Blood leaves the venous reservoir (*1*) to the roller or centrifugal pump and then is pumped through the heat exchanger (*2*) and the membrane oxygenator (*3*). The resistance to flow through the membrane oxygenator usually requires blood to be actively pumped through it unlike the bubble oxygenator. The water inlet and outlet for the heat exchanger (*4*) used in most CPB systems to warm or cool the patient's blood is demonstrated. The heat exchanger is usually located just proximal to the oxygenator to minimize the risk of releasing microbubbles of gas from the blood, which could occur if the blood is warmed after being saturated with gas. Water (cool or warm) passes on one side and blood or perfusate usually countercurrently on the other side of a stainless steel (or less frequently aluminum) interface with heat transfer by conduction. Blood is then pumped into the oxygenator which has a gas supply of oxygen, usually air, and possibly anesthetic vapor or carbon dioxide where gas exchange occurs. Arterialized blood then leaves the oxygenator (*5*) to enter the systemic circulation. (*Courtesy of* Sorin Biomedical, Irvine, CA.)

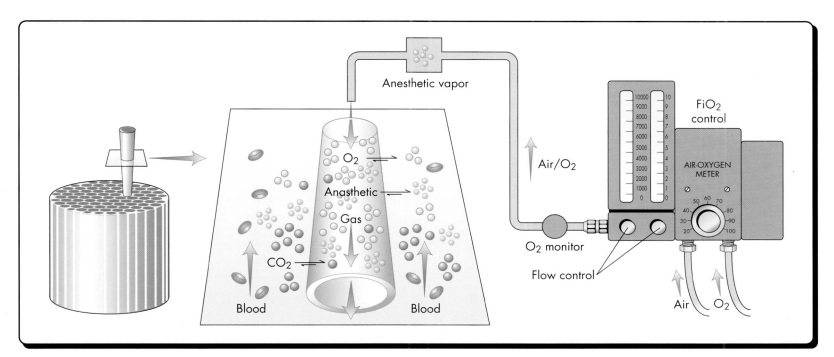

Figure 9-7. Gas exchange in a membrane oxygenator. A blood-outside and gas-inside parallel hollow fiber membrane oxygenator is shown. An air-oxygen blender controls the FIO_2 delivered to the membrane oxygenator and therefore the oxygen partial pressure gradient between the gas and blood phases, thus altering the total amount of oxygen transfer by diffusion through the membrane and ultimately the PaO_2. Arterial $PaCO_2$ is independently controlled by the gas flow (L/min) through the oxygenator, which is often referred to as the "sweep rate." Higher rates of gas flow (not containing CO_2) remove more CO_2 from the inner membrane surface establishing a diffusion gradient from the blood to the inside of the membrane decreasing the $PaCO_2$. An anesthetic vaporizer may be placed in the circuit to provide a set concentration of vapor to the membrane surface where it diffuses into the blood of the patient.

The membrane is composed of a gas permeable material,
polypropylene or silicone rubber, which physically separates the blood from the gas. Membranes made of silicone are nonporous, whereas membranes made of polypropylene are microporous. Most modern membrane lungs have small pores that allow a direct blood-gas interface at the initiation of CPB. However, during CPB a thin protein layer rapidly covers the hollow fibers to form a molecular membrane. This "lack" of a direct blood-gas interface is a major difference between bubble oxygenators and membrane oxygenators allowing gentler handling of blood and a lower rate of hemolysis.

Current membranes have a surface area of approximately 2 to 4 m^2, significantly less than the human lung, but compensate for the reduced area by an increased contact or transit time of the blood with the membrane. The membrane configuration may be fan-folded, coiled, or shaped into hollow capillary tubes as seen in the figure.

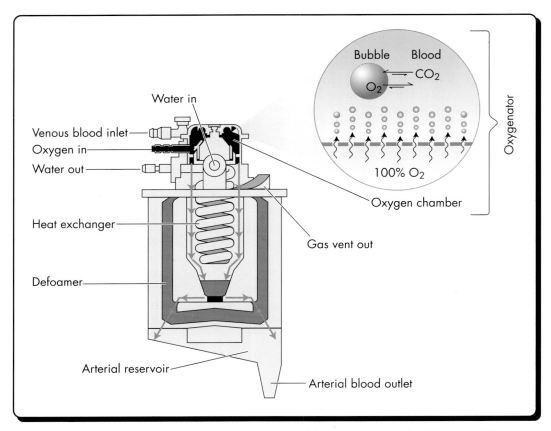

Figure 9-8. Bubble oxygenator. Although the bubble oxygenator ("bubbler") is efficient, has a simple design, is easy to prime, and is less expensive than the membrane oxygenator, it may produce more gaseous microemboli, tend to cause more trauma to the formed blood elements especially when the duration of CPB is prolonged, and therefore is used less than 10% of the time for CPB [6]. There are three main compartments in the bubble oxygenator: the oxygenation section is first, followed by the defoamer-debubbler, and then the arterial reservoir. Most "bubblers" include an integral heat exchanger within the inflow or oxygenator chamber. Venous blood drains by gravity through the bubble oxygenator which offers a much lower resistance to flow than the membrane oxygenator allowing it to be placed before rather than after the pump in the CPB circuit.

1) **Oxygenation:** The venous blood enters a mixing chamber, where the gas, usually 100% oxygen or mixtures of oxygen and carbon dioxide, flows through small holes in a gas dispersion plate (polycarbonate plate or a core of porous silicate) bubbling oxygen through the blood creating a direct blood-gas interface for gas exchange to occur. Mixtures of the ventilating gas that included inert gases like nitrogen would allow alterations in the FIO_2 and resultant PaO_2 but inert gas bubbles are less soluble than oxygen increasing the risk of gas emboli. Increasing the flow of gas through the dispersion plate will create more bubbles generated and the surface available for gas exchange potentially decreasing the $PaCO_2$ and increasing the PaO_2 but increasing the risk of gas emboli. The size of the bubbles also influences oxygen and carbon dioxide exchange. Smaller bubbles result in a larger surface area for oxygen exchange but are harder to eliminate in the defoamer-debubbler, and as oxygen diffuses from them, the bubbles collapse and then are not available for CO_2 exchange. Increasing the size of the bubble increases CO_2 transfer but will reduce the surface area for O_2 exchange. Usually 100% oxygen is used as the ventilating gas. It is more difficult to control O_2 and CO_2 exchange independently in the bubble oxygenator than the membrane oxygenator. 2) **Defoamer-debubbler:** Bubbling oxygen through the venous blood results in arterialized blood and foam which then passes through a polyurethane mesh sponge coated with an antifoam agent which breaks the surface tension of the bubbles causing them to collapse, releasing their contents, which are then vented from the device. 3) **Arterial reservoir:** The blood drains through the defoamer into the arterial reservoir or collecting chamber and then is pumped to the patient. This chamber compensates for inevitable flow descrepancies between the volume of blood passively returning and the volume being actively pumped out of the reservoir and also has a debubbler function by allowing residual bubbles to float to the top while blood is pumped to the patient from the bottom of the reservoir. (*Adapted from* Kane and coworkers [18a]; with permission.)

Figure 9-9. Comparison of oxygenators. Despite its expense, the membrane oxygenator is the most popular oxygenator used for CPB because it more closely imitates the natural lung and has theoretic advantages over the bubble oxygenator. Whether these advantages translate into a measurably improved clinical outcome in patients undergoing cardiac operations with relatively short perfusion times is a subject of debate [19–22].

COMPARISON OF OXYGENATORS

Factors Compared	Membrane	Bubble
Method of oxygenation	Gas transfer through membrane	Direct contact of gas and blood
Control of blood gases	Independent control O_2 and CO_2	Lack of independent control O_2 and CO_2
	Titrate FIO_2 to desired PaO_2	100% FIO_2—High PaO_2
Gaseous/particulate emboli	Less	More
Blood trauma	Less	More
Popularity	++++	+
Expense	$$	$
Clinical outcome	? Better for CPB >2 h	?No difference

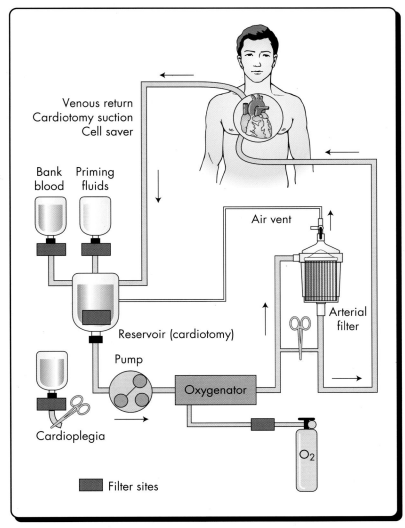

Figure 9-10. Filtration in the CPB circuit. CPB performed without filters on infusion lines is associated with embolization of thousands of gas, microbiologic, and nonbiologic particles to the body, with the lungs and the brain of special concern. In an attempt to reduce the number of these emboli, filters may be used on cardiotomy lines, integrated in cardiotomy and venous reservoirs and bubble oxygenators, for preparation of cardioplegic solutions and pre-bypass prime, and for preparation of blood products [6,23]. Filters on gas lines supplying the oxygenator may remove bacteria from the medical gas supply. Arterial micropore filtration is used more than 90% of the time in clinical practice [6]. The arterial filter should have a self-venting or continuous purge line to the cardiotomy reservoir that allows the escape of air bubbles that rise to the top of the arterial filter. A bypass safety line goes around the filter and remains clamped unless the arterial filter clogs. Arterial inflow pressure should be measured before using the arterial filter. The ideal filter should be biocompatible, offer minimal resistance to flow, and eliminate bubbles, aggregates, nonfunctional cells, and other debris without affecting functional blood components. There are two primary types of microfilters used for CPB: depth filters and screen filters. A depth filter is composed of packed fibers of Dacron that offers a tortuous wetted surface and filters by impaction and absorption. A screen filter is made of a woven mesh of polyester fibers with specific pore sizes in the mesh. Both fibers make effective bubble and particle traps. The use of microfiltration on the arterial line, in the cardiotomy reservoir, on gas lines supplying the oxygenator, and during the infusion of banked blood into the cardiotomy reservoir has been recommended [23]. Leukocyte-depleting filters should probably be used in cytomegalovirus-negative transplant recipients and pediatric patients.

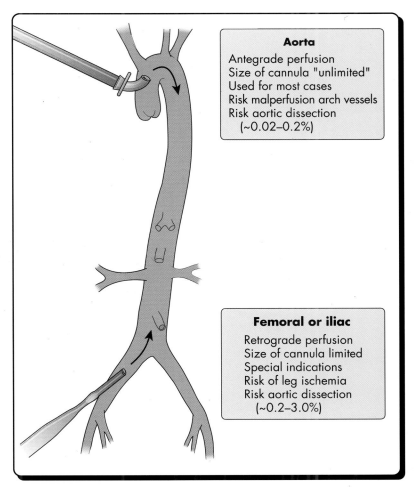

Figure 9-11. Arterial cannulation. Oxygenated blood is returned to the patient from the CPB circuit through an arterial cannula which is usually located in the ascending aorta, occasionally in the femoral artery, and rarely in other sites such as the subclavian artery [24]. Arterial cannulas may be made with right-angled tips or straight tips. They may be wire-reinforced and with support rings to aid in fixation and prevent introduction of too great a length of the cannula into the aorta. Arterial cannulas should provide adequate flow (about 2.5 to 3 L/m^2/min) without an excessive pressure gradient across the cannula ($\leq$100 mm Hg) which could result in increased hemolysis. The portion of the aortic cannula in the aorta is the narrowest part of the entire CPB circuit and should be as short as possible and of adequate diameter to meet these flow and pressure characteristics.

The site for cannulation is selected based on the operation planned and quality of the aortic wall. Epivascular or transesophageal echocardiography [25] may be used to facilitate selection of an aortic cannulation site free of calcification or atheromatous disease in an attempt to reduce the risk of dislodgement of this material which could result in stroke. Other complications of aortic cannulation include aortic dissection, often diagnosed by high CPB arterial-line pressure, decreased venous return and blue discoloration of the aorta, and abnormal cerebral perfusion if the arch vessels are accidentally cannulated. Indications for femoral arterial cannulation include presence of an ascending aortic aneurysm, severe atheromatous disease or calcification of the ascending aorta, unstable patients where cannulation is accomplished under local anesthesia before induction of anesthesia, during reoperations when bleeding complications occur during reentry, or when antegrade dissection occurs during ascending aortic cannulation. Retrograde arterial dissection and limb ischemic complications may complicate femoral arterial cannulation. Occlusive disease of the femoral and iliac vessels is a contraindication for femoral arterial cannulation.

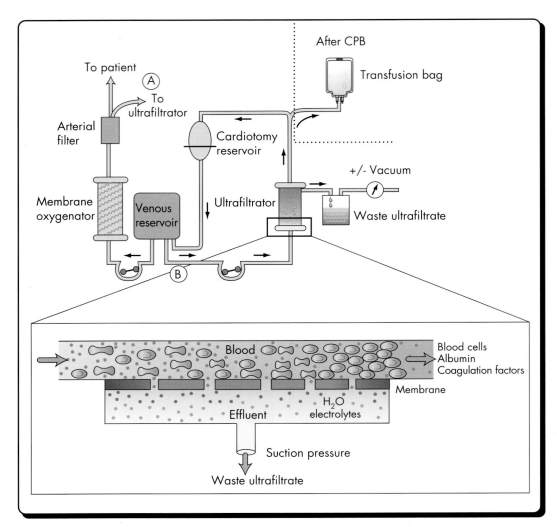

Figure 9-12. Hemofiltration and CPB. Ultrafiltration can be used during CPB [26] to increase the patient's hematocrit without transfusion by removing excess plasma water caused by preoperative cardiac failure, perioperative intravenous fluid administration, crystalloid prime in the CPB circuit, and cardioplegia solutions. The ultrafiltrator is composed of semipermeable hollow capillary fibers that function as membranes allowing the separation and removal of the aqueous phase of blood without removal of the cellular elements, albumin, or clotting factors. Blood is diverted to pass through the fibers usually from the arterial side of the main pump (*A*) or from the venous reservoir using an accessory pump (*B*). Blood is pumped along the inside of the hollow fiber, with the outside of the hollow fiber open to siphon drainage or negative pressure created by a vacuum force. The hydrostatic pressure forces water, electrolytes, and low-molecular-weight solutes (those less than 20,000 Da) through the membrane creating an ultrafiltrate with a similar composition to glomerular filtrate, which is discarded. Some heparin is removed when ultrafiltration is used during CPB and thus adequacy of heparinization should be closely monitored.

Hemofiltration may be performed after CPB to concentrate the pump blood before it is given back to the patient. Unlike the centrifugation and washing techniques of saving red blood cells, ultrafiltration preserves plasma proteins, intravascular coagulation factors, and platelets [27]. Ultrafiltration during CPB may reduce postoperative edema, raise hematocrit, and improve hemostasis [28]. It may be especially useful for managing fluid overload in patients with renal failure, to reduce pulmonary dysfunction after CPB by decreasing the amount of extravascular lung fluid, and for CPB in infants and children [29]. (*Adapted from* Nakamura [27a]; *with permission.*)

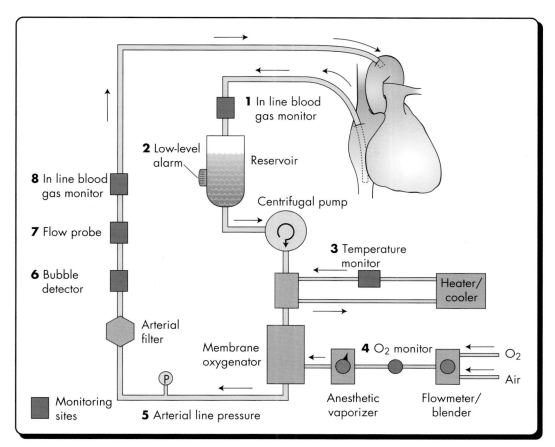

Figure 9-13. Monitoring the CPB circuit. Equipment-related damaging events involving the CPB machine generate a significant portion of adverse outcomes [8]. The CPB circuit should be vigilantly monitored [30,31] throughout cardiopulmonary bypass. An in-line continuous system for measuring blood gases in the venous (*1*) and arterial (*8*) lines is available. Monitoring the venous blood gases and oxygen saturation permits rapid assessment of the global balance of oxygen supply and demand. Blood gases may be monitored by systems that use direct sampling from the circuit and conventional blood-gas machine technology, by a sensor that uses dyes that fluoresce at intensities that vary with the concentration of the parameters measured, and by optical measurement techniques. A light source with a photodetector or an ultrasonic level detector (*2*) may be used to monitor the amount of blood in the reservoir. It may automatically stop the arterial pump or activate an audible alarm to alert the perfusionist to slow or stop the arterial pump and correct the etiology of the reduced reservoir volume before the reservoir is completely emptied and air potentially pumped into the arterial circuit. The water temperature of the fluid entering the heat exchanger (*3*), and the blood temperature proximal (venous) and distal (arterial) to the heat exchanger should be monitored (not shown). An oxygen analyzer should be placed in the gas supply to the oxygenator (*4*) to help prevent the delivery of a hypoxic gas mixture. The pressure in the arterial line should be monitored (*5*) after the pump but before the arterial line filter. Obstruction of the arterial line or arterial line filter, malposition of the arterial cannula, and aortic dissection may be detected by an increase in pressure at this monitoring site. Air or bubble detectors are placed after the arterial pump and may use a light source–photodetector system. Because the output of a centrifugal pump is pressure–dependent (*ie*, potentially increasing output with decreased afterload and decreased output with increased afterload), flow monitoring (*7*) is required. Blood flow is typically monitored by ultrasonic (Doppler) or electromagnetic methods. Monitoring of anticoagulation and cardioplegia line pressure and temperature is not shown. All of these monitors cannot substitute but must be used in concert with a vigilant perfusionist, anesthesiologist, and cardiac surgeon.

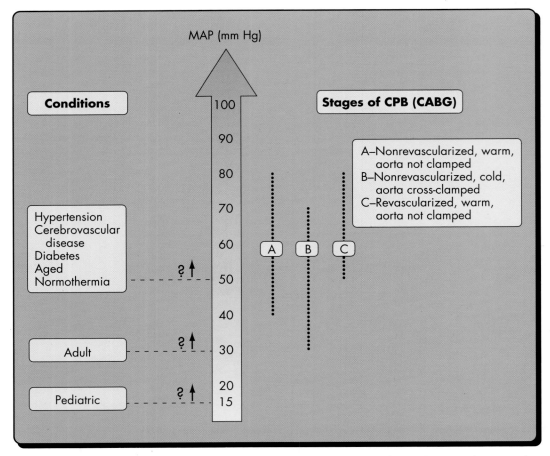

Conditions

Hypertension
Cerebrovascular
  disease
Diabetes
Aged
Normothermia

Adult

Pediatric

MAP (mm Hg)

100
90
80
70
60
50
40
30
20
15

Stages of CPB (CABG)

A–Nonrevascularized, warm,
  aorta not clamped
B–Nonrevascularized, cold,
  aorta cross-clamped
C–Revascularized, warm,
  aorta not clamped

A   B   C

Figure 9-14. Target mean arterial pressure (MAP) and CPB. Factors that may be considered when determining a target MAP during CPB for an individual patient are shown. The adequacy of perfusion of the brain [32] and heart are of particular interest.

Pressure-flow autoregulation in the brain remains intact with a MAP between 15 and 80 mm Hg during moderate hypothermic CPB using alpha-stat blood gas management in children [33]. However, autoregulation is disrupted with profound hypothermia and after deep hypothermic circulatory arrest. Children have a very compliant vasculature and it is not uncommon for the MAP to be low (20 to 40 mm Hg) despite pump flow rates that may be about two to three times that of adults. The systemic temperature, pump flow, and individual patient conditions (*ie*, aortopulmonary collaterals) must be taken into account when determining "acceptable" MAP during CPB. Indices of perfusion other than flow and MAP, such as urine output, acid-base balance, mixed venous oxygen saturation in the venous return line, and rate of cooling or warming should be monitored.

In adults, pressure-flow autoregulation is intact at a MAP as low as 30 mm Hg if alpha-stat arterial blood gas management is employed during hypothermic, nonpulsatile CPB [34,35]. Aging and the presence of coexisting disease may alter the "safe" target MAP during CPB. Although cerebral autoregulation is intact in the elderly [36], increasing atherosclerosis with occult cerebrovascular disease may place the aged at an increased risk for cerebral injury during CPB. Hypertension may be associated with a shift of the pressure-

flow autoregulatory curve to the right and left ventricular hypertrophy. A higher MAP on CPB may be required to ensure adequate perfusion of the brain and the endocardium of the hypertrophied heart. Insulin-dependent diabetic patients placed on CPB have evidence of impaired metabolism and flow autoregulation [37] with decreased jugular venous oxygen saturation during rewarming from CPB. The presence of extra- and intracranial obstructive vascular disease may also warrant maintaining a higher MAP during CPB.

It is typical for the MAP to decrease with initiation of CPB because the crystalloid prime doesn't contain endogenous catecholamines and has a low viscosity. During early CPB for myocardial revascularization surgery, the heart is empty with a reduced oxygen requirement but is still beating and is perfused from the aorta. The MAP is usually maintained at 40 to 50 mm Hg or higher, although patients with altered cerebral autoregulation, myocardial hypertrophy, or critical coronary stenosis may require an even higher MAP. During cold CPB with the aorta cross-clamped, the blood pressure is often permitted to decrease to as low as 30 to 40 mm Hg. High systemic arterial pressures during this stage may be associated with increased noncoronary collateral blood flow into the heart, warming of the heart, and washing out of the cardioplegia solution with reduced myocardial protection from ischemia. Before termination of CPB when the heart is revascularized, reperfused, and warm, it is common to maintain the MAP higher than during hypothermic CPB but slightly lower than values desired after CPB.

MAP during CPB is usually manipulated by altering systemic vascular resistance by the administration of vasoconstricting α-adrenergic agonists (*ie*, phenylephrine) or vasodilators (*ie*, anesthetics, nitroprusside) rather than altering pump flow. "Safe" lower limits and the most appropriate management of MAP during CPB remain controversial. CABG—coronary artery bypass graft.

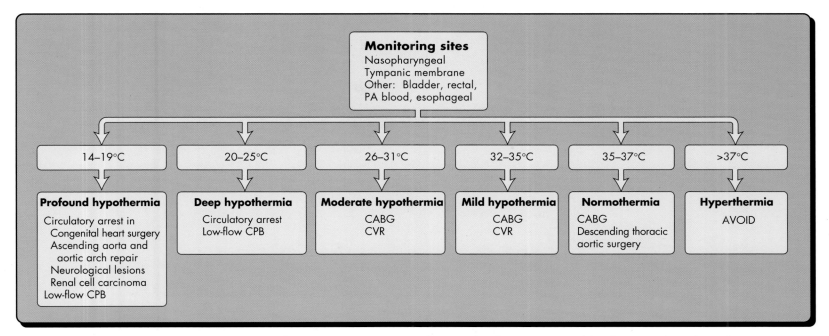

Figure 9-15. Temperature during CPB. Hypothermia (<35°C) is used empirically as the primary strategy to limit ischemic organ damage especially of the heart and brain during CPB. However, the mechanism(s) by which hypothermia attenuates the process or processes leading to irreversible loss of cellular function during ischemia is incompletely understood [38]. The neuroprotective benefits of a hypothermic versus normothermic bypass temperature management strategy for coronary revascularization, the most common use of CPB, are unproved. The reduction in total body oxygen consumption and potential organ protective effect accomplished with hypothermia must be weighed against the potential deleterious effects (*eg,* altered coagulation, decrease in blood flow to all organs, increased peripheral vascular resistance, increased viscosity, endocrine alterations and acid-base disturbances) when selecting the "optimal" temperature for perfusion.

Nasopharyngeal and tympanic membrane temperature may best reflect cerebral temperature during CPB. The bladder temperature can be affected by the rate of urine flow, rectal probes can be insulated by feces, and pulmonary artery blood (PA) and esophageal temperature probes may be influenced by ice or cold saline solutions in the chest used for myocardial protection.

The commonly accepted categorical definitions of hypothermia [39] are listed. Moderate and mild hypothermia are frequently used for coronary artery bypass graft (CABG) and cardiac valve replacement or repair (CVR) surgery. When circulatory arrest is used in adults or children, the temperature should be measured in several different sites that reflect cerebral temperature, should usually be less than 20°C, and additional cooling time after achieving the desired core temperature should be considered before initiating circulatory arrest [40]. It is not uncommon for the CPB perfusate temperature to exceed 37°C during rewarming from hypothermic temperatures. Cerebral hyperthermia (>37°C) may occur quite commonly, could exacerbate ischemic cerebral injury, and should be avoided [41].

Protocols for cooling and rewarming vary between institutions and the ideal is unknown at this time.

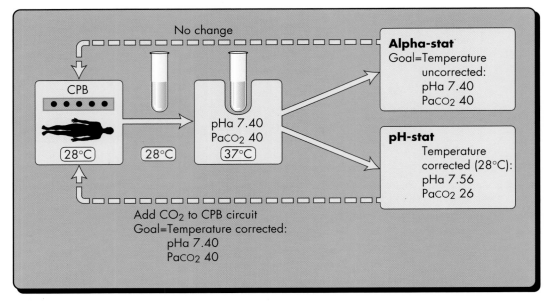

Figure 9-16. Blood gas management during CPB. Controversy exists regarding the most desirable method of blood gas management ("alpha-stat" versus "pH-stat") during hypothermic cardiopulmonary bypass and has focused primarily on the brain and whether either strategy has the potential to reduce neurologic injury after cardiac procedures [42,43]. With alpha-stat blood gas management, blood is taken from a hypothermic patient (*ie*, 28°C), placed in the arterial blood gas (ABG) machine, warmed to 37°C to provide a measurement at a standard temperature, and the ABG report is uncorrected for the patient's actual body temperature. The sweep rate (liters of gas delivered to the oxygenator per minute) may be manipulated to meet the goal of a temperature-*uncorrected* pH of 7.40 and $PaCO_2$ of 40 mm Hg. Carbon dioxide is not added to the circuit. In this patient, if the uncorrected pH was 7.40 and $PaCO_2$ 40 mm Hg no changes in gas flow to the oxygenator would need to be made. If pH-stat blood gas management were used in this same patient, blood would be sampled while hypothermic, placed in the ABG machine, and warmed to 37°C as with alpha-stat. However, the blood gas is "corrected" for the patient's actual body temperature using a nomogram to find the expected change in pH and $PaCO_2$ at this level of hypothermia and reported. Because of the increased CO_2 solubility at 28°C the corrected ABG would demonstrate a "respiratory alkalosis" with an increased pH ($\approx$ 7.56) and decreased $PaCO_2$ ($\approx$ 26 mm Hg). Carbon dioxide is then added to the oxygenator of the CPB circuit with the goal of maintaining a temperature-*corrected* pH of 7.40 and $PaCO_2$ of 40 mm Hg.

Poikilothermic animals tend to maintain electrochemical neutrality and hence "proper" functional charge ratio of intracellular enzymes and other proteins and intermediary metabolites during increasing levels of hypothermia by what appears to be a progressive and increasing physiologically appropriate "alkalosis." A key protein buffer in humans is the imidazole group of the amino acid histidine. The degree of buffer dissociation is expressed as alpha, where alpha is the proportion of imidazoles that have dissociated and lost a proton. Hence the alpha-stat approach aims to maintain a constant dissociation state of this amino acid buffer and transmembrane pH gradient helping to preserve optimum metabolic activity and enzyme function. The pH-stat method mimics that of hibernating mammals and produces a relative hypercarbia and acidemia compared with the alpha-stat method.

ARTERIAL BLOOD GAS PH MANAGEMENT DURING CPB

Factors Compared	Alpha-Stat	pH-Stat
Temperature		
Normothermia	No changes	No changes
Hypothermia		
Goal	Temperature-uncorrected pH 7.40, Pa_{CO_2} 40 mm Hg	Temperature-corrected pH 7.40, Pa_{CO_2} 40 mm Hg
Management	Sweep rate	CO_2 added to CPB circuit
CNS		
CBF	Supply = demand	Supply > demand
Autoregulation	Intact	Impaired
Heart	?Benefit	?Detrimental
Hb Oxygen Affinity		
Moderate hypothermia	Increased (p50 ≈ 12 mm Hg)	?Theoretic benefit
Adult CPB	Usual	Rare
Pediatric CPB	Usual	Rare
		?Improved CNS cooling
Outcome	?	?

Figure 9-17. The differences between alpha-stat and pH-stat arterial blood gas pH management during CPB are compared. No changes in arterial blood gas pH management are required when normothermic temperatures are used. The relative differences between the two strategies are dependent on the degree of hypothermia. Carbon dioxide dilates the cerebral vasculature. The cerebral vasodilation of pH-stat management is thought to result in loss of cerebral autoregulation and greater cerebral blood flow (CBF) levels during CPB. There are multiple air and particulate emboli present in the CPB circuit and delivered to the patient during CPB. Excessive or luxuriant CBF with pH-stat management might result in greater delivery of these emboli to the brain. Cerebral autoregulation is maintained during alpha-stat management.

The acid-base management technique during hypothermic CPB may be of relatively little importance with regard to the effect on the heart. Although it has been suggested that alpha-stat management may improve subendocardial blood flow, contractility, and fibrillation threshold [44], current clinical trials find no advantage [42].

One rationale for using pH-stat management is to counter the leftward shift of the oxyhemoglobin dissociation curve resulting from hypothermia which increases the affinity of hemoglobin for oxygen potentially decreasing tissue oxygenation. However, because dissolved oxygen increases and there is reduced total systemic and cerebral oxygen consumption with hypothermia, adequate tissue oxygen delivery becomes significantly less dependent on oxyhemoglobin kinetics.

During hypothermic CPB for both adults and children, the alpha-stat management strategy is used almost exclusively, although it is unknown if either blood gas management strategy leads to better outcome with regard to key organ systems (*ie*, brain, heart, kidneys). However, the increased CO_2 with pH-stat management results in cerebral vasodilation and increased CBF which may improve cerebral cooling and therefore hypothermic brain protection in infants and children at specific risk for cerebral ischemia during CPB and deep hypothermic circulatory arrest [45]. CNS—central nervous system.

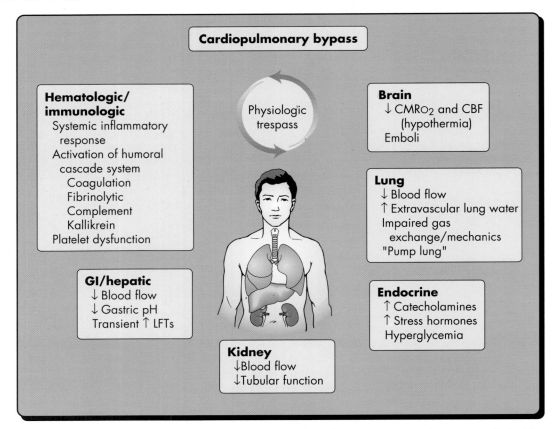

Figure 9-18. Systemic effects of CPB. CPB is a physiologic trespass with many undesirable systemic effects. Interaction between the cellular and humoral components of blood with the foreign surfaces of the extracorporeal circuit and mechanical trauma to blood elements causes activation of multiple humoral systems including the coagulation and fibrinolytic system, complement system (inflammatory reaction [46]), and kallikrein system (increased vascular permeability). Platelet number and function is often decreased after CPB. Severe gastrointestinal (GI) complications after CPB are rare (<1%) and if they occur are usually associated with postoperative low cardiac output syndrome. However, transient elevations in liver function tests (LFTs), decreased gastric pH, and decreased GI organ blood flow have been documented. The cerebral circulation must autoregulate cerebral blood flow (CBF) in the face of nonphysiologic alterations in systemic flow (*ie*, nonpulsatile), pressure, oxygen content (*ie*, hemodilution), and temperature during CPB and is subjected to air and particulate emboli. Changes in pulmonary gas exchange (*ie*, increased extravascular lung water, impaired gas exchange) and mechanics (reduced compliance) after cardiac surgery with CPB may occur, but respiratory failure requiring prolonged ventilatory support is rare and related to preoperative pulmonary dysfunction, duration of CPB, and postoperative hemodynamic status. A small number of patients develop a postperfusion lung syndrome ("pump lung") with similar pathology and clinical course as adult respiratory distress syndrome. As with other sources of stress, CPB causes increases in serum catecholamine levels and other "stress hormones" (cortisol, glucagon, growth hormone, antidiuretic hormone). Glycogenolysis and gluconeogenesis are enhanced and the effects of insulin are reduced, frequently resulting in hyperglycemia. Renal blood flow and tubular function are decreased during CPB, and postoperative "renal failure" as defined by increases in blood urea nitrogen and creatinine has an incidence of up to 30%. However, renal failure requiring dialysis is uncommon (in the range 1% to 5%), occurs more frequently in the elderly, and is often associated with preexisting renal dysfunction, long duration of CPB, and postoperative low-output syndrome. The absence of significant postoperative morbidity related to CPB depends primarily on each particular patient's ability to compensate for the physiologic derangements induced by extracorporeal oxygenation and perfusion.

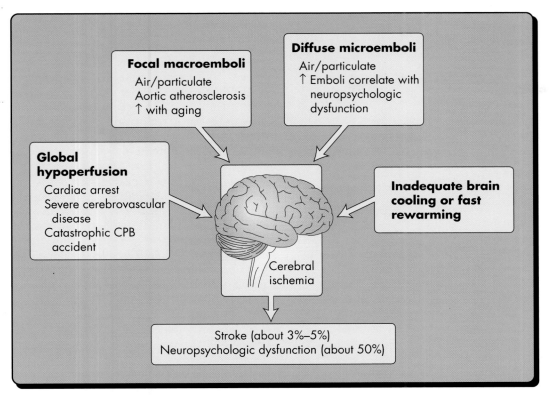

Figure 9-19. Neurologic injury and CPB. Potential mechanisms of brain injury during cardiac surgery with CPB are demonstrated [32]. Global and regional cerebral hypoperfusion are rarely a primary mechanism of neurologic injury in adults. Obvious causes of global or regional hypoperfusion include perioperative cardiac arrest, major pump accidents (*ie*, oxy-genator failure, arterial cannulation site excluding perfusion of cerebral vessels), and severe cerebrovascular disease (*ie*, bilateral internal carotid artery occlusion). Inadequate or uneven brain cooling prior to low-flow CPB or circulatory arrest and fast rewarming from hypothermic temperatures (*ie*, brain >37°C) may result in global or regional cerebral hypoperfusion and cerebral injury. Global hypoperfusion may be the primary mechanism of neurologic injury in children where hypothermic circulatory arrest is used. Embolization of the cerebral vasculature by microemboli (air, plastic, calcific particles, platelet aggregates) or macroemboli (large air bubbles, atheromatous debris from aortic plaques or cardiac valvular lesions, and intracardiac thrombi) are believed to be a major factor in the genesis of post-CPB neurologic injury. Transcranial and carotid Doppler reveal that the brain is subjected to showers of emboli throughout CPB. The number of emboli detected correlates with postoperative neuropsychologic dysfunction. The incidence of frank stroke after CPB is ≈ 3% to 5%. The incidence of subtle neurologic and neuropsychologic dysfunction in the early postoperative period approaches 50% or more but is often only identified on extensive neuropsychologic testing.

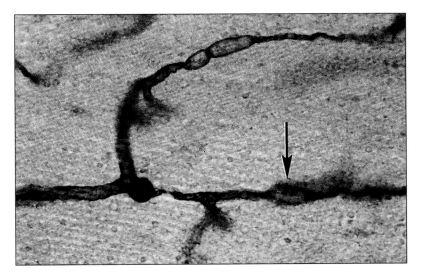

Figure 9-20. Small capillary and arteriolar dilatations (SCADs). SCADs distributed throughout the cerebral vasculature have recently been demonstrated in the brains of patients dying after cardiac surgery [47]. These lesions were demonstrated in cerebral capillaries of patients or animals only after either CPB or proximal aortic instrumentation. It is speculated that the SCADs represent histologic evidence of embolic material (air or fatty deposits) in the cerebral capillaries. (*From* Moody and coworkers [47]; with permission.)

NEUROPROTECTION AND CPB

Factor	Precaution/Protective Measure
Increased risk	
Elderly	
Heavily calcified atherosclerotic aorta	
?Genetic markers	
Cerebrovascular disease	
Carotid artery disease	Symptomatic → Benefit CEA
	Asymptomatic → ?Benefit CEA
Surgical technique	
Cannulation methods	TEE/epiaortic scan guided
	?Femoral cannulation
Aortic cross-clamp	TEE guided
De-airing	
Perfusion technique	
Membrane oxygenator	
Arterial filter	
MAP	?> 30 mm Hg with moderate hypothermia
	?> 50–70 mm Hg with at-risk population
ABG pH management	?Effect on outcome
Temperature	Mild hypothermia
	Avoid hyperthermia (> 37°C)
Hematocrit	?Optimal
Pump flow	?Optimal
Anesthetic management	
Anesthetic choice	?Effect on outcome
Thiopental	No benefit in CABG surgery
	?Benefit in valvular heart surgery
Monitoring techniques	Possible benefit: TCD, jugular venous oximetry, EEG
Pharmacologic protection	?Future

Figure 9-21. Neuroprotection and CPB. Perioperative factors that may affect the incidence of neurologic injury after CPB are demonstrated. Advanced age, severe aortic atherosclerotic disease, genetic markers (apolipoprotein E-e4), and severe cerebrovascular disease are associated with an increased risk of postoperative neurologic dysfunction after CPB [48]. Patients with symptomatic carotid artery disease who are to undergo cardiac surgery with CPB probably benefit from carotid endarterectomy (CEA). Whether the CEA should be performed as a staged or combined procedure is yet to be determined. Transesophageal echocardiography (TEE) may be used to "de-air" the heart after open ventricle procedures and alone or with epiaortic sonography to select an aortic cannulation site "free" of atheroma or calcification potentially reducing the chance of embolization. Alternative arterial cannulation sites may be used when a very heavily calcified (ie, "porcelain") or atherosclerotic aorta is identified. Membrane oxygenators generate fewer emboli than bubble oxygenators and arterial filters reduce the number of emboli delivered to the patient. The optimal mean arterial pressure (MAP), arterial blood gas (ABG) pH management strategy (alpha-stat versus pH-stat), perfusion temperature, hematocrit, and pump flow may vary depending on the clinical situation and are a matter of current debate. The best anesthetic technique with regard to neurologic outcome has not been identified. Thiopental decreases cerebral blood flow and cerebral metabolism and is a cerebrovasoconstrictor. It has no benefit as a neuroprotective agent for modern coronary artery bypass graft surgery. Whether it has any benefit for valvular heart surgery is controversial. Although prevention of perioperative neurologic injury continues to be the focus of investigations, new pharmacologic methods (eg, 21-aminosteroids, α-amino–3-hydroxy–5-methyl–4-isoxazole, postsynaptic excitatory neurotransmitter (AMPA) receptor antagonists) may be used in the future to reduce cellular injury associated with neurologic insults that occur during cardiac surgery with CPB. EEG—electroencephalogram; TCD—transcranial Doppler.

MYOCARDIAL PRESERVATION: A CONTINUUM

Pre-CPB	Cross-clamp off	Cross-clamp on	Reperfusion
Optimize myocardial oxygen supply and demand	Optimize CPP	Cardioplegia-induced electromechanical arrest	Maintain or reinstitute cardioplegic arrest (first 10 min)
	Optimize Hb	± Myocardial hypothermia	Provide O_2/substrates for aerobic metabolism
	Avoid ventricular distention	Avoid ventricular distention	Avoid ventricular distention
	Avoid ↑HR, ↑inotropy	↓ Aortic cross-clamp time	Maintain relative hypocalcemia (first 5–10 min)
			Initial reperfusate: warm, ↑ osmolality, not acidotic, ± oxygen and hydroxyl free radical scavengers
			Initial CPP low then increased

Figure 9-22. Myocardial preservation. Myocardial preservation during cardiac surgery and CPB should be thought of as a continuum beginning before CPB and continuing throughout the reperfusion period and beyond. Techniques and interventions to optimize myocardial energy supply and demand before CPB include reducing anxiety with adequate premedication; supplemental oxygen administration; appropriate preoperative use of vasodilators and β-blockers; immediate assessment and treatment of tachycardia, hypertension and myocardial ischemia; and maintenance of coronary perfusion pressure by adjusting the depth of anesthesia and the use of vasoconstrictors (*eg*, phenylephrine) if necessary. With initiation of CPB and before application of the aortic cross-clamp, substrate delivery to the myocardium should be optimized by maintaining coronary perfusion pressure (CPP) and avoiding extreme hemodilution. Tachycardia, increased inotropy, ventricular distention, and ventricular fibrillation increase myocardial oxygen demands and should also be avoided. The goal is to have a substrate-repleted, oxygenated myocardium before arrest. During CPB and with the aorta cross-clamped there is no coronary blood flow. Reducing myocardial energy demands and the time that the myocardium is not perfused (aortic cross-clamp time) then becomes the primary focus. Normothermic electromechanical arrest by the intermittent or continuous administration of a hyperkalemic cardioplegia solution decreases myocardial oxygen consumption by about 90%, whereas cardiac cooling (*ie*, cardioplegia, topical and systemic hypothermia) plays a lesser role in reducing myocardial energy demands. The cardioplegia solution should provide a favorable metabolic milieu by providing metabolic substrate (oxygen, glucose), removing and buffering acid produced by the myocardium, and maintaining myocardial arrest.

Several factors have been shown to be important during the early reperfusion period: Reducing early metabolic requirements by chemical cardioplegic arrest during the first 10 minutes and by maintaining the heart in an empty, beating state for approximately 20 to 30 minutes before it is required to work against a load, providing oxygen and substrate for metabolic replenishment and aerobic metabolism, avoiding hypercalcemia, and maintaining a low coronary perfusion pressure (30 to 50 mm Hg) for a short time to avoid endothelial cell damage and swelling that can result from high perfusion pressures after ischemia. The initial reperfusate is often warmed, alkaline, and may contain oxygen or hydroxyl free radical scavengers (*eg*, mannitol). The ultimate goal is the preservation of ventricular function. HR—heart rate.

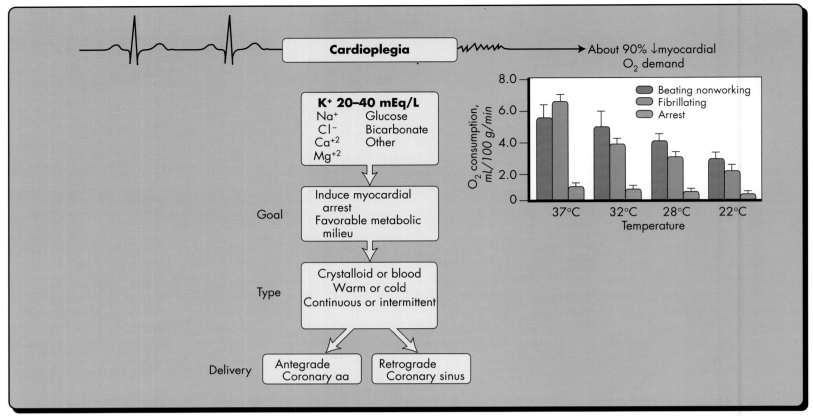

Figure 9-23. Cardioplegia and CPB. Oxygen consumption of the heart is reduced by approximately 90% with electromechanical arrest by the administration of a hyperkalemic cardioplegia solution and only a relatively smaller reduction is accomplished by cooling the heart [49]. Following initiation of CPB and application of the aortic cross-clamp, the myocardium is perfused through the coronary arteries (antegrade) or via the coronary sinus (retrograde) with a potassium-rich crystalloid or blood cardioplegia solution abolishing action potentials and arresting the heart in diastole. Although the exact composition of the cardioplegia solution varies among institutions, the essential elements are similar. The potassium concentration is usually kept below 50 mEq/L and its purpose is to maintain cardiac arrest. The sodium concentration (100 to 120 mEq/L) is less than that in plasma because ischemia tends to increase intracellular sodium content. A small amount of calcium is needed to maintain cellular integrity. If the myocardium is perfused with a calcium-free cardioplegia solution, reperfusion with calcium may cause membrane damage, cell swelling, and contracture ("calcium paradox"). Magnesium may control an excessive influx of calcium into the cell. Glucose, aspartate, or glutamate may be added to enhance substrate availability. A buffer, usually sodium bicarbonate, is necessary to prevent excessive accumulation of acid metabolites. Osmolality is adjusted with albumin or mannitol resulting in an iso-osmolar or slightly hyperosmolar solution. Other additives may include vasodilators (nitroglycerin, calcium channel antagonists), lidocaine, procaine, glucocorticoids, glucose and insulin, and blood. Blood improves oxygen delivery, has a superior buffering capacity, contains endogenous free radical scavengers, provides natural oncotic pressure, and is often mixed with crystalloid cardioplegia. The question of whether blood or crystalloid cardioplegia is best and under what circumstances each should be used is controversial. However, blood cardioplegia is considered superior for reperfusion of the acutely ischemic myocardium.

During CPB, the cardioplegia solution may be crystalloid or blood, administered intermittently or continuously, and delivered antegrade or retrograde. There is decreased delivery and risk of ventricular distention in patients with aortic insufficiency when the antegrade delivery route is used. Moreover, in the presence of severe coronary artery disease, there may be poor distribution of the cardioplegia solution distal to coronary stenoses. Retrograde cardioplegia alone or with antegrade cardioplegia is often used in these clinical scenarios. (*Adapted from* Buckberg [49a]; with permission.)

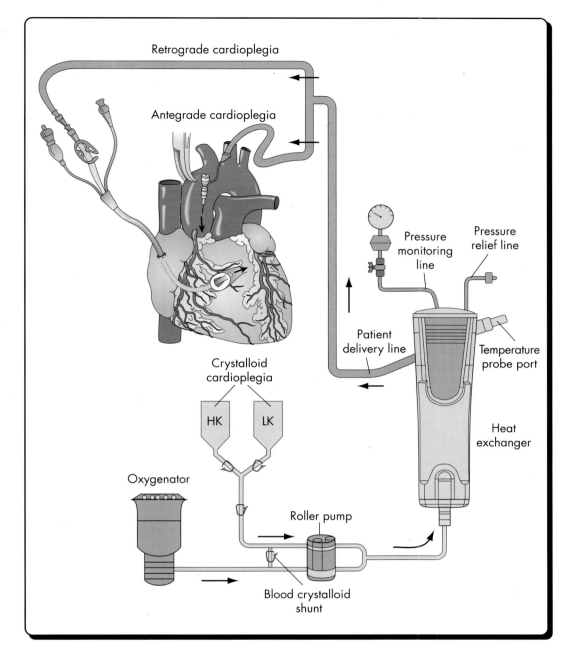

Figure 9-24. Cardioplegia delivery system. A modern cardioplegia delivery system is demonstrated. Oxygenated blood may be diverted from the oxygenator of the CPB circuit and mixed with a high potassium (HK)–containing crystalloid cardioplegia solution for induction of electromechanical arrest or with a low potassium (LK)–containing cardioplegia solution. The ratio of blood to crystalloid may be varied and the solution is pumped via a roller pump to a heat exchanger for warming or cooling before administration. The line pressure and temperature of the cardioplegia solution is monitored. Perfusion of the myocardium may be antegrade through the coronary arteries or retrograde through a catheter in the coronary sinus. The retrograde catheter is usually placed before CPB through the right atrial wall and into the coronary sinus. Evidence of successful cannulation of the coronary sinus includes dark blood (secondary to the high oxygen extraction of the heart) returning from the catheter, visualization of the catheter in the coronary sinus by transesophageal echocardiography, and intravascular pressure monitoring. During retrograde perfusion, a pressure of 30 to 50 mm Hg is desirable.

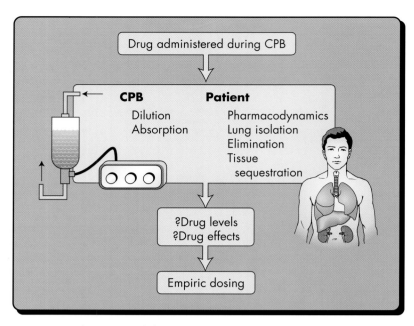

Figure 9-25. Drugs administered during CPB. Significant changes may occur in pharmacokinetics and pharmacodynamics of drugs administered during CPB [50]. With initiation of CPB the blood volume is rapidly diluted by the priming volume of the pump resulting in a reduction in total drug level. However, there is usually little change in nonprotein-bound drug (active form) concentration, likely due to a concurrent decrease in plasma proteins with hemodilution. Large amounts of drugs such as fentanyl, insulin, and nitroglycerin can be bound in vitro to oxygenators, plastic tubing, and other CPB equipment. However, there are large tissue stores available to replace lost drug and the amounts lost under normal clinical conditions are probably much lower than that observed in vitro. Hypothermia, electrolyte shifts, and an altered hormonal state may change the responsiveness of target organs to a given plasma concentration of a drug (pharmacodynamics). Basic drugs (fentanyl, propranolol) administered before CPB or during partial CPB may be "trapped" in the lung during total CPB when the lung is not perfused to be later released to the systemic circulation with resumption of ventilation and perfusion of the lung. Hypothermia (decreased enzymatic activity) and decreased hepatic and renal blood flow during CPB may significantly alter drug metabolism and excretion. Peripheral tissues that bind drug administered before CPB may be relatively poorly perfused during hypothermic cardiopulmonary bypass sequestering or "trapping" the drug until rewarming. Outcome studies have not demonstrated a "best" anesthetic technique for cardiac surgery with CPB and anesthetic agents may be administered by bolus or infusion during CPB. Opioids, benzodiazepines, propofol, and inhalational anesthetics (*eg,* isoflurane) administered via a temperature- and flow-compensating vaporizer placed in the gas inlet line to the oxygenator are frequently used during CPB. If nitrous oxide is used during the pre-bypass period, it should be discontinued prior to initiation of CPB. Nitrous oxide could enlarge air emboli that occur during CPB. It may be prudent to discontinue the volatile anesthetic prior to separation from CPB to minimize the potential for myocardial depression. The washout of isoflurane [51] is rapid (about 75% removed within 15 min) when the vaporizer is turned off during CPB.

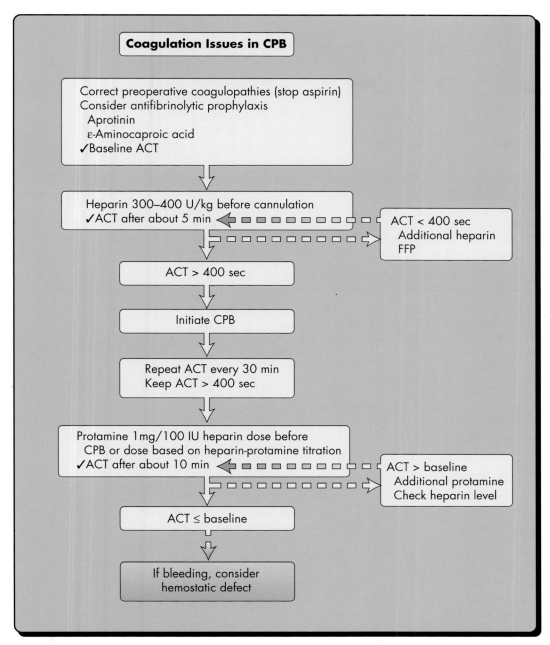

Coagulation Issues in CPB

Correct preoperative coagulopathies (stop aspirin)
Consider antifibrinolytic prophylaxis
  Aprotinin
  ε-Aminocaproic acid
✓Baseline ACT

↓

Heparin 300–400 U/kg before cannulation
✓ACT after about 5 min   ◄─ ▫▫▫▫▫▫▫▫▫▫ ── ACT < 400 sec
                         ─ ▫▫▫▫▫▫▫▫▫▫ ─➤ Additional heparin
                                          FFP

↓

ACT > 400 sec

↓

Initiate CPB

↓

Repeat ACT every 30 min
Keep ACT > 400 sec

↓

Protamine 1mg/100 IU heparin dose before
  CPB or dose based on heparin-protamine titration
✓ACT after about 10 min ◄─ ▫▫▫▫▫▫▫▫▫▫ ── ACT > baseline
                         ─ ▫▫▫▫▫▫▫▫▫▫ ─➤ Additional protamine
                                          Check heparin level

↓

ACT ≤ baseline

↓

If bleeding, consider
hemostatic defect

Figure 9-26. Coagulation issues in CPB. The biomaterial surface of the CPB circuitry is largely responsible for initiating thrombus formation without adequate anticoagulation. A simplified algorithm for anticoagulation and its reversal for the management of most cardiac surgical cases using CPB is shown. (See Chapter 10 for a complete discussion of coagulation issues). Cardiac surgery is performed safely in most patients receiving aspirin; however, operative blood loss and transfusion requirements may be increased. In high-risk patients (*ie*, redo operations), prophylactic antifibrinolytic prophylaxis should be considered in an attempt to decrease blood loss and transfusion requirements after CPB. After measuring a baseline activated coagulation time (ACT) and before cannulation, intravenous heparin should be administered to achieve an ACT greater than or equal to 400 seconds. If the ACT is not adequately prolonged by the initial dose of heparin (300 to 400 U/kg), additional heparin may be administered after considering technical reasons (mislabeled syringe, heparin not injected intravenously, reduced heparin activity) for the cause. Antithrombin III, the plasma factor necessary for heparin's anticoagulant effect, may be decreased (hereditary or acquired via preoperative administration of heparin) requiring the restoration of antithrombin III levels with transfusion of fresh-frozen plasma (FFP). Aprotinin prolongs the ACT as measured by celite activation method but the kaolin ACT is much less affected. Aprotinin should not be considered to have a heparin sparing action.

After the termination of CPB, anticoagulation is reversed by the administration of protamine which binds to heparin by an ionic interaction, inactivating it. The protamine dose is usually based on the initial dose of heparin before CPB or less frequently extrapolated from a previously constructed heparin dose-response curve [52]. An ACT value after protamine administration that remains abnormal may be due to incomplete heparin neutralization requiring more protamine, technical errors, or, less commonly, other hemostatic abnormalities. A heparin level, although infrequently performed, may detect residual unneutralized heparin.

ADULT VS PEDIATRIC CPB

Variable	Adult	Pediatric
Physiology		
Temperature, °C	≈ 28–37	15–37
Hemodilution	↑	↑↑–↑↑↑
Pump Flow, *mL/kg/min*	≈ 50–65	0–200
MAP, *mm Hg*	≥30	≥15–20
$PaCO_2$, *mm Hg*	≈ 30–40	≈ 20–80
CPB circuit		
Cannulation site		
Arterial	Aorta/femoral artery	Varies
Venous	Right atrium/femoral vein	Varies
Pump	Centrifugal > roller	Roller > centrifugal
Oxygenator	Membrane > bubble	Membrane >> bubble
Priming solutions	Crystalloid	Crystalloid/colloid/blood
Ultrafiltration	Useful	Very useful

Figure 9-27. Adult versus pediatric CPB. CPB techniques for infants and children differ significantly from adults [53]. A wide range of patient sizes and blood flow requirements precludes the standardization of pediatric perfusion circuitry. Infants and children have small circulating volumes, high oxygen consumption, and presence of congenital heart disease with shunts and aortopulmonary collateral circulation. They are exposed to biologic extremes, including temperature (*ie*, profound hypothermia), hemodilution (3 to 15 times that of an adult), low perfusion pressures, wide variations in perfusion flow rates (*ie*, from circulatory arrest to low-flow CPB to higher flow than adults at comparable temperatures) and lower $PaCO_2$ at deep and profound hypothermia when using alpha-stat management or increased $PaCO_2$ with pH-stat arterial blood gas pH management. Cannulation sites may vary depending on congenital heart disease anatomy. Because the ratio of priming volume to extracellular fluid volume is high, the priming solution for the pump frequently contains colloid solutions and blood. Ultrafiltration or hemoconcentration may be particularly useful in neonates and infants to reduce homologous blood transfusion, reduce pulmonary dysfunction after CPB, and improve cerebral blood flow and metabolism. Perfusion may be with a roller pump or centrifugal pump and oxygenation by either membrane or bubble oxygenators. Although there is a high degree of heterogeneity in clinical practice, membrane oxygenators and roller pumps may be used more frequently [18]. MAP—mean arterial pressure.

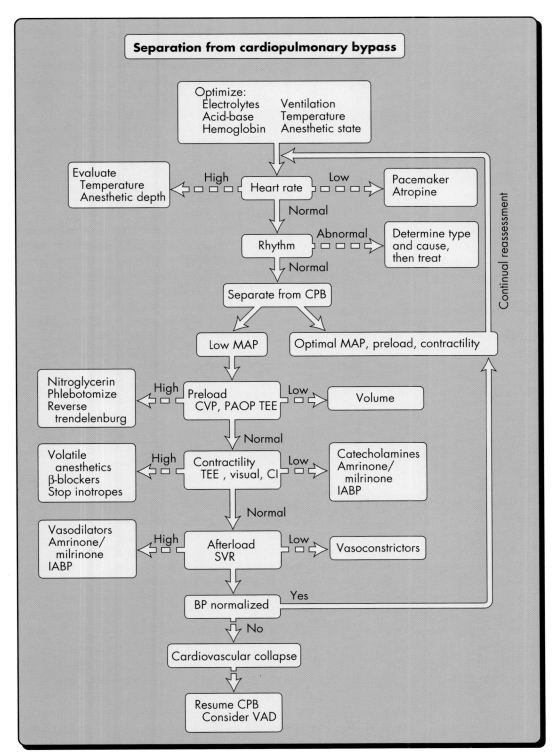

Figure 9-28. Algorithm for separation from CPB. Before separation from CPB, oxygenation, ventilation, oxygen-carrying capacity, metabolic factors, anesthetic state, and heart rate and rhythm should be optimized. Following separation from CPB, if mean arterial pressure (MAP) is low, preload, contractility, and afterload may need to be altered pharmacologically or otherwise to normalize the MAP. If the blood pressure cannot be normalized by these measures, cardiovascular deterioration is unresponsive to maximal inotropic therapy, and no immediate reversible cause can be identified, then reinstitution of CPB will be necessary and a ventricular-assist device (VAD) may be required. BP—blood pressure; CI—cardiac index; CVP—central venous pressure; PAOP—pulmonary artery occlusion pressure; SVR—systemic vascular resistance; TEE—transesophageal echocardiography. (*Adapted from* Bowering and Levy [53a]; with permission.)

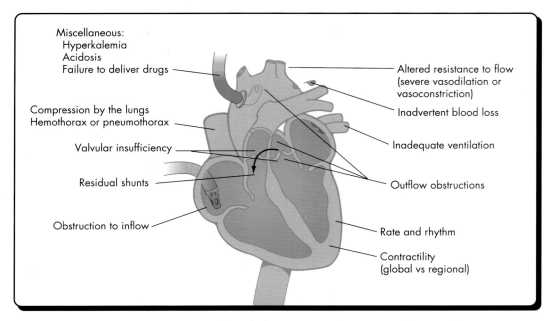

Figure 9-29. Factors that may result in failure to wean from CPB. The anesthesiologist should confirm adequacy of ventilation and oxygenation, correct metabolic factors (*eg*, hyperkalemia, acidosis), and confirm that inotropic drugs are being delivered intravascularly and at the desired dose. Transesophageal echocardiography (TEE) may be used to diagnose global or regional myocardial dysfunction. Potential etiologies of global myocardial dysfunction include inadequate myocardial protection, hyperkalemia, and administration of negative inotropes. If regional myocardial dysfunction is present, the possibility of inadequate myocardial perfusion through the graft(s) following coronary artery bypass graft surgery should be considered. Preload may be decreased secondary to inadvertent blood loss, obstruction to venous inflow from compression by the lungs and high peak airway pressures, and technical factors related to the venous cannula. Reduced preload may be suggested by a low central venous pressure, empty-appearing heart (seen on TEE or by visual inspection), or increased return to the venous reservoir via vents, suctions, or cannulas. Dysrhythmias, very low or high systemic vascular resistance, and residual shunts may cause difficulties. If the patient cannot be weaned from CPB after the potential causes have been addressed, CPB should be continued and mechanical support with an intra-aortic balloon pump (IABP) or ventricular assist device (VAD) may be required. (*Adapted from* Michelsen and Shanewise [54]; with permission.)

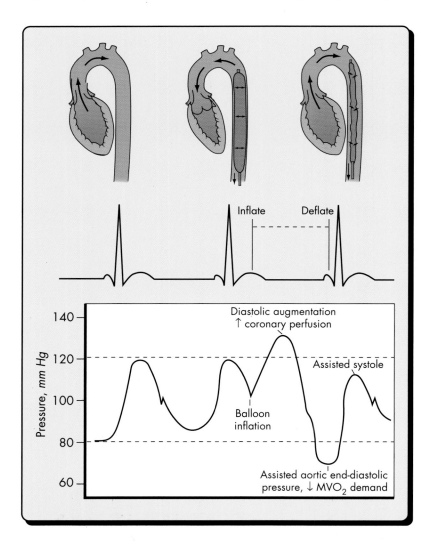

Figure 9-30. Intra-aortic balloon pump (IABP). Intra-aortic balloon counterpulsation with an IABP is the type of circulatory assistance most commonly used and is the first mechanical device that is employed to support but not take over the full function of the failing left ventricle. Anesthesiologists often encounter its use in patients who have difficulty separating from CPB. The balloon is usually placed via the femoral artery and positioned in the descending thoracic aorta just distal to the origin of the left subclavian artery. It is rapidly inflated at the beginning of diastole just after the aortic valve closes increasing volume in the aorta and hence, augmenting diastolic pressure and coronary perfusion pressure, thus potentially increasing coronary blood flow. The balloon is deflated during systole, reducing the volume and pressure in the aorta thereby reducing impedance to left ventricular (LV) ejection and systolic pressure. LV output is increased reducing residual volume in the left ventricle and LV end-diastolic pressure, which is reflected as a decrease in left atrial and pulmonary artery pressures, and myocardial oxygen consumption. If an IABP was placed preoperatively, pumping may be continued but at a decreased volume, stopped, or used to generate pulsatile flow in combination with a mechanical pump during CPB. If cardiopulmonary resuscitation with chest compressions becomes necessary with an IABP in place, the balloon may be left in the inflated position to act as an internal aortic occluder to potentially improve coronary and cerebral perfusion. The IABP is relatively contraindicated in patients with aortic regurgitation, aortic aneurysms, aorto- or aortoiliac grafts, aortoiliac occlusive disease, and sepsis.

SUGGESTED MANAGEMENT OF MASSIVE SYSTEMIC AIR EMBOLISM DURING CPB

1. Stop arterial pump immediately, and clamp both venous and arterial lines.
2. Place patient in the steep Trendelenburg position.
3. Remove aortic cannula and vent air out.
4. De-air arterial line and cannula.
5. Insert arterial cannula into SVC cannula (if one present and after excluding all air); otherwise into the SVC through a stab wound. Snare SVC cannula (if present; otherwise clamp SVC) between cannula and the right atrium and initiate retrograde SVC perfusion.
   a. Flow rate 1–2 L/min/70 kg
   b. Perfusate temperature 20°–24°C
   c. For 1–3 min or until no more froth is seen to egress from the aorta
   d. Anesthesiologist should temporarily compress the carotids during the later phase of retrograde perfusion (to purge air from vertebral system).
6. Resume antegrade hypothermic (20°–22°C), pulsatile (if available) perfusion for about 45 min at higher-than-usual pressure (high flow, vasoconstrictors, intermittent clamping of descending aorta for 2–3 min).
7. Express coronary air.
8. Consider retrograde IVC perfusion.
9. Consider giving the following:
   a. Methylprednisone, 2–4 g/70 kg
   b. Mannitol, 25 g
   c. Barbiturates (pentobarbital 10 mg/kg or pentothal 16 mg/kg)
   d. Low-molecular-weight dextran.
10. Maintain on 100% O_2 for at least 6 h postoperatively.
11. Initiate hyperbaric therapy, if available and patient's condition permits

Figure 9-31. Management of massive air embolism. A suggested strategy for the management of massive systemic air embolization during CPB is summarized. Massive air embolism is one of the most common adverse events associated with CPB (occurring in 1.2 per 1000 perfusions) and its occurrence is associated with a very high rate of permanent injury or mortality (about 25%) [8]. There are many possible sources of air emboli but half result from inattention to the venous reservoir with pumping of air directly into the aortic cannula. Factors that may decrease the incidence of air emboli include CPB circuit alarms, maintaining safe volume in the venous reservoir, use of centrifugal pumps, collapsible venous reservoirs, and arterial line filters or bubble traps. (*From* Hessel [55]; with permission.) IVC—inferior vena cava; SVC—superior vena cava.

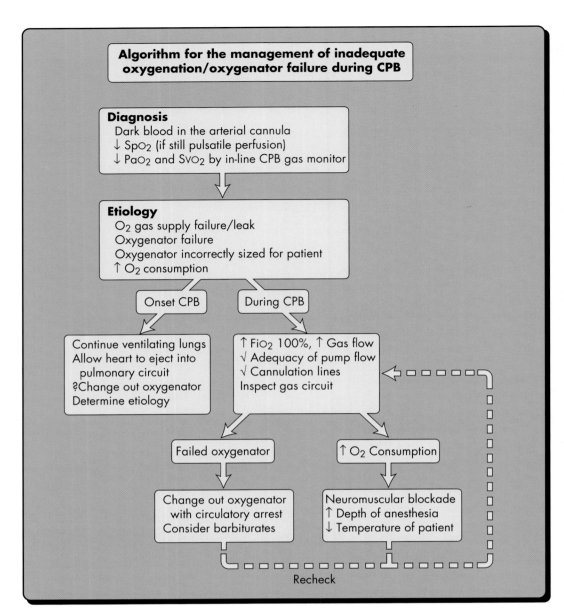

Algorithm for the management of inadequate oxygenation/oxygenator failure during CPB

Diagnosis
Dark blood in the arterial cannula
↓ SpO2 (if still pulsatile perfusion)
↓ PaO2 and SvO2 by in-line CPB gas monitor

Etiology
O2 gas supply failure/leak
Oxygenator failure
Oxygenator incorrectly sized for patient
↑ O2 consumption

Onset CPB | During CPB

Continue ventilating lungs
Allow heart to eject into pulmonary circuit
?Change out oxygenator
Determine etiology

↑ FiO2 100%, ↑ Gas flow
√ Adequacy of pump flow
√ Cannulation lines
Inspect gas circuit

Failed oxygenator | ↑ O2 Consumption

Change out oxygenator with circulatory arrest
Consider barbiturates

Neuromuscular blockade
↑ Depth of anesthesia
↓ Temperature of patient

Recheck

Figure 9-32. Algorithm for management of inadequate oxygenation during CPB. Inadequate oxygenation may be diagnosed by the visualization of dark blood in the arterial cannula, a low O_2 saturation by pulse oximetry if the patient's heart is still ejecting or pulsatile bypass is being used, or decreased PaO_2 and venous saturation values on an in-line CPB gas monitor on blood returning from the patient to the CPB machine. Potential etiologies include oxygenator failure, an oxygenator that is too small (inadequate surface area for gas exchange) for the patient, O_2 gas supply failure, or excessive O_2 consumption by the patient that might be secondary to muscle activity (shivering), increased temperature, or inadequate/light anesthesia. If this occurs at the onset of CPB before application of the aortic cross-clamp or administration of cardioplegia with ventricular standstill, continue ventilating the lungs, allow the heart to fill and eject into the pulmonary circuit, and determine the etiology of hypoxemia. If problems with oxygenation occur *during* CPB with the heart arrested, there may be little time to determine the etiology. Rapidly inspect the gas circuit for leaks, obstruction, or improper gas source; increase the FiO_2 to 100%; and check the cannulation lines and the adequacy of pump flow. If a failed oxygenator is the cause, it can be changed out in minutes with circulatory arrest. Hypothermic bypass may provide a margin of safety. Barbiturates may be administered just before circulatory arrest to reduce brain O_2 consumption and potentially provide a degree of cerebral protection. Inadequate oxygenation may be secondary to increased O_2 consumption by the patient. Shivering, increased temperature, and light anesthesia can increase O_2 requirements.

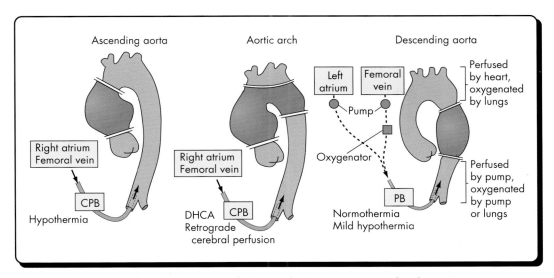

Figure 9-33. Circulatory support techniques during surgery on the thoracic aorta are shown. During repair of ascending aortic pathology, venous cannulation can usually be performed via the right atrium or occasionally the femoral vein. The arterial cannula may be placed in the upper ascending aorta if it is free of pathology, but is usually placed in the femoral artery. A proximal clamp for cardioplegia to the aortic root is not used if the aneurysm/dissection involves the proximal aorta or aortic valve. Hypothermic CPB is most commonly used although deep hypothermia and circulatory arrest are needed if the proximal arch is involved.

Repair of aortic arch pathology is usually accomplished with CPB and deep hypothermic circulatory arrest (DHCA) although individual cannulation and perfusion of cerebral vessels and retrograde perfusion of the brain via the internal jugular vein may occasionally be used. The proximal clamp is placed to arrest the heart and the distal clamp is placed at the time of circulatory arrest to isolate the arch so that the distal anastomosis can be performed. The middle clamp on the major aortic arch vessels allows en bloc attachment to the graft and is also placed at the time of circulatory arrest.

Although surgical management of descending and thoracoabdominal aortic pathology may include simple aortic cross-clamp or passive shunting (Gott shunt) with repair, CPB equipment may be used to provide distal aortic perfusion (partial bypass [PB]) with or without an oxygenator while the heart provides perfusion proximal to the aortic cross-clamp (without hypertension) with blood oxygenated by the lungs in an attempt to decrease the incidence of postoperative renal failure and paraplegia [56]. With atriofemoral bypass, blood oxygenated by the lungs is diverted from the left atria to the femoral artery via a centrifugal pump. Full anticoagulation is not required if an oxygenator is not used and the activated coagulation time (ACT) is usually maintained at about 200 seconds. Flow rates of 25 to 40 mL/kg/min are used although effective decompression of the left ventricle may occasionally require higher flow rates. With femoral vein to femoral artery bypass, blood from the femoral vein is oxygenated and pumped into the femoral artery. Similar flow rates and a distal perfusion pressure of 40 to 60 mm Hg appear adequate in most patients. Full anticoagulation and careful control of the venous return is required. Increased collection of blood in the reservoir (*ie*, reservoir level lowered) reduces inferior vena cava (IVC) flow and preload of the ventricle decreasing cardiac output, proximal aortic blood pressure, and upper body perfusion. If the venous line is clamped or the reservoir is elevated with decreased gravity drainage, IVC flow increases, filling the heart and increasing proximal aortic pressure. The lungs are continuously ventilated during either distal perfusion technique. (*Adapted from* Benumof [57]; with permission.)

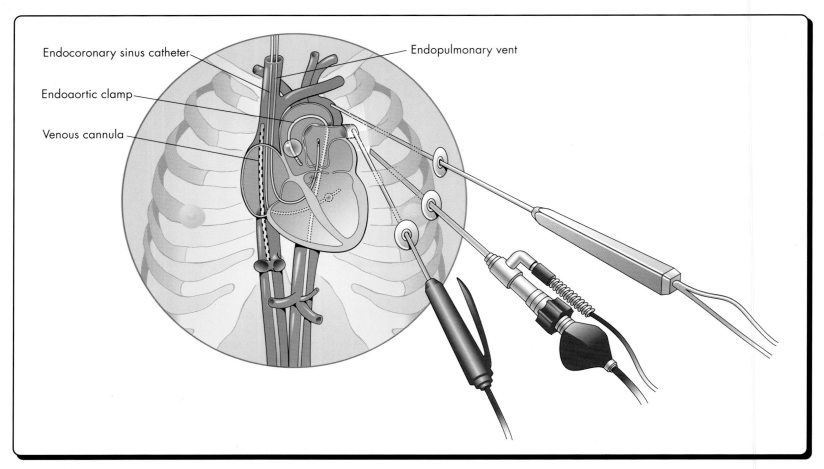

Endocoronary sinus catheter

Endoaortic clamp

Venous cannula

Endopulmonary vent

Figure 9-34. Endovascular CPB system. Minimally invasive surgical techniques have been developed to provide patients the benefits of open operations but with decreased pain and suffering. Endoscopic or "port-access" minimally invasive cardiac surgery [58] allows performance of CPB and myocardial protection with cardioplegic arrest without sternotomy or thoracotomy for coronary artery bypass graft surgery (and mitral valve replacement) but requires alterations in CPB techniques and the role of the anesthesiologist. This system uses femoral arterial and venous cannulation sites and femoral access for placement of an endoaortic balloon occlusion catheter. Using the internal jugular vein, the anesthesiologist inserts an endopulmonary vent into the main pulmonary artery using a balloon-tipped catheter and preshaped endocoronary sinus catheter into the coronary sinus facilitated by fluoroscopy, transesophageal echocardiography, and pressure waveforms. Cardioplegia delivery may be antegrade via the aorta or retrograde via the endocoronary sinus catheter. Aortic occlusion is accomplished via the endoaortic balloon catheter in the proximal ascending aorta. As with cardiopulmonary support systems, drainage from the venous cannula is augmented by a centrifugal pump.

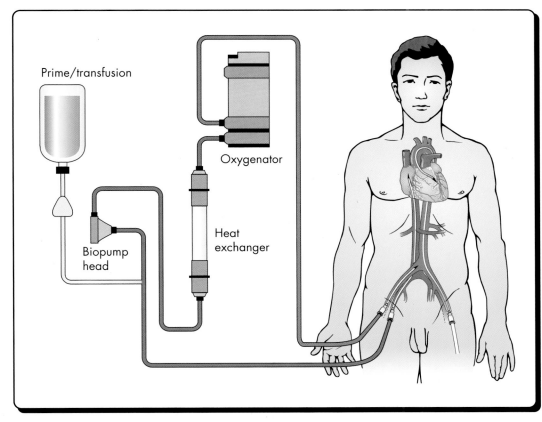

Prime/transfusion

Oxygenator

Heat
exchanger

Biopump
head

system. The blood is then warmed, oxygenated, and returned to the anticoagulated patient via the femoral artery in the presence of a heart that is still beating. CPS is occasionally used in a standby or prophylactic mode to provide systemic blood flow to supplement diminished left ventricular output anticipated during balloon inflation (coronary artery angioplasty, aortic valvotomy) in high-risk interventional cardiology procedures [59,60]. This system reduces preload and afterload and allows prolonged balloon inflations in critical coronary vessels. Unlike the intra-aortic balloon pump, CPS may effectively support the circulation in patients with severe dysrhythmias, profound ventricular dysfunction, or even cardiac arrest. It may also be used to support or provide systemic perfusion to patients who have suffered accidental hypothermia or massive pulmonary emboli and require hemodynamic assistance until initiation of some other assist device or transport to cardiac surgery and initiation of standard CPB following a failed interventional procedure. Patients with severe iliofemoral disease or an increased risk of severe bleeding complications due to concomitant anticoagulation are frequently excluded. Anesthesiologists may be consulted to provide sedation or general anesthesia for procedures using CPS.

Figure 9-35. Cardiopulmonary support (CPS) system. The CPS or "supported angioplasty" system differs from traditional cardiopulmonary bypass (CPB) systems in that blood is actively aspirated from the right atrium using a centrifugal pump rather than a gravity fill

REFERENCES

1. Lillehei CW: Historical development of cardiopulmonary bypass. In *Cardiopulmonary Bypass: Principles and Practice.* Edited by Gravlee GP, Davis RF, Utley JR. Baltimore: Williams & Wilkins; 1993:1.

2. Mora CT, ed: *Cardiopulmonary Bypass: Principles and Techniques of Extracorporeal Circulation.* New York: Springer-Verlag; 1995.

3. Gravlee GP, Davis RF, Utley JR, eds: *Cardiopulmonary Bypass: Principles and Practice.* Baltimore: Williams & Wilkins; 1993.

4. Casthely PA, Bregman D, eds: *Cardiopulmonary Bypass: Physiology, Related Complications, and Pharmacology.* Mount Kisco, NY: Futura; 1991.

5. Stammers AH, ed: Cardiopulmonary bypass: emerging trends and continued practice. *Int Anesthesiol Clin* 1996, 34(2):61–84.

6. Silvay G, Ammar T, Reich DL, et al.: Cardiopulmonary bypass for adult patients: A survey of equipment and techniques. *J Cardiothorac Vasc Anesth* 1995, 9:420–424.

7. Kurusz M, Conti VR, Arens JF, et al.: Perfusion accident survey. *Proc Am Acad Cardiovasc Perf* 1986, 7:57–65.

8. Gild WM: Risk management in cardiac anesthesia: the ASA closed claims project perspective. *J Cardiothorac Vasc Anesth* 1994, 8(1, suppl 1):3–6.

9. Lumb PD: Cardiopulmonary bypass: risk management concerns for the anesthesiologist. *J Cardiothorac Vasc Anesth* 1994, 8(1, suppl 1):7–9.

10. Reed CC, Kuruse M, Lawrence AE Jr., eds: In *Safety and Techniques in Perfusion* Stafford, TX: Quali-Med, Inc; 1992:123.

11. Bennett EV Jr, Fewel JG, Ybarra J, et al.: Comparison of flow differences among venous cannulas. *Ann Thorac Surg* 1983, 36:59–65.

12. Gravlee GP: Heparin-coated cardiopulmonary bypass circuits. *J Cardiothorac Vasc Anesth* 1994, 8:213–222.

13. Hsu L: Issues of biocompatibility: Heparin-coated extracorporeal circuit. *Int Anesthesiol Clin* 1996, 34:109–122.

14. Wheeldon DR, Bethune DW, Gill RD: Vortex pumping for routine cardiac surgery: a comparative study. *Perfusion* 1990, 5:135–143.

15. Driessen JJ, Fransen G, Rondelez L et al.: Comparison of the standard roller pump and a pulsatile centrifugal pump for extracorporeal circulation during routine coronary artery bypass grafting. *Perfusion* 1991, 6:303–311.

16. Voorhees ME, Brian BF: Blood-gas exchange devices. *Int Anesthesiol Clin* 1996, 34(2):29–45.

17. Fried DW: Performance evaluation of blood-gas exchange devices. *Int Anesthesiol Clin* 1996, 34(2):47–60.

18. Groom RC, Hill AG: Paediatric perfusion practice in North America: an update. *Perfusion* 1995, 10:393–401.

18a. Kane KM, Williams DR, Kurusz M: Cardiopulmonary circuits and design. In *A Practical Approach to Cardiac Anesthesia*, edn. 2. Edited by Hensley FA, Martin DE. Boston: Little, Brown; 1995:465–481.

19. Boonstra PW, Vermeulen FEE, Leusink JA, et al.: Hematological advantage of a membrane oxygenator over a bubble oxygenator in lung perfusion. *Ann Thorac Surg* 1986, 41:297–300.

20. Masters RG vs Bethune DW: Pro and con: Bubble oxygenators are outdated and no longer appropriate for cardiopulmonary bypass. *J Cardiothorac Anesth* 1989, 3:235–237.

21. Pearson DT: Gas exchange: Bubble and membrane oxygenators. *Semin Thorac Cardiovasc Surg* 1990, 2:313–319.

22. Utley JR, Leyland SA, Johnson HD, et al.: Correlation of preoperative factors, severity of disease, type of oxygenator and perfusion times with mortality and morbidity of coronary bypass. *Perfusion* 1991, 6:15–22.

23. Joffe D, Silvay G: The use of microfiltration in cardiopulmonary bypass. *J Cardiothorac Vasc Anesth* 1994, 8:685–692.

24. Lake CL: Controversies in the management of cardiopulmonary bypass. *Cardiothoracic and Vascular Anesthesia Updates* 1990, 1(ch. 9):1–21.

25. Konstadt SN, Reich DL, Kahn R, Biggiani RF: Transesophageal echocardiography can be used to screen for ascending aortic atherosclerosis. *Anesth Analg* 1995, 81:225–228.

26. Sutton RG: Renal considerations, dialysis, and ultrafiltration during cardiopulmonary bypass. *Int Anesthesiol Clin* 1996, 34:166–176.

27. Boldt J, Zickmann B, Fedderson B, *et al.*: Six different hemofiltration devices for blood conservation in cardiac surgery. *Ann Thorac Surg* 1991, 51:747–753.

27a. Nakamura Y, Masuda M, Toshima Y, *et al.*: Comparative Study of Cell Saver and Ultrafiltration Nontransfusion in Cardiac Surgery. *Ann Thorac Surg* 1990, 49:973–978.

28. Boldt J, Zickmann B, Czeke A, *et al.*: Blood conservation techniques and platelet function in cardiac surgery. *Anesthesiology* 1991, 75:426–432.

29. Naik SK, Elliott MJ: Ultrafiltration and pediatric cardiopulmonary bypass. *Perfusion* 1993, 8:101–112.

30. Feneck RO: Standards of monitoring. *J Cardiothorac Vasc Anesth* 1994, 8:379–381.

31. Cockroft S: Use of monitoring devices during anesthesia for cardiac surgery: a survey of practices at public hospitals within the United Kingdom and Ireland. *J Cardiothorac Vasc Anesth* 1994, 8:382–385.

32. Schell RM, Kern FH, Greeley WJ, *et al.*: Cerebral blood flow and metabolism during cardiopulmonary bypass. *Anesth Analg* 1993, 76:849–865.

33. Greeley WJ, Ungerleider RM, Kern FH, *et al.*: Effects of cardiopulmonary bypass on cerebral blood flow in neonates, infants, and children. *Circulation* 1989, 80(suppl I):I-209–I-215.

34. Govier AV, Reves JG, MeKay RD, *et al.*: Factors and their influence on regional cerebral blood flow during nonpulsatile cardiopulmonary bypass. *Ann Thorac Surg* 1984, 38:592–600.

35. Murkin JM, Farrar JK, Tweed WA, *et al.*: Cerebral autoregulation and flow/metabolism coupling during cardiopulmonary bypass: the influence of $PaCO_2$. *Anesth Analg* 1987, 66:825–832.

36. Newman MF, Croughwell ND, Blumenthal JA, *et al.*: Effect of aging on cerebral autoregulation during cardiopulmonary bypass: association with postoperative cognitive dysfunction. *Circulation* 1994, 90(suppl II):II-243–II-249.

37. Croughwell ND, Lyth M, Quill T, *et al.*: Diabetic patients have abnormal autoregulation during cardiopulmonary bypass. *Circulation* 1990, 82(suppl IV):407–412.

38. Mora Mangano, C: Cardiac surgery and central nervous system injury: The importance of hypothermia during cardiopulmonary bypass. In Neuroprotection. Edited by Blanck TJJ. *Society of Cardiovascular Anesthesiologists Monograph*; 1997:197–237.

39. Taylor CA: Surgical hypothermia. *Pharmacol Ther* 1988, 38:169–200.

40. Hindman BJ, Dexter F: Estimating brain temperature during hypothermia. *Anesthesiology* 1995, 82:329–330.

41. Mora CT, Henson MB, Weintraub WS, et al.: The effect of temperature management during cardiopulmonary bypass on neurologic and neuropsychologic outcomes in patients undergoing coronary revascularization. *J Thorac Cardiovasc Surg* 1996, 112:514–522.

42. Bashein G, Townes BD, Nessly ML, et al.: A randomized study of carbon dioxide management during hypothermic cardiopulmonary bypass. *Anesthesiology* 1990, 72:7–15.

43. Prough DS, Stump DA, Troost BT: $PaCO_2$ management during cardiopulmonary bypass: intriguing physiologic rationale, convincing clinical data, evolving hypothesis? *Anesthesiology* 1990, 72:3–6.

44. Swain JA, White FN, Peters RM: The effect of pH on the hypothermic ventricular fibrillation threshold. *J Thorac Cardiovasc Surg* 1984, 87:445–451.

45. Kirshbom PM, Skaryak LR, DiBernardo LR, et al.: pH-stat cooling improves cerebral metabolic recovery after circulatory arrest in a piglet model of aortopulmonary collaterals. *J Thorac Cardiovasc Surg* 1996, 111:147–157.

46. Hall RI, Stafford Smith M, Rocker G: The systemic inflammatory response to cardiopulmonary bypass: pathophysiological, therapeutic, and pharmacological considerations. *Anesth Analg* 1997, 85:766–782.

47. Moody DM, Bell MA, Challa VR, et al.: Brain microemboli during cardiac surgery or aortography. *Ann Neurol* 1990, 28:477–486.

48. Newman MF, Croughwell MD, Blumenthal JA, et al.: Predictors of cognitive decline after cardiac operation. *Ann Thorac Surg* 1995, 59:1326–1330.

49. Rosenkranz ER: Myocardial preservation. In *Cardiac Anesthesia*. Edited by Estafanous FG, Barash PG, Reves JG. Philadelphia: JB Lippincott; 1994:293–324.

49a. Buckberg GD: Recent Progress in Myocardial Protection During Cardiac Operations. In *Cardiac Surgery*, edn 2. Edited by McGoon DC. Philadelphia: FA Davis; 1987:291.

50. Rosow CE: Pharmacokinetic and pharmacodynamic effects of cardiopulmonary bypass. In *Cardiopulmonary Bypass*. Edited by Gravlee GP, Davis RF, Utley JR. Baltimore: Williams & Wilkins; 1993:207–232.

51. Henderson JM, Nathan JH, Lalande M, et al.: Washin and washout of isoflurane during cardiopulmonary bypass. *Can J Anaesth* 1988, 35:587–590.

52. Bull BS, Huse WN, Brauer FS, Korpman RA: Heparin therapy during extracorporeal circulation II: the use of a dose response curve to individualize heparin and protamine dosage. *J Thorac Cardiovasc Surg* 1975, 69:685–689.

53. Groom RC, Akl BF, Albus R, Lefrak EA: Pediatric cardiopulmonary bypass: a review of current practice. *Int Anesthesiol Clin* 1996, 34:141–163.

53a. Bowering J, Levy JH: The Postcardiopulmonary Bypass Period: Asystems Approach. In *A Practical Approach to Cardiac Anesthesia*, edn. 2. Hensley FA, Martin DE, eds. Boston: Little, Brown; 1995:232–245.

54. Michelson LG, Sharewise JS: Discontinuation of Cardiopulmonary Bypass. In *Cardiopulmonary Bypass*: Principles and Techniques of Extracorporeal Circulation. Edited by Mora C. New York: Springer-Verlag; 1995:281–297.

55. Hessel EA: Cardiopulmonary Bypass Equipment and Circulation Assist Devices. In *Cardiac Anesthesia*. Edited by Estafanous FG, Barash PG, Reves JG. Philadelphia: JB Lippincott; 1994:241–292.

56. O'Connor CJ, Rothenberg DM: Anesthetic considerations for descending thoracic aortic surgery: Part II. *J Cardiothorac Vasc Anesth* 1995, 9:734–747.

57. Benumof JF: Anesthesia for Emergency Thoracic Surgery. In *Anesthesia for Thoracic Surgery*. Edited by Benumof JL. Philadelphia: WB Saunders; 1987:375–404.

58. Stevens JH, Burdon TA, Peters WS: Port-access coronary artery bypass grafting: a proposed surgical method. *J Thorac Cardiovasc Surg* 1996, 111:567–573.

59. Urbanek P, Bock H, Vicol C: Percutaneous cardiopulmonary support (PCPS). *Cardiology* 1994, 84:216–221.

60. McErlean ES, Cross JA, Booth JE: Percutaneous cardiopulmonary bypass support: a new approach to high-risk angioplasty. *Crit Care Nurs Clin North Am* 1992, 4:347–357.

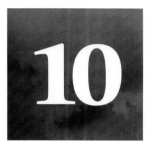

The Coagulation System and Cardiac Surgery

Thomas F. Slaughter

Nearly 45 years have elapsed since the first successful application of cardiopulmonary bypass (CPB) for cardiac surgery by Gibbon in 1953 [1]. During the interim, advances in surgical and anesthetic techniques, accompanied by increased understanding of the pathophysiology of extracorporeal circulation, have reduced the mortality associated with cardiac surgery to extraordinarily low levels. Despite these impressive accomplishments, however, excessive bleeding continues to frequently complicate otherwise successful cardiac surgery.

Management of hemostasis during CPB is complicated by the need to suppress coagulation during the period of extracorporeal circulation, and then rapidly reverse the process to achieve a normal hemostatic response immediately after completion of CPB. Although an effective anticoagulant in most situations, heparin has proved inadequate at eliminating extracorporeal-mediated thrombogenesis. In fact, within minutes of initiating CPB, each major component of the hemostatic system—plasma coagulation, platelet function, and fibrinolysis—has been adversely impacted by interactions between the blood and artificial surfaces of the CPB circuit.

Increasing recognition of complications, both infectious and immunologic, accompanying blood transfusions lends a sense of urgency to understanding the pathophysiologic mechanisms underlying the coagulopathy accompanying cardiac surgery. Given the rapid evolution of noninvasive surgical techniques, the long-term viability of CPB as an adjunct to cardiac surgery will likely be limited. However, insights gained from hemostatic research of CPB remains crucial to further progress in the technologies of hemodialysis, extracorporeal membrane oxygenation (ECMO), and biomaterials research. Recent advances in the understanding of hemostatic dysfunction at the molecular level suggest that effective countermeasures to the physiologic trespass of extracorporeal circulation will be attainable in the near future.

PHYSIOLOGY OF NORMAL HEMOSTASIS

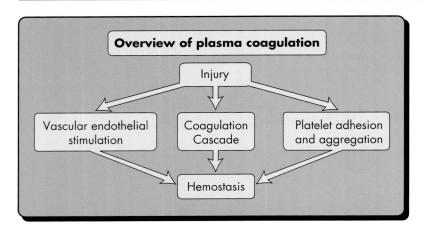

Figure 10-1. Overview of plasma coagulation. The normal hemostatic reaction to a vascular injury involves an integrated response among plasma coagulation proteins, platelets, and the vascular endothelium culminating in the formation of a stable hemostatic plug.

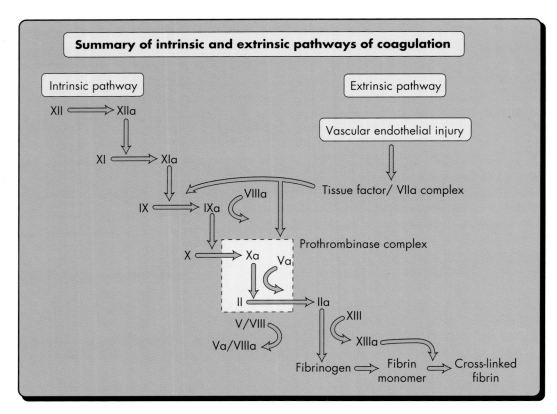

Figure 10-2. Intrinsic and extrinsic pathways of coagulation. Plasma coagulation consists of intrinsic and extrinsic components, each of which is capable of activating the common pathway to generate fibrin clot [2]. Intrinsic and extrinsic pathways converge to activate factor X, thereby initiating the common pathway. Factor Xa converts prothrombin (factor II) to thrombin, and thrombin converts fibrinogen to fibrin clot. Cofactors Va and VIIIa are essential to formation of coagulation factor activation complexes that accelerate clot formation. The importance of these cofactors is perhaps best evidenced by an example of nature: deficiency of factor VIII results in the bleeding disorder, hemophilia A. (*From* Slaughter [3]; with permission.)

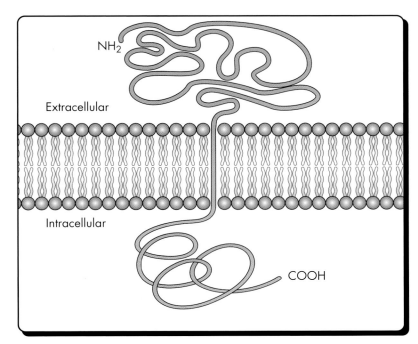

Figure 10-3. Structure of tissue factor. Tissue factor is an integral membrane lipoprotein with intracellular, transmembrane, and extracellular domains [4]. Under normal conditions, tissue factor is not expressed by tissues in contact with the plasma. However, vascular endothelial cells and monocytes may be induced to express tissue factor by inflammatory mediators such as thrombin and endotoxin. Recent evidence suggests that tissue factor and the extrinsic pathway of coagulation are the primary mediators of *in vivo* coagulation [5]. The intrinsic pathway of coagulation appears to amplify and propagate the coagulation process after initiation by tissue factor. (*Adapted from* Nemerson [6]; with permission.)

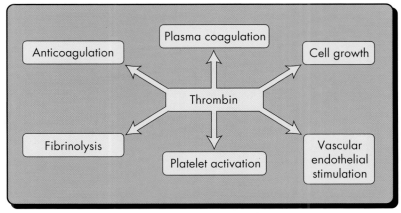

Figure 10-4. Physiologic roles of thrombin. Thrombin generation represents the key regulatory step in the hemostatic process. In addition to the recognized role of generating fibrin clot from fibrinogen, thrombin also activates platelets and provides a positive feedback mechanism to activate factor XI, factor XIII, and cofactors V and VIII. Furthermore, thrombin interacts with the vascular endothelium to express tissue factor [7] and to release von Willebrand factor and plasminogen activator inhibitor-1 (PAI-1) [8]. In addition to these procoagulant functions, thrombin simultaneously down-regulates clot formation by inducing the release of tissue plasminogen activator (t-PA) [9], prostacyclin (PGI$_2$), and nitric oxide [10], from vascular endothelial cells. Also, thrombin binds thrombomodulin on the vascular endothelium, leading to activation of the anticoagulant, protein C [11]. Finally, thrombin is a potent mitogen, resulting in the migration and growth of vascular smooth muscle cells.

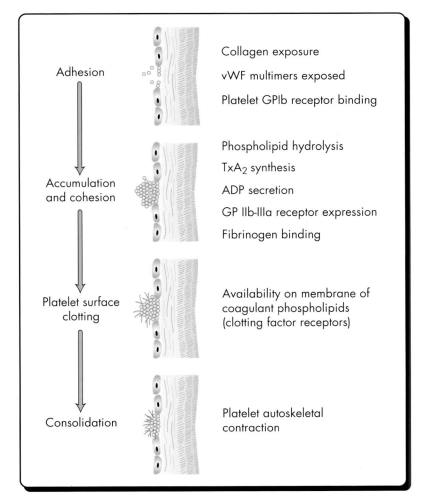

Figure 10-5. Overview of the platelet response in coagulation. The platelet plays a crucial role in clot formation by delivering hemostatically active proteins to the site of thrombosis, by adding to the structural integrity of the clot, and by providing a phospholipid surface on which plasma coagulation may occur. A typical response to vascular injury, with exposure of the extracellular matrix, would begin with platelet adhesion to exposed collagen [12]. Interaction of the platelet with collagen results in platelet activation, with the biochemical formation and release of hemostatically active proteins. Thromboxane (Tx) and adenosine diphosphate (ADP) released from adhering platelets attract and activate additional platelets, leading to the accumulation of a platelet mass [13]. Structural changes on the platelet surface provide a phospholipid template on which activation complexes assemble to generate fibrin and form an interconnected platelet fibrin clot [14]. Finally, contraction of the platelet cytoskeleton begins the process of consolidation and resolution of the clot. GP—glycoprotein; vWF—von Willebrand factor. (*Adapted from* Rappaport [15]; with permission.)

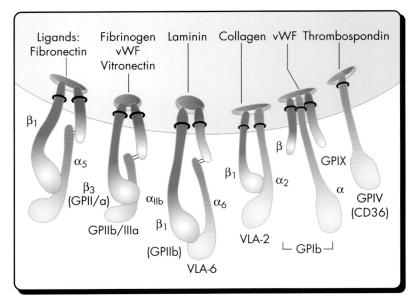

Figure 10-6. Platelet surface receptors. The platelet surface contains a variety of glycoprotein receptors, each of which binds a distinctive set of substrate ligands. Each receptor subtype varies in number from a few hundred to several thousand receptor sites per platelet. Glycoprotein surface receptors are essential for normal adhesion and activation of the platelet [16]. Activation of the platelet generally occurs after an agonist binds to a specific surface receptor triggering the activation of membrane-bound guanosine triphosphate-binding proteins and initiating an intracellular cascade culminating in the activation of numerous intracellular phosphorylases and proteases. GP—glycoprotein; VLA—very late antigens. (*From* Hawiger [17]; with permission.)

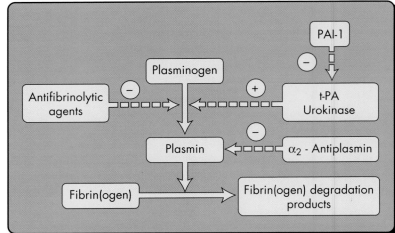

Figure 10-7. Overview of fibrinolysis. The fibrinolytic system characterizes the biochemical process by which the fibrin clot is degraded *in vivo*. The proteolytically active mediator of fibrinolysis is the enzyme plasmin. Under normal conditions, tissue plasminogen activator (t-PA) released from the vascular endothelium activates plasminogen to form plasmin [18]. A second plasminogen activator, urokinase, is generated by the urinary tract; however, this pathway accounts for only a small fraction of the fibrinolytic activity present in plasma. Each step in the fibrinolytic pathway is regulated by specific inhibitory proteases. Plasminogen activator inhibitor-1 (PAI-1) inhibits the activity of both t-PA and urokinase. PAI-1, an acute-phase reactant, is released from both the α-granules of platelets and the vascular endothelium. The major inhibitor of plasmin is the serine protease inhibitor (serpin), α_2-antiplasmin. Both t-PA and plasmin are relatively resistant to inhibition when bound to fibrin; this characteristic, as well as the presence of high plasma concentrations of protease inhibitors, limits the propagation of fibrinolytic activity beyond the clot. (*From* Slaughter [3]; with permission.)

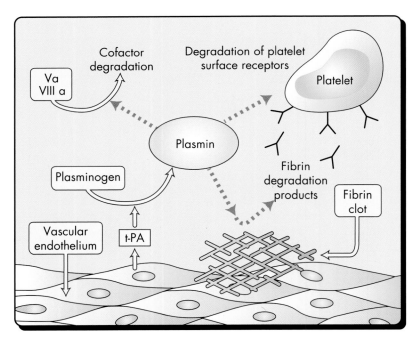

Figure 10-8. The effects of fibrinolysis on hemostasis. In addition to degradation of the fibrin clot itself, plasmin acts to suppress clot formation by a number of additional mechanisms. Fibrin degradation fragments act as anticoagulants by suppressing both fibrin polymerization and platelet aggregation. Furthermore, the protease-sensitive domain of platelet glycoprotein receptors is susceptible to plasmin degradation, resulting in loss of the receptor. Both of the cofactors, Va and VIIIa, are susceptible to proteolytic degradation by plasmin [19]. Loss of the cofactors limits the formation of membrane-bound activation complexes, thereby suppressing plasma coagulation. t-PA—tissue plasminogen activator.

PATHOPHYSIOLOGIC EFFECTS OF CARDIOPULMONARY BYPASS ON HEMOSTASIS

ADVERSE HEMOSTATIC EFFECTS OF CPB

Coagulation factors

Hemodilution
Protein denaturation
Deposition onto extracorporeal surfaces
Hypothermia
Consumptive coagulopathy

Fibrinolysis

Vascular endothelial (t-PA) release

Platelet dysfunction

Quantitative deficiencies
   Hemodilution
   Hepatic sequestration
Qualitative deficiencies
   Activation and clearance
   Fibrinolytic degradation of surface receptors

Figure 10-9. Cardiopulmonary bypass (CPB) circuit. Multiple components of the CPB circuit contribute to hemostatic dysfunction following cardiac surgery [20]. Mixing of the patient's blood with the crystalloid priming volume during initiation of CPB results in hemodilution of plasma proteins and platelets. Artificial surfaces of the CPB circuit, oxygenator membranes, and arterial line filters bind plasma proteins, including fibrinogen, resulting in subsequent fibrin generation and platelet adhesion and activation. The air-fluid interfaces associated with the cardiotomy suction and reservoir result in protein denaturation and further activation of coagulation. Finally, cooling during the period of CPB impairs the activity of both coagulation enzymes and platelets. LV—left ventricular. (*From* High and coworkers [21]; with permission.)

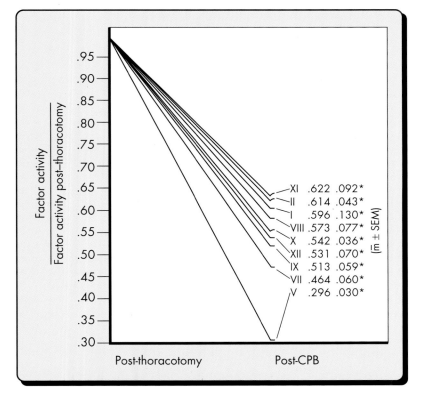

Figure 10-10. Reductions in plasma coagulation factors following cardiopulmonary bypass (CPB). Significant reductions in plasma concentrations of coagulation proteins occur with initiation of CPB. Hemodilution accounts for the major portion of these declines; however, adhesion of proteins to the artificial surfaces of the CPB circuit and consumption of coagulation factors resulting from activation of coagulation contribute. The reduction in plasma concentrations of coagulation factors rarely achieves levels traditionally associated with increased bleeding risk, and no correlation has been noted between reductions in coagulation factors during CPB and postoperative bleeding [22]. (*From* Kalter and coworkers [23].)

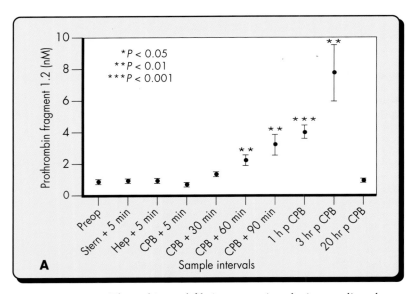

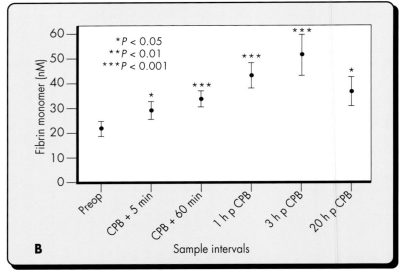

Figure 10-11. Thrombin and fibrin generation during cardiopulmonary bypass (CPB). **A,** Prothrombin fragment 1.2 (F1.2) is an activation peptide generated during the formation of thrombin. Despite the administration of relatively large concentrations of heparin before initiation of CPB, both thrombin and fibrin continue to be generated throughout the period of CPB [24]. One explanation for this finding is the limited efficacy of heparin to inhibit thrombin bound to fibrin. **B,** The development of specific thrombin inhibitors may provide a more effective means to inhibit activation of coagulation during cardiac surgery [25]. (*From* Slaughter and coworkers [24]; with permission.)

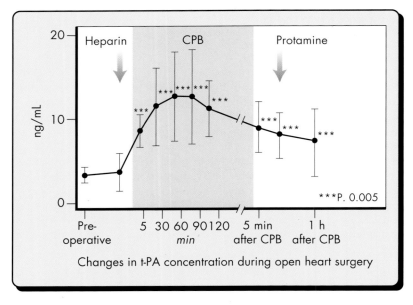

Figure 10-12. Generation of tissue plasminogen activator (t-PA) during cardiopulmonary bypass (CPB). Although the mechanism remains unclear, CPB is associated with increased release of t-PA from the vascular endothelium [26]. As many as two-thirds of patients experience increased fibrinolytic activity during CPB, with rapid resolution of the fibrinolytic state following the completion of surgery [27]. Thrombin stimulates vascular endothelial release of t-PA [28], and the failure to suppress thrombin generation during CPB may contribute to perioperative fibrinolysis. (*From* Tanaka and coworkers [29]; with permission.)

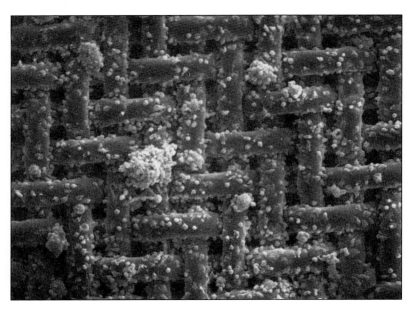

Figure 10-13. Activation of platelets during cardiopulmonary bypass (CPB). Fibrinogen, bound to the artificial surfaces of the CPB circuit, provides innumerable substrate binding sites for platelet adhesion and activation. Considerable evidence exists to suggest that activation of platelets occurs during CPB [30]. In fact, one investigation using flow cytometric techniques demonstrated that as many as 29% of total circulating platelets are in an activated state during CPB [31]. Prior to clearance from the circulation, activated platelets provide a phospholipid surface on which plasma coagulation may be propagated. (Electron micrograph of arterial filter following CPB.) (*From* Kurusz asnd Butler [32]; with permission.)

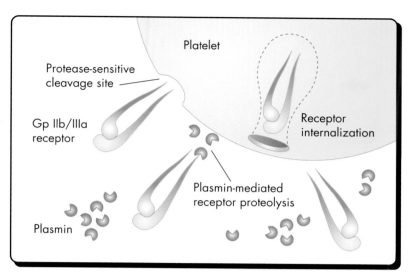

Figure 10-14. Loss of platelet surface receptors during cardiopulmonary bypass (CPB). The extracellular portion of platelet surface receptors contains protease-sensitive domains susceptible to plasmin-mediated cleavage. Evidence exists to suggest that platelet surface receptors are down-regulated during CPB [33]. Whether this results from internalization of the receptor or protease-mediated degradation of the receptor remains unclear. Some authors have postulated that fibrinolytic degradation of platelet receptors may account for platelet dysfunction following CPB. However, other investigations suggest that platelet biochemical pathways and platelet surface receptors are unaffected by CPB and that platelet dysfunction associated with CPB results from extrinsic factors in the platelets' environment, such as heparin [34]. This remains a controversial subject, and the mechanisms underlying platelet dysfunction during CPB will require further investigation. GP—glycoprotein.

PHARMACOLOGIC MANIPULATION OF COAGULATION

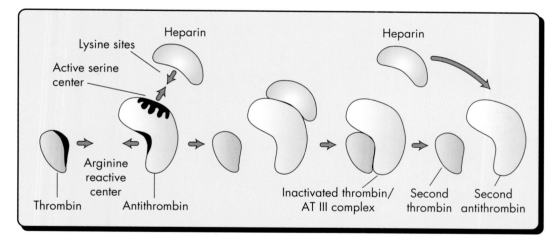

Figure 10-15. Biochemical structure of heparin. Heparin is comprised of heterogeneous sulfated mucopolysaccharide chains containing alternating subunits of uronic acid and glucosamine [35]. Unfractionated commercial heparin is obtained by the purification of bovine lung or porcine intestinal mucosa, and contains heparin molecules with molecular weights ranging from approximately 3000 to 35,000 D. The pharmokinetic and anticoagulant properties of heparin vary depending on the molecular weight of the constituent molecules. (*From* Rosenberg and Bauer [36]; with permission.)

Figure 10-16. Mechanism of action of heparin. Heparin acts as a catalyst to promote the anticoagulant activity of the antithrombin molecule [37]. Heparin binds antithrombin producing a conformational change which facilitates the binding of antithrombin to select serine proteases involved in coagulation. The heparin–antithrombin III (AT III) complex irreversibly inactivates factors IXa, Xa, XIa, and XIIa. Heparin also catalyzes the inhibition of thrombin by way of heparin cofactor II, although the *in vivo* importance of this reaction remains unclear. Following inactivation of the serine protease, heparin is released to catalyze additional antithrombin molecules.

Figure 10-17. Variables affecting physiologic response to heparin.

VARIABLES AFFECTING PHYSIOLOGIC RESPONSE TO HEPARIN

Pharmacokinetic variables

Age
Sex
Weight

Pharmacodynamic variables

Plasma protein concentrations
    Antithrombin
    Platelet factor 4
    Histidine-rich glycoprotein
Ongoing thrombosis
Heparin-associated antibodies

Figure 10-17. Variables affecting physiologic response to heparin.

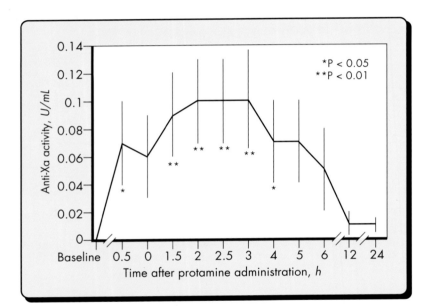

*P < 0.05
**P < 0.01

Figure 10-18. Heparin rebound. Heparin rebound refers to the condition in which anticoagulant activity recurs following apparently successful neutralization of heparin at the conclusion of cardiopulmonary bypass (CPB). This figure demonstrates the recurrence of heparin activity, as measured by anti-Xa activity, in the hours following completion of CPB. Administration of blood from the CPB circuit following protamine administration is a common mechanism for recurrence of heparin anticoagulation in the postoperative period. Recent evidence suggests a more subtle mechanism for heparin rebound relating to the molecular heterogeneity of unfractionated heparin. Release of heparin bound to plasma proteins occurs at variable times during the postoperative period dependent upon the binding affinity associated with specific heparin molecules [38]. Heparin activity, resulting from release of protein-bound heparin, has been observed as long as 6 hours after heparin neutralization. (*From* Teoh and coworkers [38]; with permission.)

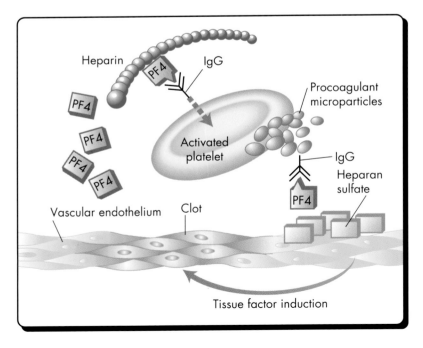

Figure 10-19. Heparin-associated thrombocytopenia. A subset of patients with prior heparin exposure develop antibodies to a protein complex comprised of heparin and platelet factor 4 (PF4) [39]. Reexposure of these patients to heparin may result in the formation of immune complexes that are capable of activating platelets [40] and stimulating vascular endothelial tissue factor expression [41]. Despite the frequent occurrence of thrombocytopenia in these patients, bleeding complications rarely occur. These patients are at particular risk for arterial thrombotic complications and all sources of heparin, including heparin-bonded vascular catheters, must be meticulously avoided in this patient population [42]. (*From* Slaughter and Greenberg [42]; with permission.)

ALTERNATIVE ANTICOAGULANTS FOR THE PATIENT WITH HEPARIN-ASSOCIATED ANTIBODIES

Drug	Source	Chemical structure	Mechanism of action	Cross-reactivity with heparin antibodies
Low-molecular-weight heparins	Porcine and bovine mucosa extract; synthetic	Glycosaminoglycans; mean MW 4–6.5 kD	Inhibits factor Xa > thrombin	Yes; 90%
Heparinoid	Porcine mucosa extract	Mixture of heparan, dermatan, and chondroitin sulfates	Inhibits factor Xa > thrombin	Yes; 10%
Ancrod	Malayan pit viper venom extract	"Thrombin-like" enzyme	Proteolysis of fibrinogen	No
Argatroban	Synthetic	Arginine analogue	Thrombin active site inhibitor	No
Hirudin	Leech salivary gland extract	66-amino-acid polypeptide	Thrombin active site inhibitor	No
Hirulog	Synthetic	Hirudin-derived peptide	Thrombin active site inhibitor	No
Iloprost	Synthetic	Prostacyclin analogue	Adenylyl cyclase activator	No; limited anticoagulant efficacy
Aspirin	Synthetic	Acetylsalicylic acid	Cyclooxygenase inhibitor	No; limited anticoagulant efficacy

Figure 10-20. Alternative anticoagulants to heparin. (*From* Slaughter and Greenberg [42]; with permission.)

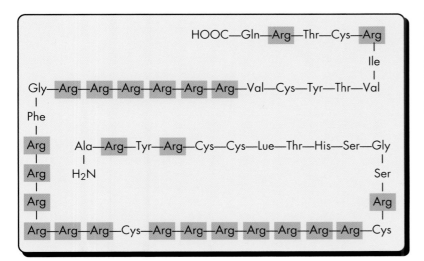

Figure 10-21. Structure of protamine. Protamine is a highly cationic protein, derived from the purification of salmon sperm, with the ability to neutralize the anticoagulant activity of heparin. The mechanism of inhibition is that of a simple acid-base reaction. The highly anionic nature of heparin, attributable to the predominance of sulfated side-groups, results in a "salting out" reaction. (*From* Horrow [43]; with permission.)

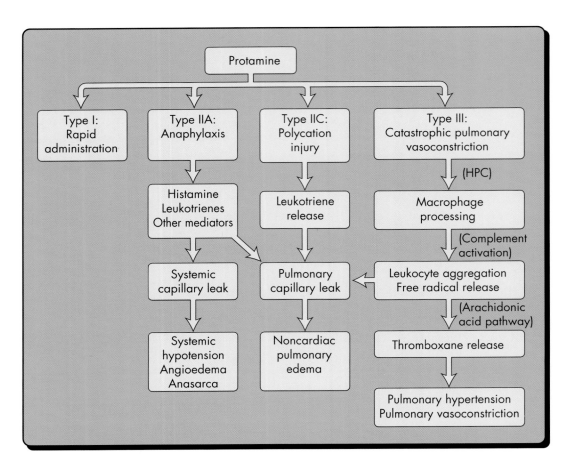

Figure 10-22. Adverse reactions associated with protamine. Adverse reactions associated with protamine administration are generally one of three types [44]. First, rapid administration of protamine results in vasodilation. Vasodilation in this setting has traditionally been attributed to cationic displacement of histamine from mast cells. However, recent evidence suggests that nitric oxide generation, resulting from protamine interactions with the vascular endothelium, may play a contributory role [45]. A second type of reaction results from anaphylactoid responses in patients hypersensitized to protamine or protamine-like molecules [46]. Finally, catastrophic pulmonary vasoconstriction rarely has been described in patients receiving protamine. The mechanism underlying this reaction remains unclear, but may involve alterations in prostanoid metabolism within the pulmonary vasculature [47]. Slow administration of protamine appears useful in limiting the incidence of hypotension associated with heparin neutralization. Several alternative agents for the neutralization of heparin are currently in clinical trials. HPC—heparin protamine complexes. (*From* Horrow [48]; with permission.)

Figure 10-23. Alternatives to administration of protamine.

ALTERNATIVES TO PROTAMINE

Forego heparin neutralization—associated with increased bleeding
Platelet factor 4—clinical trials ongoing
Heparinase—clinical trials ongoing
Hexadimethrine—potential renal toxicity

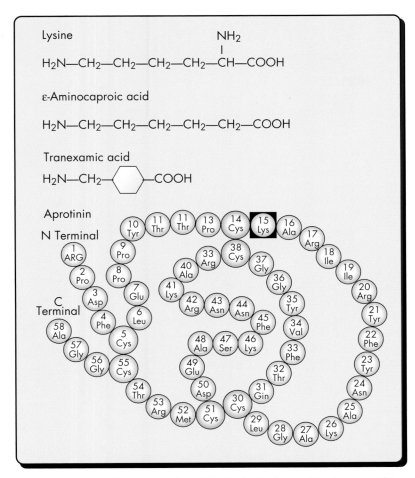

Lysine

$$H_2N\text{---}CH_2\text{---}CH_2\text{---}CH_2\text{---}CH_2\text{---}\overset{\overset{\displaystyle NH_2}{\displaystyle |}}{CH}\text{---}COOH$$

ε-Aminocaproic acid

$$H_2N\text{---}CH_2\text{---}CH_2\text{---}CH_2\text{---}CH_2\text{---}CH_2\text{---}COOH$$

Tranexamic acid

$$H_2N\text{---}CH_2\text{---}\bigcirc\text{---}COOH$$

Aprotinin

N Terminal

C Terminal

Figure 10-24. Structure of antifibrinolytic drugs. To date, antifibrinolytic drugs have proved the most effective hemostatic agents available for use in patients undergoing cardiac surgery. Randomized prospective trials demonstrate 30% to 50% reductions in bleeding in patients receiving antifibrinolytics before initiation of cardiopulmonary bypass [49]. ε-Aminocaproic acid and tranexamic acid are synthetic lysine analogues that inhibit the generation of plasmin as well as the binding of plasmin to the fibrin clot. Aprotinin is a broad-spectrum serine protease inhibitor that directly binds and inhibits plasmin, kallikrein, and a variety of other serine proteases. (*Modified from* Horrow [48].)

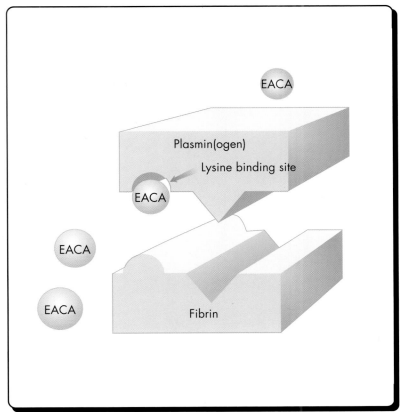

Figure 10-25. Mechanism of action of the synthetic antifibrinolytic drugs. The synthetic antifibrinolytic drugs interact at lysine binding sites within plasmin [50]. Binding of plasmin to fibrin is competitively inhibited, thereby limiting fibrinolytic degradation of the clot. The synthetic antifibrinolytics also interfere with the binding of plasminogen to fibrin, a necessary precursor step in the synthesis of plasmin. EACA—ε-aminocaproic acid. (*From* Slaughter [3]; with permission.)

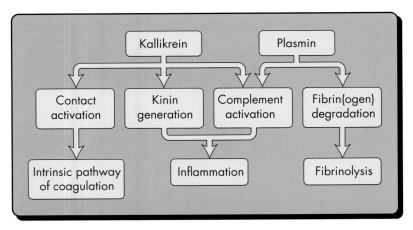

Figure 10-26. Mechanism of action of aprotinin. In addition to direct inhibition of plasmin and the fibrinolytic pathway, aprotinin impairs a number of additional protease-mediated pathways that may contribute to inflammatory events associated with cardiac surgery [51]. Inhibition of kallikrein, a component of the contact activation complex, may contribute to reductions in complement and cell activation in the postoperative period. Recent evidence further suggests that aprotinin administration may be associated with reductions in thrombin and fibrin generation in patients undergoing cardiac surgery [52]. Clearly, inhibition of the intrinsic pathway, as mediated by kallikrein, interferes with monitoring heparin anticoagulation by both the activated coagulation time and the activated partial thromboplastin time.

MONITORING ANTICOAGULATION DURING CARDIAC SURGERY

Functional measures of coagulation
  ACT
  High-dose thrombin time
  Heparin management test
Monitoring heparin concentration
  Automated heparin-protamine titration
Viscoelastic measures of coagulation
  Thromboelastogram
  Sonoclot

Figure 10-27. Monitoring anticoagulation during cardiac surgery. Currently available point-of-care instruments suitable for monitoring heparin anticoagulation in the perioperative setting may be broadly considered to fall into one of three categories. Functional measures of coagulation, *eg,* the activated coagulation time (ACT) [53], measure the time necessary for a sample of whole blood to form a clot. Generally, a contact activator of coagulation such as celite or kaolin is contained within the sample collection chamber to speed the time to clot formation. The major advantage of the functional measures of coagulation is that they provide an assessment of a particular patient's ability to form a clot in whole blood at the time of the test. In con-trast, heparin-protamine titration tests exploit the fact that protamine directly inhibits heparin, on a milligram for milligram basis, to calculate the heparin concentration present in a sample of whole blood [54]. The advantage of these systems is that extraneous factors such as hemodilution, temperature, or aprotinin therapy do not significantly affect determination of heparin concentration. Maintenance of a pre-calculated heparin concentration during cardiopulmonary bypass has been suggested to provide a better method of suppressing thrombin generation in this setting [55]. However, one must consider that heparin-protamine titration provides no data regarding the patient's intrinsic ability to form a clot. For example, the use of heparin-prota-mine titration following administration of heparin to a patient with antithrombin deficiency will indicate that a normal heparin concentra-tion has been achieved; however, functional measures of coagulation performed concurrently would demonstrate that the patient has not achieved an anticoagulated state.

Viscoelastic monitors of coagulation constitute the least widely used measure for monitoring anticoagulation during cardiac surgery. Viscoelastic instruments provide a global measure of clot formation in whole blood from the initiation of clotting to subsequent lysis of the clot [56]. Viscoelastic monitors provide a unique real-time measure of fibrinolysis, and there is some evidence to suggest that these monitors are useful in differentiating surgical bleeding from a coagulopathy fol-lowing cardiac surgery [57]. However, the qualitative component of the data interpretation and the failure of viscoelastic measures to cor-relate with more standardized laboratory-based tests of coagulation have limited acceptance of this form of monitoring.

LIMITATIONS OF CURRENTLY AVAILABLE MONITORS

Monitor	Ease of use	Functional measure of anticoagulation	Cost
ACT	+	Yes	$
HiTT	–	Yes	$$
HMT	+	Yes	$$
Automated prota-mine titration	±	No (Heparin concentration)	$$$
Viscoelastic methods	–	Yes	$$$

Figure 10-28. Limitations of currently available monitors. ACT—activated coagu-lation time; HiTT—high-dose thrombin time; HMT—heparin management test.

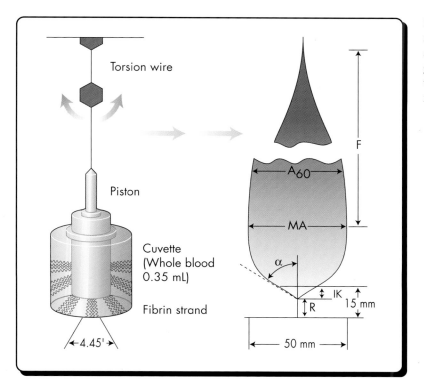

Figure 10-29. Structural components of the thromboelastogram and normal measured parameters. α—α angle, 40°–60°; A60—amplitude after 60 min; A60/MA—whole blood clot lysis index, greater than 0.85; F—whole blood clot lysis time, > 300 min; K—3 to 7 min; MA—maximum amplitude; R—reaction time, 7.5 to 15 min. (*From* Tuman and coworkers [58]; with permission.)

REFERENCES

1. Gibbon JH Jr: Application of a mechanical heart and lung apparatus to cardiac surgery. *Minn Med* 1954, 37:171.

2. Furie B, Furie BC: Molecular and cellular biology of blood coagulation. *N Engl J Med* 1992, 326:800–806.

3. Slaughter TF: The coagulation system and cardiac surgery. In *Cardiac Anesthesia: Principles and Clinical Practice*. Edited by Estafanous FG, Barash PG, Reves JG, *et al*. Philadelphia: JB Lippincott; 1994:621–633.

4. Camerer E, Kolsto, Prydz H: Cell biology of tissue factor, the principal initiator of blood coagulation. *Thromb Res* 1996, 81:1–41.

5. Gailani D, Broze GJ: Factor XI activation in a revised model of blood coagulation. *Science* 1991, 253:909–912.

6. Nemerson Y: The tissue factor pathway of blood coagulation. In *Hemostasis and Thrombosis: Basic Principles and Clinical Practice*, edn 3. Edited by Colman RW, Hirsh J, Marder VJ, Salzman EW. Philadelphia: JB Lippincott; 1994:81–93.

7. Bartha K, Brisson C, Archipoff G, *et al*.: Thrombin regulates tissue factor and thrombomodulin mRNA levels and activities in human saphenous vein endothelial cells by distinct mechanisms. *J Biol Chem* 1993, 268:421–429.

8. Gelehrter TD, Sznycer-Laszuk R: Thrombin induction of plasminogen activator inhibitor in cultured endothelial cells. *J Clin Invest* 1986, 77:165–169.

9. Levin EG, Marzec U, Anderson J, Harker LA: Thrombin stimulates tissue plasminogen activator release from cultured human endothelial cells. *J Clin Invest* 1984, 74:1988–1995.

10. DeMey JG, Claeys M, Vanhoulte PM: Endothelium-dependent inhibitory effects of acetylcholine, adenosine triphosphate, thrombin and arachidonic acid in the canine femoral artery. *J Pharmacol Exp Ther* 1982, 222:166–173.

11. Esmon CT: The roles of protein C and thrombomodulin in the regulation of blood coagulation. *J Biol Chem* 1989, 264:4743–4746.

12. Weiss H: Platelet physiology and abnormalities of platelet function. Parts 1 and 2. *N Engl J Med* 1975, 293:531–541:580–588.

13. Kroll MH, Schafer AI: Biochemical mechanisms of platelet activation. *Blood* 1989, 74:1181–1195.

14. Kalafatis M, Swords NA, Rand MD, *et al*.: Membrane-dependent reactions in blood coagulation: role of the vitamin K–dependent enzyme complexes. *Biochim Biophys Acta* 1994, 1227:113–129.

15. Rappaport SI: *Introduction to Hematology*, edn 2. Philadelphia: JB Lippincott; 1987:439.

16. George JN, Shattil SJ: The clinical importance of acquired abnormalities of platelet function. *N Engl J Med* 1991, 324:27–39.

17. Hawiger J: Adhesive interactions of blood cells and the vascular wall. In *Hemostasis and Thrombosis: Basic Principles and Clinical Practice*, edn 3. Edited by Colman W, Hirsh J, Marder VJ, Salzman EW. Philadelphia: JB Lippincott; 1994:762–796.

18. Vassalli JD, Sappino AP, Belin D: The plasminogen activator/plasmin system. *J Clin Invest* 1991, 88:1067–1072.

19. Omar MN, Mann KG: Inactivation of factor Va by plasmin. *J Biol Chem* 1987, 262:9750–9755.

20. Woodman RC, Harker LA: Bleeding complications associated with cardiopulmonary bypass. *Blood* 1990, 76:1680–1697 .

21. High KM, Williams DR, Kurusz M: Cardiopulmonary bypass circuits and design. In *The Practice of Cardiac Anesthesia*, edn 2. Edited by Hensley Jr FA, Martin DE. Boston: Little, Brown; 1995:468.

22. Gelb AB, Roth RI, Levin J, *et al*.: Changes in blood coagulation during and following cardiopulmonary bypass: lack of correlation with clinical bleeding. *Am J Clin Pathol* 1996, 106:87–99.

23. Kalter RD, Saul CM, Wetstein L, *et al*.: Cardiopulmonary bypass: associated hemostatic abnormalities. *J Thorac Cardiovasc Surg* 1979, 3:427–435.

24. Slaughter TF, LeBleu TH, Douglas Jr, JM, *et al*.: Characterization of prothrombin activation during cardiac surgery by hemostatic molecular markers. *Anesthesiology* 1994, 80:520–526.

25. Weitz JI, Hudoba M, Massel D, *et al*.: Clot-bound thrombin is protected from inhibition by heparin-antithrombin III but is susceptible to inactivation by antithrombin III-independent inhibitors. *J Clin Invest* 1990, 86:385–391.

26. Stibbe J, Kluft C, Brommer EJP, *et al*.: Enhanced fibrinolytic activity during cardiopulmonary bypass in open-heart surgery in man is caused by extrinsic (tissue-type) plasminogen activator. *Eur J Clin Invest* 1984, 14:375–382 .

27. Chandler WL, Fitch JCK, Wall MH, *et al.*: *Thromb Haemost* 1995, 74:1293–1297.

28. Levin EG, Marzec U, Anderson J, *et al.*: Thrombin stimulates tissue plasminogen activator release from cultured human endothelial cells. *J Clin Invest* 1984, 74:1988–1995.

29. Tanaka K, Takao M, Yada I, *et al.*: Alterations in coagulation and fibrinolysis associated with cardiopulmonary bypass during open heart surgery. 1989, 3:181–188.

30. George JN, Picket EB, Saucerman S, *et al.*: Platelet surface glycoproteins: studies on resting and activated platelets and platelet microparticles in normal subjects and observations in patients during adult respiratory distress syndrome and cardiac surgery. *J Clin Invest* 1986, 78:340–348.

31. Rinder CS, Bohnert J, Rinder HM, *et al.*: Platelet activation and aggregation during cardiopulmonary bypass. *Anesthesiology* 1991, 75:388–393.

32. Kurusz M, Butler BD: Embolic events and cardiopulmonary bypass. In *Cardiopulmonary Bypass: Principles and Practice*. Edited by Gravlee GP, Davis RF, Utley JR. Baltimore: Williams & Wilkins; 1993:280.

33. Musial J, Niewiarowski S, Hershock D, *et al.*: Loss of fibrinogen receptors from the platelet surface during simulated extracorporeal circulation. *J Lab Clin Med* 1985, 105:514–522.

34. Kestin AS, Valeri RC, Khuri SF, *et al.*: The platelet function defect of cardiopulmonary bypass. *Blood* 1993, 82:107–117.

35. Hirsh J: Heparin. *N Engl J Med* 1991, 324:1565–1574.

36. Rosenberg RD, Bauer KA: Prothrombinase generation and the regulation of coagulation. In *Thrombosis and Hemorrhage*. Edited by Loscalzo J, Schafer AI. Boston: Blackwell Scientific Publications; 1994:25.

37. Pratt CW, Church FC: Antithrombin: structure and function. *Semin Hematol* 1991, 28:3–9.

38. Teoh KHT, Young E, Bradley CA, *et al.*: Heparin binding proteins: contribution to heparin rebound after cardiopulmonary bypass. *Circulation* 1993, 88(part 2):420–425.

39. Amiral J, Bridey F, Dreyfus M, *et al.*: Platelet factor 4 complexed to heparin is the target for antibodies generated in heparin-induced thrombocytopenia. *Thromb Haemost* 1992, 68:95–96.

40. Warkentin TE, Hayward PCM, Boshkov LK, *et al.*: Sera from patients with heparin-induced thrombocytopenia generate platelet-derived microparticles with procoagulant activity: An explanation for the thrombotic complications of heparin-induced thrombocytopenia. *Blood* 1994, 11:3691–3699.

41. Cines DB, Tomaski A, Tannenbaum S: Immune endothelial-cell injury in heparin-associated thrombocytopenia. *N Engl J Med* 1987, 316:581–589.

42. Slaughter TF, Greenberg CS: Heparin-associated thrombocytopenia and thrombosis: implications for perioperative management. *Anesthesiology* 1997, 87:667–675.

43. Horrow J: Management of coagulation and bleeding disorders. In *Cardiac Anesthesia*, edn 3. Edited by Kaplan J. Philadelphia: WB Saunders; 1993:951–994.

44. Horrow JC: Protamine allergy. *J Cardiothorac Anesth* 1988, 2:225–242.

45. Raikar GV, Kisamochi K, Raikar BL: Nitric oxide inhibition attenuates systemic hypotension produced by protamine. *J Thorac Card Surg* 1996, 111:1240–1246.

46. Weiss ME, Nyhan D, Peng Z, *et al.*: Association of protamine IgE and IgG antibodies with life-threatening reactions to intravenous protamine. *N Engl J Med* 1989, 320:886–892.

47. Montalescot G, Lowenstein E, Ogletree ML, *et al.*: Thromboxane receptor blockade prevents pulmonary hypertension induced by heparin-protamine reactions in awake-sheep. *Circulation* 1990, 82:1765–1777.

48. Horrow JC: Heparin reversal of protamine toxicity: have we come full circle? *J Cardiothorac Anesth* 1990, 4:539–542.

49. Slaughter TF, Greenberg CS: Antifibrinolytic drugs and perioperative hemostasis. *Am J Hematol* 1997, 56:32–36.

50. Hoylaerts M, Lijnen HR, Collen D: Studies on the mechanism of antifibrinolytic action of tranexamic acid. *Biochim Biophys Acta* 1981, 673:75–85.

51. Royston D: High-dose aprotinin therapy: a review of the first five years' experience. *J Cardiothorac Vasc Anesth* 1992, 6:76–100.

52. Dietrich W, Dilthey G, Spannagl M, *et al.*: Influence of high-dose aprotinin on anticoagulation, heparin requirement, and celite- and kaolin-activated clotting time in heparin-pretreated patients undergoing open-heart surgery. *Anesthesiology* 1995, 83:679–689.

53. Hattersly PC: Activated coagulation time of whole blood. *JAMA* 1966, 196:436.

54. Perkins HA, Osborn JJ, Hurt R, *et al.*: Neutralizing of heparin *in vivo* with protamine: a simple method of estimating the required dose. *J Lab Clin Med* 1956, 48:223–226.

55. Despotis GJ, Joist JH, Hogue CW, *et al.*: More effective suppression of hemostatic system activation in patients undergoing cardiac surgery by heparin dosing based on heparin blood concentrations rather than ACT. *Thromb Haemost* 1996, 76:902–908.

56. Tuman KJ, Spiess BD, McCarthy RJ, *et al.*: Comparison of viscoelastic measures of coagulation after cardiopulmonary bypass. *Anesth Analg* 1989, 69:69–75.

57. Spiess BD, Tuman KJ, McCarthy RJ, *et al.*: Thromboelastography as an indicator of post-cardiopulmonary bypass coagulopathies. *J Clin Monit* 1987, 3:25–30.

58. Tuman KJ, Spiess BD, McCarthy RJ, *et al.*: Effects of progressive blood loss on coagulation as measured by thromboelastography. *Anesth Analg* 1987, 66:856–863.

Postoperative Intensive Care of the Cardiothoracic Patient

Andrew K. Hilton and Christopher C. Young

Postoperative intensive care of the cardiothoracic patient encompasses a variety of surgical procedures, each with unique potential problems and management strategies. It is not possible to describe completely the spectrum of intensive care support required for all cardiothoracic patients. The emphasis here is on adult cardiac surgery, as cardiac patients with or without ischemic heart disease represent the majority of admissions to the cardiothoracic intensive care. The common postoperative problems and their management are addressed.

To some extent postoperative intensive care management is a continuation of intraoperative care and many of the problems that were identified intraoperatively may remain to be managed in the postoperative period. However, the patient's postoperative course also represents a complex interaction between the patient's presenting illness and associated comorbidities and the consequences and complications of surgery, anesthesia, and cardiopulmonary bypass. A continuum of expected physiologic changes occurs even in the apparently uncomplicated patient; these must be understood and deviations from the norm recognized.

Respiratory and cardiac abnormalities following cardiac surgery are common. Most patients are ventilated for at least 4 to 6 hours postoperatively, although this varies depending on the patient, procedure performed, and the institutional practice. These patients may be extubated uneventfully, but abnormal lung mechanics and gas exchange persist for at least several days. This predisposes some patients to further respiratory complications and prolongs their stay in the intensive care unit. Common postoperative cardiovascular events temporally range from the nadir of reversible myocardial dysfunction and vasodilation associated with rewarming, to atrial tachyarrhythmias on postoperative day 2 or 3. At any time less frequent but more serious problems, such as the various causes of low cardiac output syndrome and perioperative myocardial infarction, can occur. Although many monitoring and diagnostic modalities are available, early identification and characterization of these problems still remains a challenge to any physician.

Minor reversible changes occur in most organ systems following cardiac surgery and cardiopulmonary bypass. For example, coagulation abnormalities; fluid, electrolyte, and acid-base derangements; and slight elevation of liver function tests are nearly always demonstrable. When clinically significant, these organ system complications have an cumulative impact on postoperative mortality. Unfortunately, postoperative stroke, acute renal failure, and major gastrointestinal complications are not rare. No uniformly adopted or unequivocally proved preventive strategies have been defined, and postoperative management is often just supportive.

Models for the assessment of perioperative risk have been proposed and may allow better quantification of the risks of surgery, as well as use of perioperative resources. Risk assessment facilitates the stratification of patients for "fast track" surgery. Given present economic constraints, the need to decrease the length of the patient's stay in the intensive care unit has been emphasized and can result in substantial cost savings. The thrust of this approach has been through early extubation and the performance of postoperative care according to predefined care maps.

However, preoperative risk prediction alone ignores the dynamic changes associated with intraoperative events and the patient's postoperative clinical behavior. The patient's risk assessment must be continuous throughout the perioperative period so that deviations from the expected path can be recognized and the patient's care altered accordingly. This recognition, as well as the performance of all aspects of postoperative intensive care, are best achieved when the clinician understands and anticipates the temporal pattern and extent of the normal postoperative pathophysiologic changes.

ASSESSMENT AND MONITORING

PATIENT ASSESSMENT ON ARRIVAL AT THE ICU

Assessment Area	Information Gained
Demographic data	Patient name, age, and brief history
Surgery	Operation performed
	Problems encountered
Anesthesia	Anesthetic agents
	Problems encountered
	Airway anatomy and difficulty
	Size of endotracheal tube
	Access to central circulation and difficulty
	Available peripheral venous access
Cardiopulmonary bypass	Problems encountered
	CPB time
	Aortic cross-clamp time
	Events during weaning off CPB
Respiratory management	Tidal volume, rate, and F_{IO_2}
	Most recent ABG values
	Plans for awakening and extubation
Cardiovascular management	Hemodynamic monitoring used
	Rate, rhythm, blood pressure, and CO
	Optimal filling pressures
	Current vasoactive drug infusions and titration plans
	Pacemaker and antiarrhythmic drugs
Fluid and electrolyte management	Fluid and blood products administered
	Urine output
	Hematocrit, potassium, base deficit, and pH
	Availability of blood products
Perioperative antibiotics	Type, last dose, planned dosing schedule

Figure 11-1. Assessment of the cardiothoracic patient in the intensive care unit (ICU). Postcardiac surgery ICU management is often predicted by the events occurring in the operating room. The immediate problems to be addressed in the ICU may be the same as those that occurred in the operating room and the strategies to deal with them may have already been explored and defined. Hence, continuing care in the ICU is optimized by a succinct, relevant perioperative history, taking into account pertinent surgical, anesthetic, and cardiopulmonary bypass (CPB) procedures and events. ABG—arterial blood gases; CO—cardiac output. (*Adapted from* Higgins and coworkers [1]; with permission.)

ICU ADMISSION INVESTIGATIONS AND TESTS

Test	Information Gained
Physical examination and bedside assessment	
Auscultation of breath sounds	Exclude endobronchial intubation, pneumo/hemothorax, pulmonary edema.
Auscultation of heart sounds	Assess presence of new murmurs, prosthetic valve function; subsequent muffling may indicate tamponade.
Palpation of peripheral pulses	May provide rapid assessment of CO/SV; absence may indicate acute arterial pathology dissection and/or occlusion especially if IABP present.
Degree of peripheral vasoconstriction	Assessment of perfusion adequacy of CO; staging of rewarming.
Level of anesthetic depth	Guide to timing of extubation; awake but paralyzed patient may cause hemodynamic perturbation.
Chest tube drainage	Bleeding/hemostatic defects; may indicate need for surgical exploration.
Core body temperature	Adequacy of CO.
Chest x-ray	Assess position of endotracheal tube, central lines/hemodynamic catheters, nasogastric tubes, etc., and any related complications. Exclude pneumo/hemothorax. Changes to width of mediastinum. Presence of atelectasis, pulmonary edema.
12-Lead ECG	Record baseline changes for later comparison. Diagnosis of arrhythmias and perioperative infarction.
Blood Chemistry	
Arterial blood gases	Adequacy of gas exchange and ventilator management. Acid-base status.
Mixed venous blood gases	Calibrate oximetric PA catheter if used; assessment of adequacy of peripheral gas exchange and perfusion.
Electrolytes	Abnormalities to K, Mg, and Ca common and may need to be corrected.
BUN and creatinine	Assess perioperative renal function.
Glucose	Abnormalities, especially hyperglycemia common; may require further management.
Complete blood count	Assess hemodilution; provide guide to correcting anemia and/or thrombocytopenia, if indicated.
Coagulation profile	Laboratory coagulation abnormalities common after CPB; may provide guide to treatment if clinical coagulation abnormalities present.

Figure 11-2. After cardiac surgery a range of biochemical and hematologic tests, as well as a chest radiograph and electrocardiogram (ECG) are performed in order to quantify expected perturbations (eg, changes to hematocrit) and to exclude any complications associated with surgery, anesthesia, and cardiopulmonary bypass (CPB). Many of these tests are repeated at regular intervals, depending on the patient's condition and institutional practice. However, it should not be forgotten that the most immediate information at hand is that disclosed by a directed physical examination, which in some circumstances (eg, hypoxia associated with right mainstem bronchus intubation) may direct the performance of critical measures before any definitive investigations can be performed (eg, chest radiograph). BUN—blood urea nitrogen; CO—cardiac output; IAPB—intra-aortic balloon pulsation; PA—pulmonary artery; SV—stroke volume.

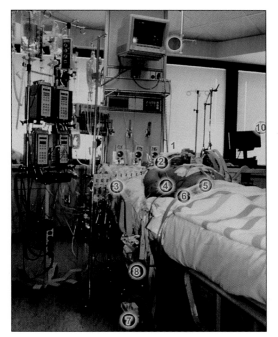

Figure 11-3. Patient monitoring in the intensive care unit. Monitoring of the postcardiac surgery patient is usually a direct continuation of that used intraoperatively. The monitors used depend on the patient's perioperative cardiorespiratory status and events, as well as institutional practice. Indicated in the figure are the common monitoring modalities and other machines attached to the patient. 1) Endotracheal tube with end-tidal CO_2 monitor; 2) central venous access via sheath introducer—in this case, a pulmonary artery catheter is present for measurement of central venous pressure, pulmonary artery pressure, pulmonary artery wedge pressure, cardiac output, and core temperature; 3) transducers for measurement of central pressures, as well as for radial arterial line for direct measurement of systemic pressure; 4) pacemaker box attached to epicardial leads; 5) mediastinal and pleural drainage tubes attached to 7) drainage/suction system; 6) pulse oximeter; 8) urinary catheter and collection system; 9) monitor screen for display of continuous electrocardiography, respiratory and hemodynamic measurements and waveforms; 10) ventilator monitoring screen for display of ventilatory parameters and respiratory mechanics.

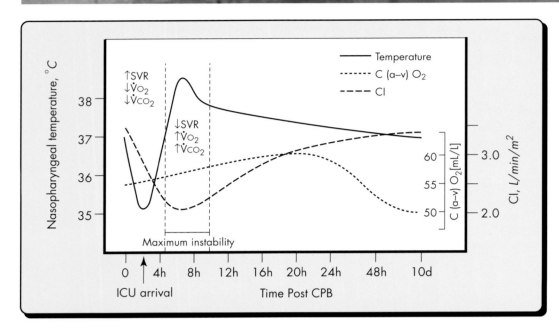

Figure 11-4. Overview of pathophysiology following cardiac surgery. Key to the management of the post–cardiac surgery patient is an understanding of the evolution of the "normal" pathophysiologic changes that accompany cardiopulmonary bypass. Not only is this important in the way it directs the management of the routine patient but it also allows identification of possible life-threatening deviations from the expected course. Subsequent management can then be altered accordingly. Of particular note is the instability associated with the first 6 to 8 hours, a time associated with rewarming and possible temperature overshoot, vasodilatation, impaired gas exchange, and the nadir of cardiac function. $C(a-v)_2$—arterial-venous oxygen content difference; CI—cardiac index. (*Adapted from* Sladen [2]; with permission.)

RESPIRATORY CHANGES

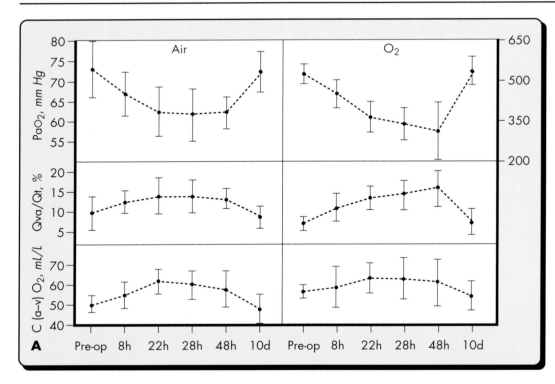

Figure 11-5. Respiratory changes following cardiopulmonary bypass (CPB). Impairment in the efficiency of pulmonary gas exchange is a common and expected sequelae to CPB. **A,** Changes are seen in arterial oxygen tension (PaO$_2$), venous admixture, or intrapulmonary shunt ($\dot{Q}va/\dot{Q}t$), and arteriovenous oxygen content difference, from preoperative values through the early postoperative period and on to postoperative day 10. Note that these changes often continue beyond a week postoperatively.

(*Continued on next page*)

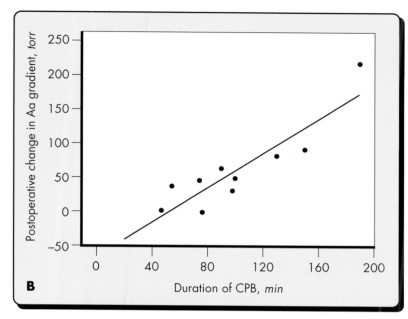

B

Figure 11-5. (*Continued*) B, Relationship is shown between the severity of postoperative respiratory dysfunction (as measured by alveolar-arterial oxygen gradient, P[A-a]o$_2$) and the duration of CPB. The causes of these changes are probably multifactorial, but changes in lung volume and subsequent $\dot{V}/\dot{Q}$ mismatching are strongly implicated. The role of pulmonary endothelial dysfunction secondary to bypass-induced "systemic inflammatory response" remains to be fully defined. (Panel A *from* Kirklin and Barratt-Boyes [3]; with permission; panel B *from* MacNaughton and coworkers [4]; with permission.)

CAUSES OF POSTOPERATIVE RESPIRATORY DYSFUNCTION

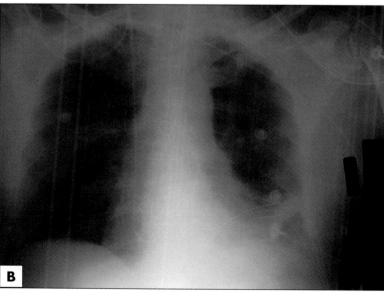

Impaired gas exchange
  Intrapulmonary shunt (low $\dot{V}/\dot{Q}$ units)
    Atelectasis
    Pulmonary edema
    Infection
  Extrapulmonary shunt
    Cyanotic congenital heart disease
  Alveolar dead space (high $\dot{V}/\dot{Q}$ units)
    Hypovolemia
    Excessive PEEP
    Decreased pulmonary blood flow
    Pulmonary embolism
Decreased central respiratory drive
  General anesthesia
  Opioid analgesia
  Perioperative cerebral insult
Decreased respiratory muscle function
  Pain (incision, chest tubes)
  Persistent neuromuscular blockade
  Obesity
  Age
  Decreased respiratory muscle perfusion secondary to decreased
    cardiac output
  Phrenic nerve injury
Exacerbation of chronic lung disease
  Increase in airway resistance
  Increased secretions
  Pneumonia/acute bronchitis

Figure 11-6. Causes of postoperative respiratory dysfunction. The causes of post–cardiac surgery respiratory dysfunction are multifactorial. The most significant causes in any particular instance are related to the presence and interaction of preoperative respiratory disease with the effects of anesthesia and surgery on respiratory mechanics and gas exchange, the duration of cardiopulmonary bypass, and subsequent management and complications in the intensive care unit. PEEP—positive end-expiratory pressure; $\dot{V}/\dot{Q}$—ventilation/perfusion ratio. (*Adapted from* Antman [5]; with permission.)

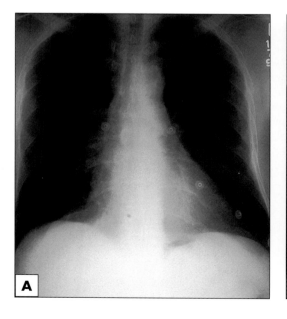

A

B

Figure 11-7. Atelectasis after cardiopulmonary bypass. Abnormalities on chest radiograph are common after cardiac surgery and, in the uncomplicated case, follow a typical evolution. A, Preoperative posteroanterior chest radiograph in a patient with no history of significant pulmonary disease. B, Immediate postoperative chest radiograph following uncomplicated coronary artery bypass graft. (*Continued on next page*)

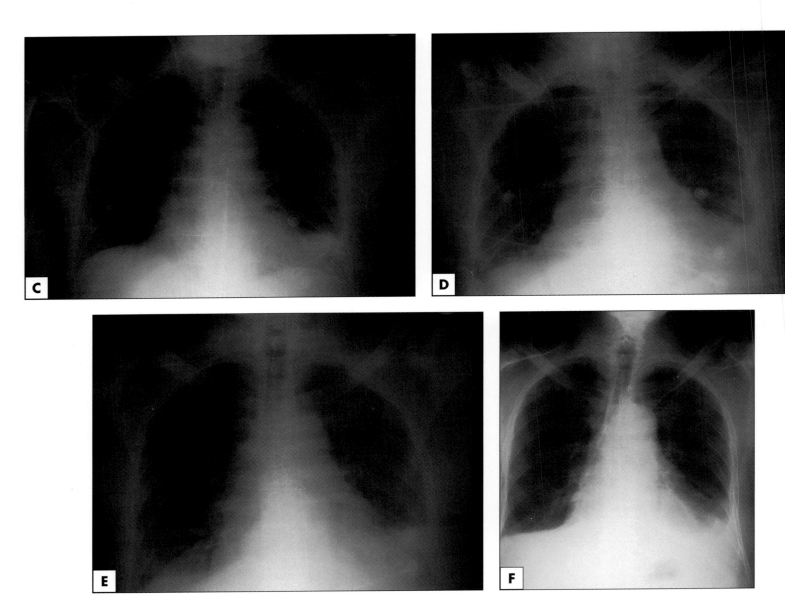

Figure 11-7. (*Continued*) Note presence of endotracheal tube, intravascular catheters, and mediastinal and left pleural tubes. Pleural effusion and decreased volume at the left base is already present. C, Postoperative day 1. Patient is extubated; similar changes are seen at the left base as were seen earlier. D, Postoperative day 2. Intravascular catheters and drainage tubes have been removed.

Further loss of lung volume is shown, particularly at the left base. E, Postoperative day 3: Retrocardiac density and loss of definition of diaphragm and pleural angle at the left base. F, Postoperative day 4. Some restoration of lung volume, but atelectasis and small effusion remain at the left lung base.

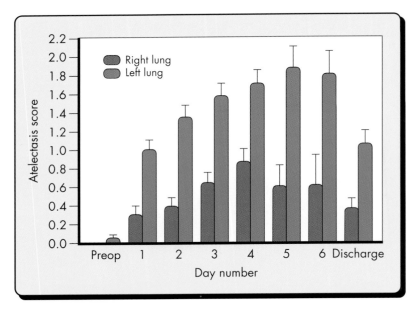

Figure 11-8. Atelectasis scores before and after cardiac surgery. Atelectasis scores for right (*hatched bars*) and left (*open bars*) lungs for preoperative and postoperative days 1 to 6. Atelectasis scoring system: 0, no atelectasis; 1, plate-like atelectasis; 2, mild lobar collapse; 3, moderate lobar collapse; 4, complete lower lobe collapse. (*From* Wilcox and coworkers [6]; with permission.)

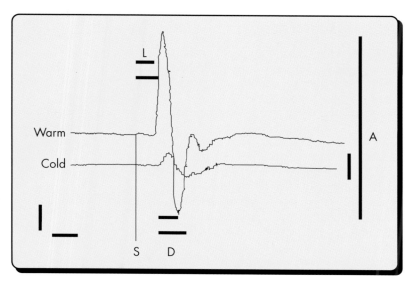

Figure 11-9. Diaphragmatic temperature during cardiac surgery. Cold injury to the phrenic nerve(s) with subsequent diaphragmatic dysfunction has long been thought to be contributory to postcardiac surgery atelectasis, although its relative significance remains unclear and controversial. In particular, the application of ice slush to the heart during aortic cross-clamping has been incriminated. However, even mild systemic hypothermia may impair diaphragmatic function, with implications as to the timing of extubation (*eg*, fast track surgery) in relation to the level and stability of core body temperature postoperatively. The figure shows a representative example of two evoked compound action potentials recorded directly from the left diaphragm using needle electrodes, in response to pulses of magnetic stimulation to the left phrenic nerve in one patient. Recordings were made at two diaphragmatic temperatures: first, cold (approximately 31°C) and 12 minutes later, warm (approximately 36°C). A—amplitudes of the warm and cold conditions; D—durations between the first deflection and the peak on the second wave; L—latency (the *bars* represent the latencies between the stimulus and the first deflection in "cold" and "warm" conditions); S—stimulus artifact. On the bottom left hand corner, horizontal bar = 10 ms and vertical bar = 0.2 mV. (*From* Mills and coworkers [7]; with permission.)

ROUTINE VENTILATOR MANAGEMENT

$FiO_2 = 0.6$
PEEP = 5 cm H_2O
    May need to increase either if gas exchange immediately after
        CPB is very impaired
Mandatory respiratory rate 8–10/min
Tidal volume 10–12 mL/kg
    May need greater minute ventilation if significant metabolic
        acidosis is present after CPB
Pressure support 10 cm H_2O (optional)
    Available on many ventilators in combination with (S)IMV
    May need to adjust according to endotracheal tube diameter
        and MV demands of patient

Figure 11-10. Routine ventilator management. CPB—cardiopulmonary bypass; MV—minute ventilation; PEEP—positive end-expiratory pressure; (S)IMV—(synchronized) intermittent mandatory ventilation.

EXTUBATION CRITERIA

Neurologic criteria
    Awake, cooperative, and following verbal command
    Intact airway reflexes
    Neuromuscular blockade reversed/dissipated
Cardiovascular criteria
    Stable and acceptable hemodynamics
        Sinus rate 70–100/min, or stable paced rhythm
        MAP >70 mm Hg
        CI > 2.0 L/min/m²
        PAWP < 20 mm Hg
        Svo_2 > 60%
    No significant/malignant arrhythmias
    No mechanical cardiovascular support
    Minimal chest tube drainage < 100 mL/h
Respiratory criteria
    Mechanics
        Patient comfortable, spontaneous respiratory rate < 25
        IMV rate 4 or less
        Vital capacity > 10–15 mL/kg
        Maximal inspiratory pressure > 25–30 cm H_2O
    Gas exchange
        $Pao_2 \geq 80$ with $FiO_2 \leq 0.50$
        $Paco_2 \leq 45$
        Acceptable chest x-ray
Metabolic criteria
    Fully rewarmed temperature $\geq 36.5°C$
    Absence of shivering
    pH ≥ 7.35

Figure 11-11. Extubation criteria. In the uncomplicated patient the primary criteria for extubation are the patient's level of consciousness and the satisfaction of respiratory goals, as defined in the table. However, in the more complicated patient, many other factors should be considered in the timing of extubation. For example, irrespective of satisfactory gas exchange and respiratory mechanics, extubation of a bleeding, acidotic, possibly oliguric patient clearly would be unwise. CI—cardiac index; IMV—intermittent mandatory ventilation; MAP—mean arterial pressure; PAWP—pulmonary artery wedge pressure; Svo_2—mixed venous oxygen saturation. (*Adapted from* Higgins and coworkers [1]; with permission.)

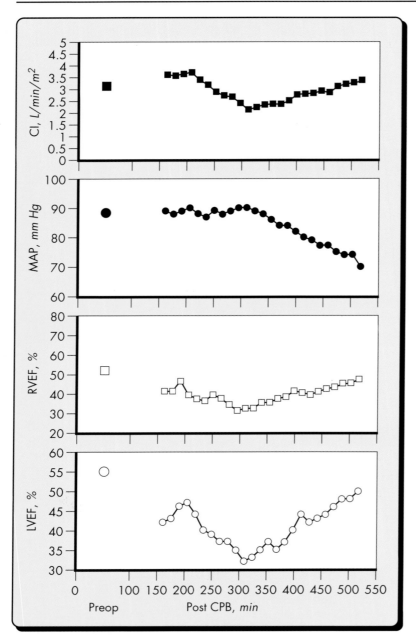

Figure 11-12. Acute reversible myocardial dysfunction following cardiac surgery. Reversible myocardial dysfunction following cardiac surgery appears to be a common occurrence, although this is not supported in all studies. Hemodynamic management of the post–cardiac surgery patient requires an appreciation of the expected changes to biventricular function in otherwise uncomplicated patients. Furthermore, in those patients with impaired myocardial function immediately following discontinuation of cardiopulmonary bypass (CPB), possible worsening dysfunction should be anticipated. The figure illustrates the evolution of hemodynamic changes in a patient treated with dobutamine and nitroprusside after coronary artery bypass surgery. Despite such treatment note the nadir of cardiac index (CI), right ventricular ejection fraction (RVEF), and left ventricular ejection fraction (LVEF) 5 hours after CPB, and their subsequent restoration by 9 hours. The mechanism of myocardial dysfunction remains unknown although reperfusion injury following cardioplegic arrest has been implicated. CI—cardiac index. (*Adapted from* Breisblatt and coworkers [8]; with permission.)

A. REDUCED PRELOAD

	Hypovolemia	Vasodilation	Cardiac tamponade
Hemodynamics			
RAP, *mm Hg*	< 8	< 8	> 15
PAWP, *mm Hg*	< 15	< 15	> 15
CI, *L/min/m²*	< 2.0	< 2.0	< 2.0
SVR, *dyne/sec/cm⁵*	> 1200	< 1000	> 1000
SVR			
Other			RAP = PAD = PAWP (within 5 mm Hg). However, postoperative tamponade is most often due to asymmetric chamber compression by clot; therefore, actual hemodynamic values depend on site of compression, volume status of patient, and ventricular function
Echocardiogram	Small LV chamber with vigorous contraction unless LV systolic dysfunction is present	Small LV chamber with vigorous contraction unless LV systolic dysfunction is present	Pericardial fluid or clot with chamber compression. May see RA and RV diastolic collapse depending on site of compression. Ventricular function may or may not be normal
Management	Intravenous fluids or blood if appropriate	Vasopressors	Volume expansion and inotropic support. Requires surgical reexploration

B. CARDIOGENIC CAUSES

	Bradycardia	LV failure	RV failure
Hemodynamics			
RAP, *mm Hg*	≤ 10	> 10	> 10
PAWP, *mm Hg*	> 15	> 20	≤ 15
CI, *L/min/m²*	< 2.0	< 2.0	< 2.0
SVR, *dyne/sec/cm⁵*	> 1200	> 1000	> 1000
Other	Hemodynamics depend up ventricular function	Filling pressures depend on whether biventricular failure is present or not	
Echocardiogram	Normal ventricle with normal systolic function. Appearance depends on underlying ventricular function	Dilated LV and LA with global and/or regional systolic wall motion abnormalities. MR may be present	Dilated RV and RA with reduced/absent systolic wall motion. TR may be present
Management	Cardiac pacing	Search for correctable lesions. Support ventricular function with inotropes. Adjust LV afterload with vasopressors or vasodilators. Reduce RV afterload with measures that increase oxygenation, maintain lung volume, and reduce hypocarbia. Mechanical assistance	

Figure 11-13. Low cardiac output (CO) and shock states. Causes of low cardiac output and/or hypotension can be pathophysiologically categorized into those due to a derangement of preload (**A**), contractility, afterload, and heart rate. Clinically it is useful to make the distinction between "noncardiogenic" and "cardiogenic" causes; the former dictates the need for volume expansion and vasopressors, while the latter might demand the use of inotropes or pacing (**B**).

(Continued on next page)

POSTOPERATIVE INTENSIVE CARE OF THE CARDIOTHORACIC PATIENT   11.9

C. SYSTEMIC INFLAMMATORY RESPONSE SYNDROME (SIRS)/SEPSIS

Hemodynamics

RAP, *mm Hg*	< 10
PAWP, *mm Hg*	< 15
CI, *L/min/m²*	≥ 2.0
SVR, *dyne/sec/cm⁵*	< 1000

Other

    Mixed venous O_2 saturation often ≥75%. Actual hemodynamic values depend on preexistent ventricular function, adequacy of volume resuscitation, and acute effects of SIRS/sepsis on vascular tone and ventricular diastolic and systolic function

Echocardiogram

    Actual chamber size and function dependent on volume status, preexistent ventricular function, and effects of circulating mediators on ventricular systolic and diastolic function. Combination of chamber size and systolic function often consistent with exaggerated CO

Management

    Optimization of volume status. Inotropic and/or vasopressor support. Antibiotics if infective cause found. Definitive surgical drainage or correction (mediastinitis, endocarditis)

Figure 11-13. (*Continued*) However, in many clinical situations there are component noncardiogenic and cardiogenic causes, which may confound diagnosis and complicate management. Tamponade and SIRS/sepsis (**C**) are particularly difficult from this perspective. These disorders are associated with abnormalities of loading conditions (tamponade in preload; sepsis in preload and afterload). Both may also be associated with, or result in, impaired contractility (*eg*, tamponade-induced hypotension with myocardial ischemia; sepsis with the release of putative myocardial depressant factors). CI—cardiac index; LA—left atrium; LV—left ventricular; MR—mitral regurgitation; PAD—pulmonary artery diastolic pressure; PAWP—pulmonary artery wedge pressure; RA—right atrial; RAP—right atrial pressure; RV—right ventricular; SVR—systemic vascular resistance; TR—tricuspid regurgitation. (*Adapted from* Antman [5]; with permission.)

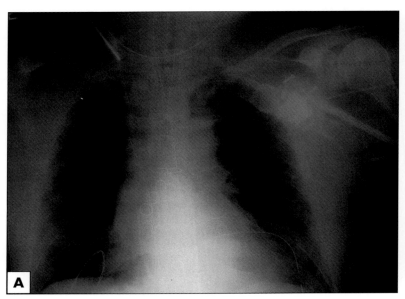

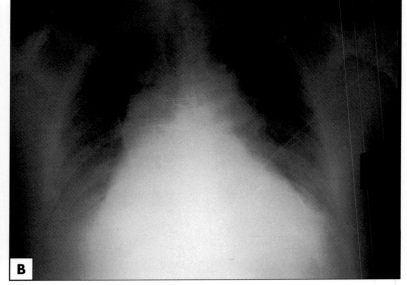

Figure 11-14. Pericardial tamponade. The presence of a pericardial effusion is detected by echocardiography in approximately 50% to 75% of patients following cardiac surgery [9]. Hemodynamically significant tamponade occurs in 0.5% to 5.8% of patients and although it often manifests early in the postoperative period, presentation may be delayed [10]. Tamponade in the setting of cardiac surgery is often associated with localized chamber compression by clot rather than a circumferential effusion with compressive forces distributed over all the chambers (*eg*, malignant pericardial effusion). This confounds the demonstration of equalization of filling pressures as a diagnostic tool. For example, right atrial (RA) compression results only in elevated RA pressure, with normal or low left-sided filling pressures.

Furthermore, if presentation is early, the patient is likely to be receiving positive pressure ventilation. In this circumstance clinical signs such as pulsus paradoxus and mitral flow variation seen with echocardiography are not applicable, as they pertain to spontaneously breathing patients. **A,** Immediate postoperative chest radiograph of a 59-year-old man following uncomplicated coronary artery bypass graft. **B,** Postoperative day 1 chest radiograph. The first 20 postoperative hours were complicated by excessive chest tube drainage of blood. Note widened mediastinum. The patient was reintubated on postoperative day 3 due to progressive respiratory failure. Transesophageal echocardiography was performed.

(Continued on next page)

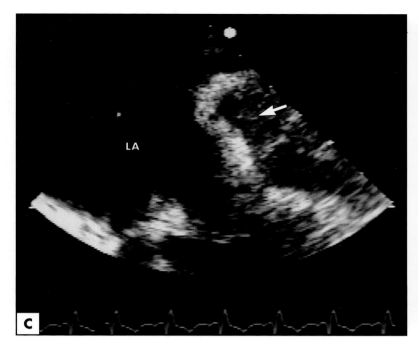

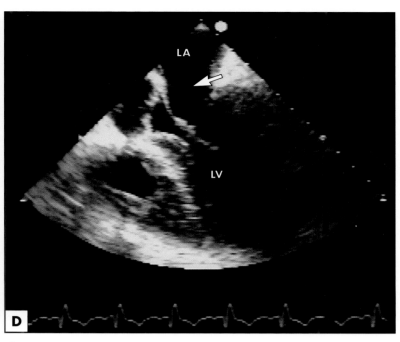

Figure 11-14. (*Continued*) C, Note large clot with left atrial compression (*arrow>*), and distortion of mitral annulus (arrowhead in D). The patient returned to the operating room for removal of the clot. He recovered without incident and was discharged home by postoperative day 7.

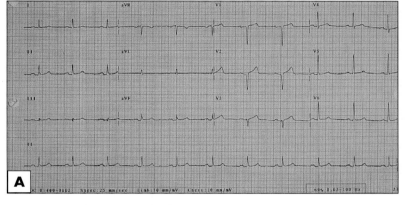

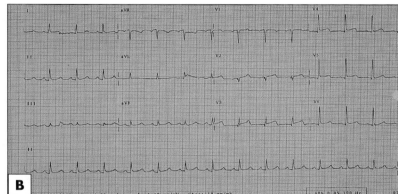

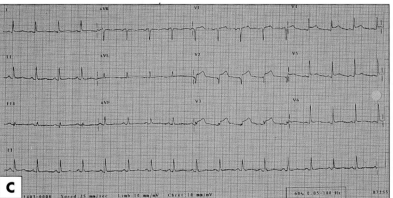

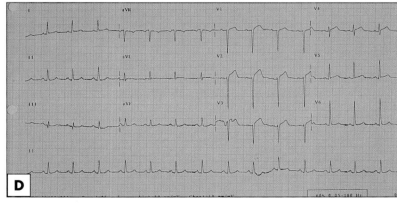

Figure 11-15. Post–cardiopulmonary bypass electrocardiogram (ECG). The postoperative ECG can be difficult to interpret due to the confounding effects of anesthesia, temperature, alterations to autonomic tone, electrolyte abnormalities, inotropic and antiarrhythmic drugs, cardiac pacing, and pericardial inflammation due to surgery and the presence of mediastinal chest tubes. In particular, this is manifested as repolarization changes resulting in abnormalities of the ST segment and T wave. A, Preoperative ECG of a 67-yearold man for elective coronary artery bypass graft (CABG), with recent anteroseptal infarction. B, Immediate postoperative (uncomplicated) ECG. Note widespread ST-segment elevation, *ie*, no specific coronary artery distribution is seen. C, Postoperative day 1: Persistent widespread ST elevation. No significant rise in creatine kinase–MB isoenzymes. D, Marked resolution of ST-segment changes; no new Q waves. The patient's postoperative course was uncomplicated.

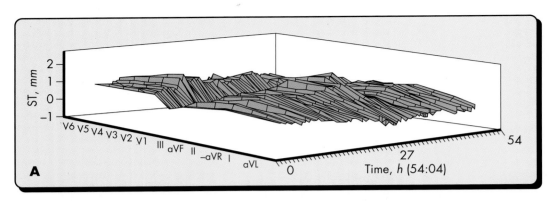

A

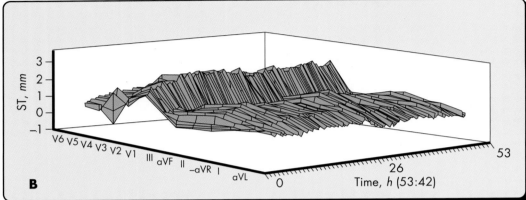

B

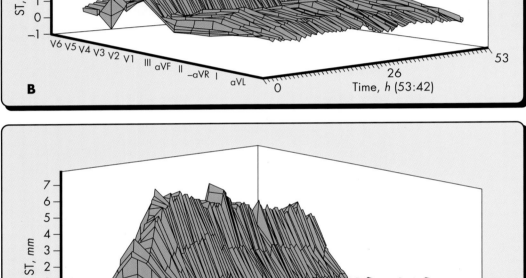

C

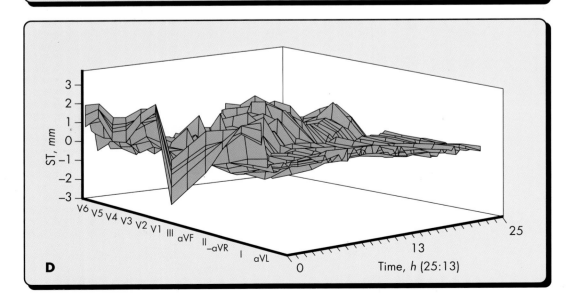

D

Figure 11-16. A–C, Continuous 12-lead ST-segment monitoring. Three representative examples from patients following uncomplicated coronary artery bypass graft (CABG). Note rapid evolution of stable, widespread ST-segment elevation. Although peak ST-segment elevation is usually only 1 to 2 mm, it may be considerably greater in apparently uncomplicated patients. Generally, these ST changes have resolved before the 30-day routine follow-up electrocardiogram. D, Continuous 12-lead ST-segment monitoring in a patient with hemodynamic instability and presumptive perioperative infarction following CABG. Note instability of ST-segment changes, with both unstable elevation and depression. (*From* Hilton and coworkers [11]; with permission.)

DIAGNOSIS OF MYOCARDIAL INFARCTION AFTER CARDIAC SURGERY

Diagnostic Finding	Comment
Symptoms	
Early (<48 h postop)	Not reliable because of residual effects of anesthesia, postoperative pain and postoperative analgesia
Late (> 48 h postop)	Potentially reliable, but confounded by incisional pain and pleuritic and pericardial pain from chest and mediastinal tubes
Electrocardiogram	
New persistent Q waves	Most reliable diagnostic finding but only if Q waves persist on serial ECGs
ST-T changes	Supportive data favoring the diagnosis of MI only if typical evolutionary pattern is observed (*see* Fig. 11-16)
Myocardial specific enzymes	
Total CK	Elevated total CK levels postoperatively may arise from multiple sources, including skeletal muscle in the thorax and calf as well as myocardium
CK-MB	Myocardial-specific CK may be released from ischemia occurring during CPB, as well as myocardial and aortic incisions made intraoperatively (*eg*, right atrium for cannulation of venae cavae). Because of the nearly universal release of CK-MB, a diagnosis of MI should not be made unless the CK-MB is significantly elevated (*eg*, > 30 U/L).
Troponins I and T	May be more specific than CK-MB in the setting of perioperative infarction with noncardiac surgery [12]. Value in the setting of cardiac surgery not established
Echocardiogram	A persistent regional wall motion abnormality is a helpful finding by comparison with a preoperative study

Figure 11-17. Diagnosis of myocardial infarction after cardiac surgery. CK—creatine kinase; CK-MB—myocardial-specific CK isoenzyme; MI—myocardial infarction. (*Adapted from* Antman [5]; with permission.)

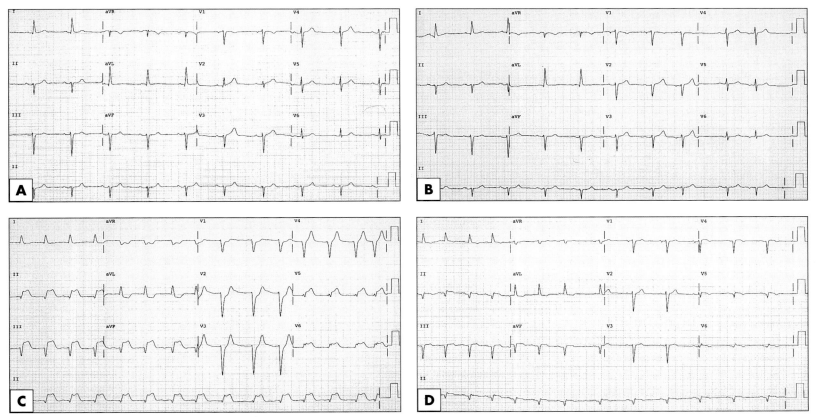

Figure 11-18. Electrocardiographic (ECG) diagnosis of myocardial infarction. **A,** Preoperative 12-lead ECG of a 78-year-old man for elective coronary artery bypass graft (CABG). **B,** Morning of postoperative day 1: Mild ST-T changes anteriorly, and occasional premature atrial complexes. **C,** Afternoon of postoperative day 1: Inferolateral ST-segment elevation with reciprocal depression in V1 and V2. Note that ST elevation is not widespread but has a specific distribution, and that ST-segment depression is present as well. Both these features contrast with the normal ST changes seen after an uncomplicated CABG. **D,** Postoperative day 4: Fully evolved Q waves consistent with inferolateral infarction. Peak level of creatine kinase—MB isoenzyme was 207 ng/mL.

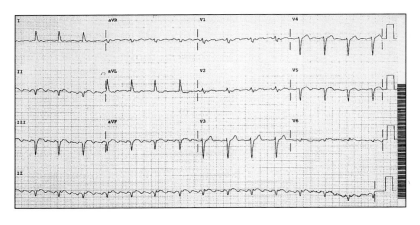

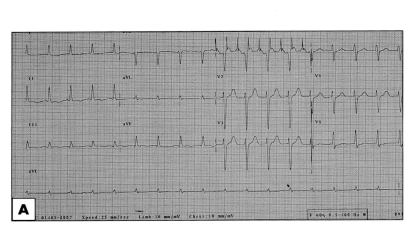

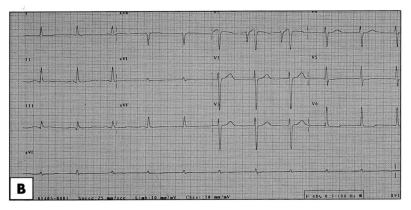

Figure 11-19. Atrial Tachyarrythmias. Atrial tachyarrythmias following cardiac surgery are common with a reported incidence ranging from 11% to greater than 50% of patients. The exact cause of these postoperative arrythmias is unknown, but may be due to pericardial inflammation, endogenous or exogenous catecholamines, autonomic imbalance, electrolyte and blood volume changes, or incomplete protection of the atria during cardioplegic arrest [13]. Although an electrocardiographic (ECG) diagnosis may be established with a one- or two-lead rhythm strip, if clinical circumstances allow, accuracy is improved if a 12-lead ECG is obtained. The ECG shown demonstrates atrial flutter with 3:1 atrioventricular block on postoperative day 3 after coronary artery bypass graft. (Note that odd-number AV conduction ratios in atrial flutter are unusual.) If the diagnosis is unclear and atrial pacing wires are still present, then an atrial ECG can be obtained and often is diagnostic.

Figure 11-20. A, Modified 12-lead electrocardiogram (ECG) with V1 lead connected to an atrial epicardial lead (unipolar atrial ECG). Perusal of other leads suggests a "nonsinus" rhythm but exact diagnosis is difficult to establish. The monopolar atrial lead clearly demonstrates atrial depolarizations consistent with atrial tachycardia with 2:1 atrioventricular block. B, Same patient as in *panel A* but the ECG was obtained after synchronized DC cardioversion. Again V1 is a monopolar atrial lead. Note exaggerated terminal negative forces in "V1" (atrial wires are attached to right atrium; left atrium depolarization follows right).

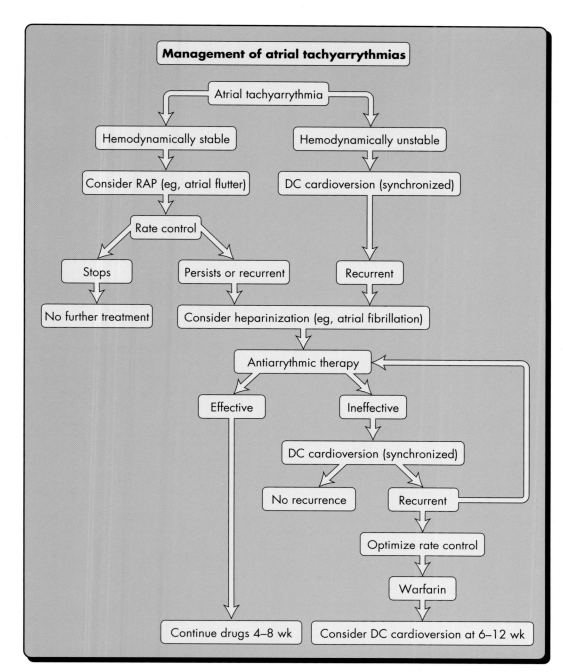

Figure 11-21. Algorithm for the management of atrial tachyarrhythmias following cardiac surgery. Stable conversion to sinus rhythm is often difficult to obtain, in which case rate control becomes the more likely achievable goal of management. Anticoagulation with heparin in the immediate postoperative patient is controversial. RAP—rapid atrial pacing. (*Adapted from* Ommen and coworkers [13]; with permission and Olshansky [14]; with permission.)

Text in figure:

Management of atrial tachyarrythmias

Atrial tachyarrythmia

Hemodynamically stable → Consider RAP (eg, atrial flutter) → Rate control

Hemodynamically unstable → DC cardioversion (synchronized)

Rate control → Stops → No further treatment

Rate control → Persists or recurrent

DC cardioversion (synchronized) → Recurrent

Persists or recurrent / Recurrent → Consider heparinization (eg, atrial fibrillation) → Antiarrythmic therapy

Antiarrythmic therapy → Effective → Continue drugs 4–8 wk

Antiarrythmic therapy → Ineffective → DC cardioversion (synchronized)

DC cardioversion (synchronized) → No recurrence

DC cardioversion (synchronized) → Recurrent → Optimize rate control → Warfarin → Consider DC cardioversion at 6–12 wk

DOSAGE OF DRUGS USED TO TREAT POSTOPERATIVE ATRIAL TACHYARRHYTHMIAS

Drug	IV bolus	IV Infusion	Oral dose
Anticoagulants			
Heparin	5000 U	Sufficient to produce aPTT 2–3 times control value	
Warfarin			Sufficient to produce INR of 2–3
Drugs to control rate			
β-Adrenergic blockers			
Esmolol	500 µg/kg	50–250 µg/kg/min	
Propranolol	1 mg every 5 min (max., 5 mg)		10–80 mg every 6–8 h
Metoprolol	5 mg every 5 min (max., 15 mg)		25–100 mg every 12 h
Atenolol	5 mg every 10 min (max., 10 mg)		50–200 mg/d
Calcium channel blockers			
Diltiazem	0.25 mg/kg	5–15 mg/h	180–360 mg/d
Verapamil	0.15 mg/kg	5 mg/h	120–480 mg/d
Digoxin	250 µg every 4h × 3–4		125–250 µg/d
Antiarrhythmic drugs			
Class IA			
Procainamide	10–15 mg/kg	1–6 mg/min	500–2000 mg twice a day
Quinidine	200–400 mg		300–600 mg three times a day
Class IC			
Flecainide	2 mg/kg		50–150 mg twice a day
Propafenone	1–2.5 mg/kg	2 mg/min	150–300 three times a day
Class III			
Amiodarone	150 mg	1000 mg/d	200–400 mg/d
Sotalol	0.2–1.5 mg/kg	0.15 mg/kg/h	80–240 mg twice a day
Ibutilide	1 mg (may repeat once)		
Magnesium	2–4 g	2–25 mg/min	

Figure 11-22. Drugs used to manage postoperative atrial tachyarrhythmias. Choice of drugs for the goals of rate control and/or arrhythmia termination or suppression are often guided by institutional preference and experience, as well as individual response to drugs. Although magnesium is included in the table, its exact role and efficacy remain uncertain, and a standardized dosing schedule remains undefined. In this setting adverse effects associated with its use are uncommon, and its potential risk-benefit ratio is appealing. aPTT—activated partial thromboplastin time; INR—international normalized ratio; IV—intravenous. (*Adapted from* Ommen and coworkers [13]; with permission.)

IATROGENIC CONSEQUENCES OF TREATING POSTOPERATIVE ATRIAL ARRHYTHMIAS

Intervention	Possible consequence
Early DC cardioversion	May only provide transient benefit; may cause bradycardia, tachycardia, and myocardial damage; requires anesthesia
Rapid atrial pacing	May be ineffective (*eg*, type II atrial flutter) or transient benefit; requires atrial pacing wires; may precipitate other arrhythmia
Drugs to control heart rate	
β-Adrenergic blockers	May cause bradycardia, hypotension, heart failure, or bronchospasm
Calcium channel blockers	May cause bradycardia or hypotension
Digoxin	Lack of efficacy; toxicity with excessive dosing
Antiarrhythmic drugs	
Class IA	Proarrhythmia; torsades de pointes, other ventricular arrhythmias; acceleration of ventricular rate; AV block; sinus bradycardia; hypotension; gastrointestinal tract upset (quinidine)
Class IC	Proarrhythmia: torsades de pointes, other ventricular arrhythmias; hypotension; bronchospasm (propafenone)
Class III	Proarrhythmia: torsades de pointes, other ventricular arrhythmias; AV block; sinus bradycardia; hypotension; pulmonary fibrosis, cirrhosis, or thyroid abnormalities (amiodarone)
Anticoagulation	Bleeding; drug interactions (warfarin)
Drug combination	Increased toxic potential
Atrial arrhythmia with poor hemodynamics (Inotropic support vs arrhythmia management)	Onset and ventricular rate related to adrenergic stimulation; correction of volume and electrolyte status, and tapering of intotropes may be more appropriate

Figure 11-23. Consequences and problems associated with the treatment of atrial postoperative arrhythmias. AV—atrioventricular. (*Adapted from* Olshansky [14]; with permission.)

NEUROLOGIC CHANGES

Figure 11-24. Differential diagnosis of neurologic deficit following cardiac surgery. CPB—cardiopulmonary bypass.

DIFFERENTIAL DIAGNOSIS OF NEUROLOGIC DEFICITS FOLLOWING CARDIAC SURGERY

Embolic
  Dislodgement of atherosclerotic/calcific plaque at site of aortic cannulation
  Microaggregate formation in CPB circuit
  Air introduced via CPB circuit or following incomplete de-airing of the ventricle
  Calcific debris from valve or valve ring
  Carotid arterial plaque dislodgement from aortic inflow cannula ("jet effect")
  Mural thrombus dislodgement
  Mechanical valve thrombus formation
  Ineffective anticoagulation before CPB initiation
Hemorrhagic
  Anticoagulation
  Uncontrolled hypertension following CPB
Ischemic
  Cerebral hypoperfusion during bypass (nonpulsatile flow)
  Cerebral hypoperfusion (shock) following CPB

ADVERSE OUTCOMES OF CORONARY BYPASS SURGERY

Type of deficit	None	Type I	Type II
Mortality, %	2	21	10
ICU, d	3	11	7
Hospital length of study, d	10	25	21
Intermediate/long-term care, %	8	47	30

Figure 11-25. Adverse outcomes of coronary artery bypass graft (CABG) surgery. At 24 US institutions 2108 patients undergoing elective CABG were prospectively analyzed for adverse neurologic outcomes. Adverse outcomes were classified as none; type I (focal): neurologic deficit or stupor/coma at discharge; or type II (global): deterioration in intellectual function, memory deficit, or seizure. Adverse neurologic outcomes occurred in 129 of 2108 patients (6.1%), evenly distributed between type I and type II deficits. The presence of any postoperative neurologic deficit was associated with a higher mortality rate, longer intensive care unit (ICU) and hospital stay, and greater frequency of discharge from hospital to intermediate- or long-term care facility when compared with patients who had no postoperative neurologic compromise. The group with type I (focal) neurologic deficit experienced more morbidity and mortality and longer ICU and hospital length of stay than those with type II (global) deficit. Factors that are predictive of type I and type II deficits are listed in Figure 11-26. All values are $P<0.001$. (*Adapted from* Roach and coworkers [15].)

VASCULAR CHANGES

PREDICTORS OF POSTOPERATIVE STROKE IN PATIENTS UNDERGOING ELECTIVE CABG

Type I
    Proximal aortic atherosclerosis
    History of neurologic disease
    Age >70 years
    Diabetes mellitus
    Hypertension
    Pulmonary disease
    Placement of intra-aortic balloon pump
Type II
    Age >70 years
    Systolic blood pressure > 180 mm Hg on admission
    Pulmonary disease
    Excessive consumption of alcohol
    Prior CABG surgery
    Dysrhythmia

Figure 11-26. Predictors of postoperative stroke in patients undergoing elective coronary artery bypass graft (CABG) surgery.

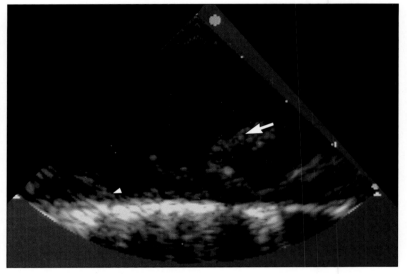

Figure 11-27. Transesophageal echocardiography (TEE) and aortic atherosclerosis. TEE demonstrates the presence of a mobile atherosclerotic plaque in the descending aorta (*arrow*) and a sessile atheroma (*arrowhead*). However, although TEE of the ascending aorta may identify similar disease, the images tend to be less satisfactory and the aortic cannulation site is often not visualized. The presence of atheromatous disease appears to be related to an increased risk of stroke and peripheral arterial embolization, presumably due to showering of emboli when the diseased portion of the aorta is manipulated. Pedunculated or mobile densities represent a higher risk for embolization.

ABNORMALITIES OF COAGULATION FOLLOWING CPB

Activation of coagulation by CPB circuit

Platelets

    Oxygenator surface induces platelet aggregation and activation; platelet number decreases intraoperatively.

    Depletion of platelet alpha granules occurs with ongoing exposure; platelet function is impaired postoperatively.

Coagulation factors

    Systemic inflammatory response syndrome (SIRS) occurs as a result of blood contacting foreign body (CPB circuit); complement, coagulation, and fibrinolytic cascades are activated.

    Consumption of coagulation factors occurs.

Hemodilution

    CPB circuit primed with several liters of crystalloid solution. Initiation of bypass results in dilution of all blood components.

Heparin

    ACT maintained > 400 s on bypass to minimize thrombus formation on circuit and reversed with protamine at end of bypass. Postoperative rewarming results in washout of residual heparin ("heparin rebound"). Diagnosed by increased ACT, PTT, or measured heparin levels. Treatment is protamine.

    Rarely, heparin induces an immune-mediated thrombocytopenia (usually on repeat exposure). Treatment includes cessation of all heparin therapy, possibly use of novel anticoagulant agents.

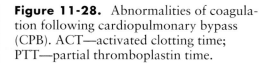

Figure 11-28. Abnormalities of coagulation following cardiopulmonary bypass (CPB). ACT—activated clotting time; PTT—partial thromboplastin time.

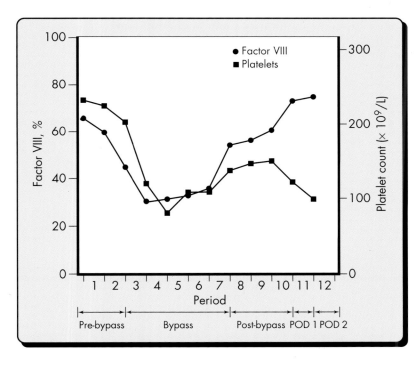

Figure 11-29. Coagulation changes in patients undergoing coronary artery bypass grafting with hypothermic cardiopulmonary bypass (CPB). Abnormalities of platelet number and coagulation factor VIII level are seen within 15 minutes of the initiation of CPB (period 4). Mean factor VIII levels declined to 30% of their preoperative values during bypass (periods 4 to 7) and recovered toward normal postoperatively (periods 8 to 12). Platelet counts declined to less than 100×10^9/L during bypass and remained low in the postoperative period, not returning to baseline levels for up to 1 week. These coagulation abnormalities recover at varying rates following discontinuation of CPB and do not correlate with the amount of postoperative bleeding present. There were no clinically relevant differences in any of the laboratory measurements of coagulation between patients with normal postoperative blood loss and those with increased blood loss. Therefore, laboratory evidence of impaired hemostatic ability is transient following bypass, is not predictive of increased postoperative blood loss and should only be used as one component in the evaluation of postoperative bleeding following CPB. POD—postoperative day. (*Adapted from* Gelb and coworkers [16]; with permission.)

RISK FACTORS FOR POSTOPERATIVE RENAL DYSFUNCTION FOLLOWING CARDIAC SURGERY

Preoperative renal dysfunction
Congestive heart failure
Extremes of age (neonates and adults > 70 y)
Prolonged CPB time (> 4 h)
Acute reduction in cardiac output
Aminoglycoside antibiotics

Figure 11-30. Risk factors for postoperative renal dysfunction following cardiac surgery.

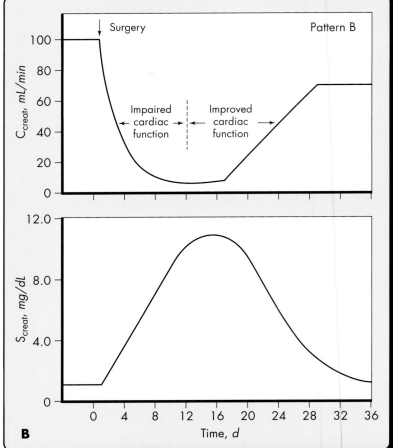

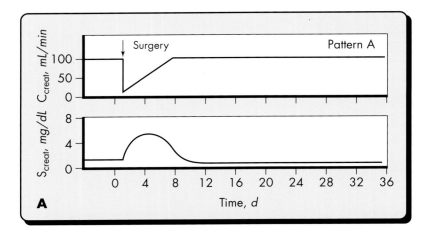

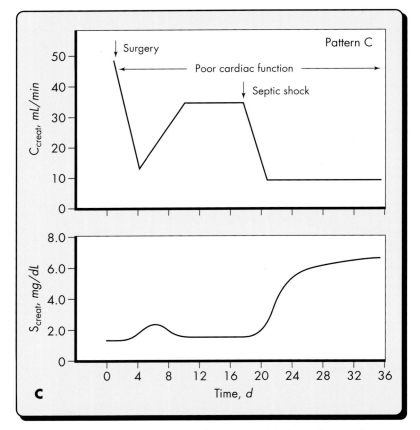

clearance (C_{creat}) over a period of approximately 1 week, which is reflected by the return of serum creatinine (S_{creat}) to its baseline level. Prognosis is generally favorable in pattern A. Pattern B: overt form. Acute renal failure is exacerbated by a period of postoperative cardiac dysfunction. Creatinine clearance continues to fall during the period of impaired cardiac function. Recovery of the decrement in creatinine clearance is delayed until cardiac function is restored on postoperative day 12. The pattern and duration of recovery of renal function often mirror the initial decrement and may take several weeks to resolve. Pattern C (protracted form): In pattern C acute renal failure is complicated by multiple episodes of renal hypoperfusion. An initial episode of postoperative cardiac dysfunction and subsequent recovery is further complicated by a second process producing renal hypoperfusion, in this case, septic shock. Some recovery of creatinine clearance occurs following the recovery of cardiac function, but a persistent low output state prevents recovery from the second insult. This may result in irreversible renal damage. (*From* Myers and Moran [17]; with permission.)

Figure 11-31. Three patterns of acute renal failure after cardiac surgery (A–C). Pattern A (abbreviated form): This pattern of acute renal failure follows an isolated ischemic insult to the kidney. An abrupt decrement in creatinine clearance occurs immediately following the insult. This is followed by a prompt but gradual rise in creatinine

GOALS FOR FLUID AND ELECTROLYTE MANAGEMENT FOLLOWING CARDIAC SURGERY

Fluid	Patients tend to have excess fluid secondary to CPB circuit priming volume. Additional fluid is used only as needed to maintain filling pressures and cardiac output during rewarming. General goal is to achieve net fluid loss in the initial 48–72 h postoperatively
Potassium and magnesium	Decrease in exchangeable potassium and magnesium invariably occurs when renal function is normal. Maintain serum potassium 4.5 ± 0.5 mEq/L and magnesium > 2.0 mEq/L to decrease incidence of cardiac arrhythmia
Glucose	Serum levels are frequently elevated (stress response, glucose-containing IV solutions). Usually doesn't require therapy unless patient is diabetic. If required, use regular insulin infusion to provide basal insulin need; subcutaneous availability is erratic in the immediate postoperative period
Calcium	Mild to moderate degrees of ionized hypocalcemia are common following cardiac surgery and generally don't require treatment. Excess calcium administration may worsen ischemic reperfusion injury
Acid/base	Mild metabolic acidosis or alkalosis is common during rewarming. These abnormalities usually don't require treatment in the absence of acute renal dysfunction

Figure 11-32. Goals for fluid and electrolyte management following cardiac surgery. CPB—cardiopulmonary bypass; IV—intravenous.

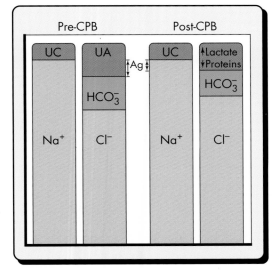

Figure 11-33. Anion gap decreases after cardiopulmonary bypass (CPB). The anion gap is calculated as

$$\text{anion gap} = \text{sodium} - (\text{chloride} + \text{bicarbonate}),$$

and in normal healthy adults is 10 ± 4 mEq/L.

The law of electrical neutrality states that the sum of positive charges in the blood must always equal the sum of negative charges present. Positive and negatively charged particles, however, include more than sodium (Na^+), chloride (Cl^-), and bicarbonate (HCO_3^-). Therefore, when unmeasured anions (UA) and unmeasured cations (UC) are considered, electrical neutrality requires:

$$Na^+ + UC = Cl + HCO_3 + UA \text{ (equation 2).}$$

Rearranging equation 2, we get

$$Na^+ - (Cl^- + HCO_3^-) = UA - UC \text{ (equation 3).}$$

Therefore, substituting equation 1 into equation 3:

$$\text{anion gap} = UA - UC.$$

Since UAs decrease following CPB, the anion gap likewise decreases [18].

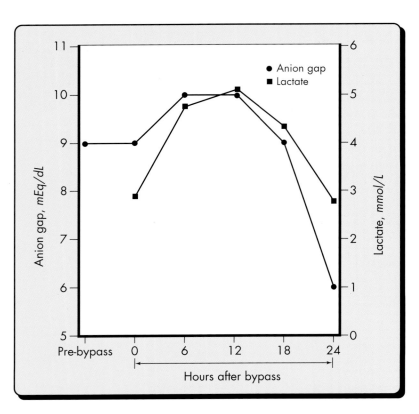

Figure 11-34. Time course of change in anion gap and lactic acid production during and after cardiopulmonary (CPB). Lactic acidosis is often seen following cardiac surgery and an increasing level of lactate postoperatively is an ominous sign indicating impaired tissue oxygen delivery. When lactate (or some other unmeasured anion) is present, the anion gap increases, *ie*, unmeasured anions outnumber unmeasured cations, and an anion gap acidosis is said to be present. Therefore, a rising lactate level can be inferred by worsening anion gap acidosis. However, during and after CPB, this traditional acid/base analysis may not hold owing to the effect of CPB on unmeasured anions, specifically, serum proteins. Serum proteins are the most important contributors to the unmeasured anion pool, and hemodilution due to CPB produces significant hypoproteinemia. Therefore institution of CPB leads to decreased plasma proteins, metabolic alkalosis, and a reduction in the anion gap (time 0). Despite significant elevation of serum lactate from onset of CPB to 12 hours after bypass, the anion gap remains in the normal range. Therefore, if significant acidosis is suspected, measurement of serum lactate is necessary [18].

GASTROINTESTINAL CHANGES

Figure 11-35. Gastrointestinal (GI) complications following cardiac surgery. GI complications requiring intervention occur in 1% to 3% of patients but are associated with high mortality rates (~50%). IV—intravenous.

GASTROINTESTINAL COMPLICATIONS FOLLOWING CARDIAC SURGERY	
Complication	**Comment**
Ileus	Most common postoperative GI complication. Conservative management is IV fluids and nasogastric decompression. May be exacerbated by postoperative narcotic therapy
Upper GI ulceration/bleeding	Increased risk with preexisting peptic ulcer disease. Minimized with antacid therapy, histamine blockers, proton pump inhibitors, or barrier protection such as sucralfate. Early enteral nutrition is protective
Lower GI bleeding	Risk factors include previous lower GI bleed, diverticular disease, and multisystem organ failure
Cholecystitis	Fever, leukocytosis, right upper quadrant tenderness: consider acalculous etiology. Treat with drainage and antibiotic therapy
Pancreatitis	Poor prognosis, particularly in the setting of multisystem organ failure. Isolated elevation of amylase (but not lipase) is common after cardiac surgery
Mesenteric ischemia	May result from low perfusion (low cardiac output, arterial dissection from intra-aortic balloon pump) or embolization of atheroma. Early identification and surgical resection necessary, but mortality remains high
Jaundice	Mild elevations of bilirubin seen in ≈ 20% of patients postoperatively. More common with valve replacement, large transfusion requirements. Markedly elevated levels. Seen with "shock liver"—prognosis extremely poor.

FEVER

FEVER FOLLOWING CARDIAC SURGERY

Noninfectious causes of fever
  Atelectasis
  Drug reaction
  Pulmonary embolism
  Postpericardiotomy syndrome
  Phlebitis
Infectious causes of fever
  Leg wound infection
  Mediastinitis
  Pneumonia
  Urinary tract infection
  Line infection
  Sinusitis
  Decubitus ulcer
  Prostatitis

Figure 11-36. Fever is the most common clinical finding in the setting of postoperative infection. The activation of the systemic inflammatory syndrome by the cardiopulmonary bypass circuit often results in low-grade temperature elevations for 4 to 5 days postoperatively, and sometimes fever persists as long as 2 weeks. Additional causes of postoperative fever are listed in the table.

FAST-TRACK CARDIAC SURGERY PROGRAM

A. STEP 1: PREOPERATIVE RISK ASSESSMENT

Risk Factor	Points	Risk Factor	Points
Emergency surgery	6	Prior vascular surgery	2
Serum creatinine > 1.9 mg/dL	4	COPD on medication	2
Serum creatinine 1.6–1.8 mg/dL	1	Hct < 34%	2
Severe LV dysfunction	3	Aortic stenosis	1
Prior cardiac operation	3	Weight < 65 kg	1
Mitral valve insufficiency	3	Diabetes on medication	1
Age > 75 g	2	Cerebrovascular disease	1
Age 65–74 y	1		
Total Score ≤ 4: proceed to Step 2: Intraoperative risk assessment (*See* Fig. 11-37B)		Total Score > 4: High-risk patient; Consider prolonged (>8 h) postoperative mechanical ventilation	

Figure 11-37. A–C, Suggested strategy for fast track management of the cardiac surgery patient. Institution of a fast track cardiac surgery program can decrease length of hospital stay and improve morbidity and mortality. Education and "buy-in" of all involved services is required for successful implementation. One aspect of fast tracking is postoperative management for early extubation. Appropriate selection of patients includes consideration of pre-, intra-, and postoperative factors.

(Continued on next page)

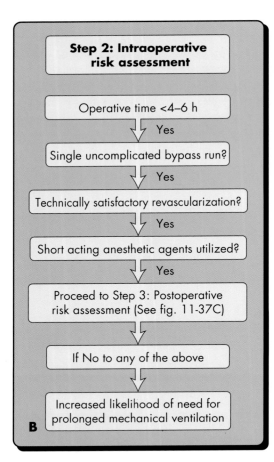

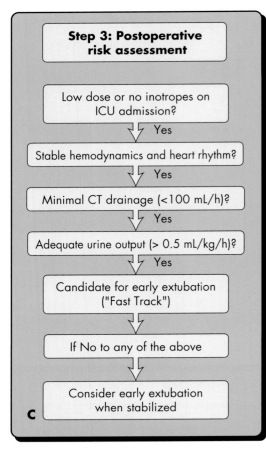

Figure 11-37. (*Continued*) As experience is gained, patients considered inappropriate for fast track management may become acceptable. COPD—chronic obstructive pulmonary disease; ICU—intensive care unit; LV—left ventricular. (Panel A *from* Higgins and coworkers [19]; with permission; panel C *from* Higgins [20]; with permission.)

REFERENCES

1. Higgins TL, Yared J-P, Ryan T: Immediate postoperative care of cardiac surgical patients. *J Cardiothorac Vasc Anesth* 1996, 10:643–658.

2. Sladen RN: Management of the adult cardiac patient in the intensive care unit. In *Acute Cardiovascular Management in Anesthesia and Intensive Care.* Edited by Ream AK, Fogdall RP. Philadelphia: JB Lippincott; 1982.

3. Kirklin JW, Barratt-Boyes BG: Postoperative care. In *Cardiac Surgery,* edn.2. New York: Churchill-Livingstone; 1992.

4. MacNaughton PD, Braude S, Hunter DN, *et al.*: Changes in lung function and pulmonary capillary permeability after cardiopulmonary bypass. *Crit Care Med* 1993, 20:1289–1294.

5. Antman EM: Medical management of the patient undergoing cardiac surgery. In *Heart Disease: A Textbook of Cardiovascular Medicine.* Edited by Braunwald E. Philadelphia: WB Saunders; 1997:1715–1740.

6. Wilcox P, Baile EM, Hards J, *et al.*: Phrenic nerve function and its relationship to atelectasis after coronary artery bypass surgery. *Chest* 1988, 93:693–698.

7. Mills GH, Khan ZP, Moxham J, *et al.*: Effects of temperature on phrenic nerve and diaphragmatic function during cardiac surgery. *Br J Anaesth* 1997, 79:726–732.

8. Breisblatt WM, Stein KL, Wolfe CJ, *et al.*: Acute myocardial dysfunction and recovery: A common occurrence after coronary bypass surgery. *J Am Coll Cardiol* 1990, 15:1261–1269.

9. Pepi M, Muratori M, Barbier P, *et al.*: Pericardial effusion after cardiac surgery: incidence, site, size, and hemodynamic consequences. *Br Heart J* 1994, 72:327–331.

10. Russo AM, O'Connor WH, Waxman HL: Atypical presentations and echocardiographic findings in patients with cardiac tamponade occurring early and late after cardiac surgery. *Chest* 1993, 104:71–78.

11. Hilton AK, Botz GH, Krucoff MW, Mark JB: Continuous 12-lead ECG fingerprint of the post–coronary artery bypass (CABG) patient [abstract]. *Anesth Analg* 1996, 82:SCA-44.

12. Adams JE, Sicard GA, Allen BT, *et al.*: Diagnosis of perioperative infarction with measurement of cardiac troponin. *N Engl J Med* 1994, 330:670–674.

13. Ommen SR, Odell JA, Stanton MS: Atrial arrhythmias after cardiothoracic surgery. *N Engl J Med* 1997, 336:1429–1434.

14. Olshansky B: Management of atrial fibrillation after coronary artery bypass graft. *Am J Cardiol* 1996, 78(suppl 8A):27–34.

15. Roach GW, Kanchuger M, Mangano CM, *et al.*: Adverse cerebral outcomes after coronary bypass surgery. *N Engl J Med* 1996, 335:1857–1863.

16. Gelb AB, Roth RI, Levin J, *et al.*: Changes in blood coagulation during and following cardiopulmonary bypass: Lack of correlation with clinical bleeding. *Am J Clin Pathol* 1996, 106:87–99.

17. Myers BD, Moran SM: Hemodynamically mediated acute renal failure. *N Engl J Med* 1986, 314:97–105.

18. Ernest D, Herkes RG, Raper RF: Alterations in anion gap following cardiopulmonary bypass. *Crit Care Med* 1992, 20:52–56.

19. Higgins TL, Estafanous FG, Loop FD, *et al.*: Stratification of morbidity and mortality outcome by preoperative risk factors. *JAMA* 1992, 267:2344–2348.

20. Higgins TL: Safety issues regarding early extubation after coronary bypass surgery. *J Cardiothorac Vasc Anesth* 1995, 9(suppl 1):24–29.

History, Practice Management, and Education

J.G. Reves and Mark F. Newman

This chapter examines the organization, scope and education required for the practice of cardiothoracic anesthesia. No chapter on the subject would be complete without a section on the history; thus, we begin with that.

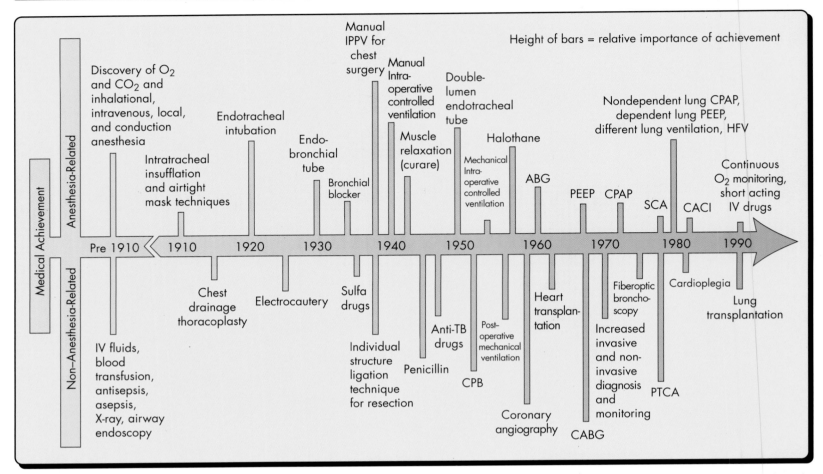

Figure 12-1. The history of cardiothoracic anesthesia is inextricably related to the surgical and technological developments as well as the many advances made in anesthesiology, critical care, and drug development. Of particular note is the development of endotracheal intubation and the use of intermittent positive pressure ventilation during open chest surgery in the 1930s. The advent of curare in 1942 and halothane in 1956 considerably facilitated both the work of surgeons and anesthesiologists. The development of extracorporeal circulation by Gibbon in 1953 was a major technological development in the emergence of cardiac surgery. Monitoring the cardiovascular and respiratory systems with invasive and noninvasive technology has also made steady improvement and assisted physicians in the care of patients intra- and postoperatively. A critical but still evolving step in the successful development of cardiothoracic surgery has been the organization and implementation of the cardiothoracic surgical team. This concept of subspecialty practice assures the close cooperation of the varied professionals required to produce optimal results. Members of this team are cardiac surgeons, cardiac anesthesiologists, perfusionists, and cardiac operating room nurses who all work in concert, each doing his particular task, all with the common goal of superlative patient care. For the best results, each member of the team should be trained in those disciplines required of cardiothoracic subspecialists, their defined roles understood, and communication constant. The creation of heart-lung (thorax) centers, using the interdisciplinary work of subspecialists in the operating room as the model, is the embodiment of this concept to improve all aspects of patient care, teaching and research. The American Board of Internal Medicine began certifying cardiologists in 1941 and the American Board of Thoracic Surgeons was founded in 1937. The Society of Cardiovascular Anesthesiologists was formed in 1978 to formalize and meet the educational needs of the emerging anesthesiologists whose practice involved cardiothoracic and vascular surgical anesthesia. Yet to come is the accreditation of training programs and ultimately certification of anesthesiologists in this anesthesia subspecialty practice: certification of cardiologists and cardiothoracic surgeons has been in place for some time. ABG—arterial blood gas; CABG—coronary artery bypass grafting; CACI—computer assisted continuous infusion; CPAP—continuous positive airway pressure; CPB—cardiopulmonary bypass; HFV—high-frequency ventilation; IPPV—intermittent positive-pressure ventilation; IV—intravenous; PEEP—positive end-expiratory pressure; PTCA-percutaneous transluminal coronary angioplasty; SCA— Society of Cardiovascular Anesthesiologists; TB—tuberculosis. (*Adapted from* Benumof [1]; with permission.)

SCOPE OF PRACTICE

PROFESSIONAL ACTIVITIES OF THE CARDIOTHORACIC ANESTHESIOLOGIST

Clinical care of cardiac and thoracic surgical patients during operation

Clinical care of cardiac and thoracic surgical transplantation patients during operation

Preoperative consultation and evaluation of patients with cardiac and pulmonary problems

Intraoperative diagnostician (transesophageal echocardiography and other modalities)

Postoperative management (intensive care and pain management)

Research (basic science and clinical)

Education

Administration

Figure 12-2. The cardiothoracic anesthesiologist is a subspecialist who concentrates professional activities in the field of cardiac and thoracic surgery. The professional activities can be categorized broadly into eight domains. Most of the activities are self-evident and need no elaboration. One role, however, has recently emerged: the cardiothoracic anesthesiologist as diagnostician [2]. This is now an important new responsibility that has developed with the technology of transesophageal echocardiography and the fact that the only person in the operating room with expertise in this diagnostic technique is usually the cardiothoracic anesthesiologist. This specialist is called upon to make decisions regarding pathology in the patient and appropriateness of the surgical repair.

OPTIMAL DESIGN OF CARDIOTHORACIC SERVICES

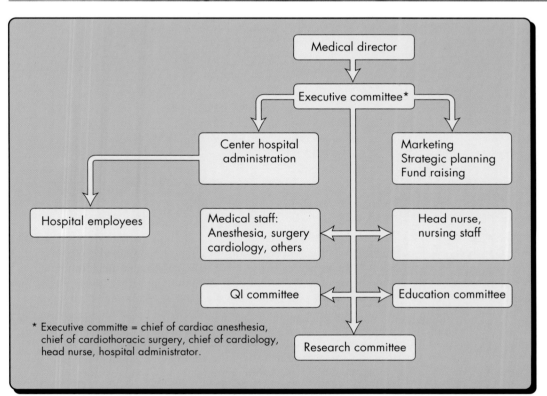

* Executive committe = chief of cardiac anesthesia, chief of cardiothoracic surgery, chief of cardiology, head nurse, hospital administrator.

Figure 12-3. Optimal design of cardiothoracic services. A striking, but very understandable change in the organization of hospitals and medical centers has been the emergence of "product lines," which generally result in the creation of "centers" or "institutes" that focus on a complete line of clinical services that span all clinical departmental services and are therefore called interdisciplinary. These programs are called by various names, such as heart center or thorax institutes or heart lung hospitals. A truly effective center has an interdisciplinary team made up of physicians, nurses, pharmacists, perfusionists, administrators, and others. These professionals work together under an organization. For the center to be effective, the members must put their programmatic concerns as the top priority and focus on improving patient care, reducing costs, and providing continuing medical education. Heart centers are often referred to as the "crown jewel" among many of the hospital's clinical programs. Communities are proud of their heart programs and use them as a means of bolstering community support. Anesthesiologists can and should seek leadership roles in these organizations. The anesthesiologist is often viewed as neutral when occasional disputes arise between cardiologists and surgeons. The hospital administrators also rely on anesthesiologists to see that operating rooms run smoothly and efficiently.

CABG/VALVE CLINICAL PATH

	Preop	Day of Surgery	Postop Day 1	Postop day 2	Postop Day 3	Postop Day 4-5
Medications	Antibiotics Sleep medication	Antibiotic	Routine medication Oxygen Wean from O_2 if saturation > 88%	Routine medication Routine laboratory tests	Routine medication Complete blood work	Routine medication Routine laboratory tests
Diet	Step I AHA NPO after MN	NPO Post extubation ice chips	Advance diet Limit fluids	Advance diet 2000 mL fluid	Advance diet 2000 mL fluids	Advance diet 2000 mL fluids
Activity	As tolerated	Extubate, cough, bedrest. Turn q 4 h	Ambulate	Pulmonary toilet, telemetry monitoring, ambulate TID	Pulmonary toilet, wound care, ambulate TID	Ambulate 5–10 min with minimal symptoms
Teaching	Detailed teaching of procedure and postoperative expectations	Review heart center postoperative plan	Wound care, constipation treatment, pain management	Wound care Increase activity Plan discharge Occupational therapy	Wound care Food/drug interactions Occupational therapy	Monitor heart rate for irregularity Cardiac rehabilitation Activity progression Driving Sexual activity
Psychological adjustment	Anticipate needs	Assess family Provide information	Assess patient and family Make realistic plans		Assess self-care needs Normalize realistic concerns Evaluate family for discharge	Evaluate patient and family comfort with discharge
Continuation of care		Anticipate discharge	Identify discharge needs Discharge from ICU	Consults if required	Case manager to assess if LOS > 5 days	Discharge or plan for prolonged care

Figure 12-4. There was a time not in the distant past when "protocol medicine" was mentioned only to be condemned. Fiercely independent physicians believed that individual practices on individual patients required individual practice management, and as a result protocols were often referred to in a derogatory manner as "cookbook medicine." This has now changed with the advent of managed care and the necessity to practice consistent, high quality, cost-effective medicine. Protocols are required to do this properly. This has been known by clinical investigators for years, who have relied on strict protocols to answer scientific questions, and now these protocols are used to govern the routine clinical practice of cardiothoracic anesthesia and surgery, cases that lend themselves to evidenced-based, guideline clinical management.

Protocols are generally euphemistically referred to as "care maps," perhaps to avoid the stigma attached to the word protocol. A care map is ideally designed by members of the center and is based on local experience and information in the literature about ideal ways to care for patients having common procedures such as coronary artery bypass surgery, valve replacement, transplantation, pneumonectomy. The team that draws up the plan must be led by a respected physician. Others on the team must represent all groups that are required to put the plan into effect: physicians, nurses, pharmacists, dietitians, physical therapists, respiratory care technicians, and so on. This team has to fashion a document that is simple, realistic, and understandable by patients and caregivers alike. It is important that a timeline be a major part of the plan so that progress of the patient can be easily measured. Space does not permit us to include examples of all care maps, but the point is that every common procedure should have a management protocol. An abbreviated example of the Duke Heart Center coronary artery surgery/valve surgery protocol (called "clinical path") is illustrated in this figure. ICU—intensive care unit; TID—three times per day.

CARDIAC ANESTHESIA PATIENT MANAGEMENT PROTOCOL

Preoperative Steps

Evaluate and visit the patient

Discuss the patient and anesthetic plan with attending (before operation)

Adequately premedicate and order anticipated supportive drips

Operative Steps

Place monitoring devices

Induce and maintain anesthesia

Anticoagulate the patient after communication with "team"

Establish adequate anticoagulation

Commence cardiopulmonary bypass after communication with team

Communicate pharmacologic interventions (including anticoagulation) with the perfusionists

Measure and communicate coagulation status, hemoglobin, and electrolyte information regularly (about every 30-45 min during CPB).

Anticipate and plan any drug or assist device needs prior to discontinuation of CPB

Discontinue CPB when the team is prepared and the patient is warm, has a stable rhythm, acceptable cardiac function, and acceptable hematocrit and electrolytes

Major pharmacologic and blood product interventions must be communicated to the team

Decisions regarding assist devices should be made conjointly with the surgeons

Report to ICU care providers should be complete

Postoperative visits should be thorough and informative for the patient and the anesthesia team

Figure 12-5. Cardiac anesthesia patient management protocol. There are very systematic and logical steps for anesthesiologists regardless of the particular patient or operation. Protocols for specific management also involve the anesthesiologist directly. These "best practices," like those put together for the hospital practices in the previous figure, should be developed by a group who are expected to abide by them. Anesthesia Best Practices not only are designed for consistent high-quality care but also have as an objective cost-effective care. When new protocols are put into place, some outcome analysis has to be performed to insure that the new protocols do not add morbidity, mortality, and hidden added costs.

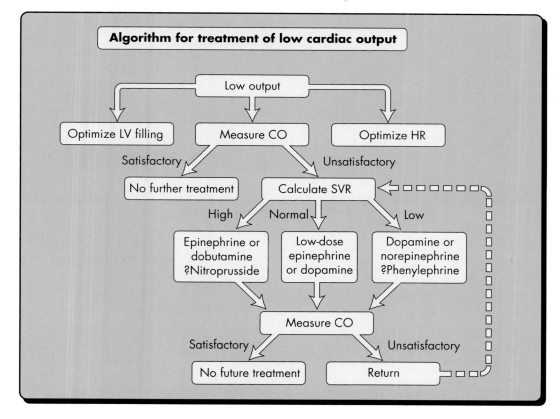

Figure 12-6. Algorithm for treatment of low cardiac output. This is a treatment protocol for improving cardiac performance that is used by the anesthesiologist. Patient management protocols used by anesthesiologist and others relate to the use of more expensive drugs like milrinone, hydroxyethyl starch, remifentanil, newer muscle relaxants, and propofol [3]. In the overall cost of a cardiac operation, drug costs for anesthesia are not a large part, but the discipline of choosing the most cost-effective approach regardless of clinical setting is increasingly going to be required in the future.

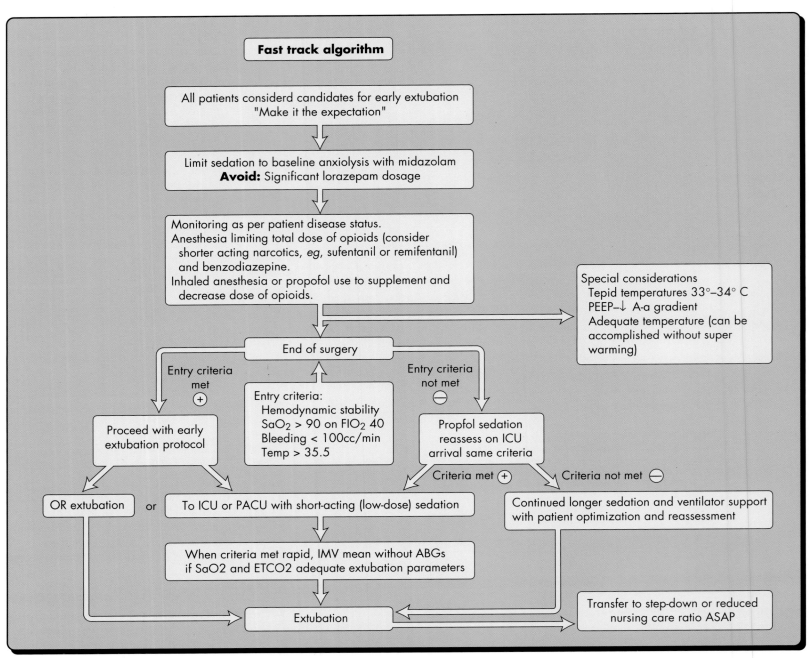

Figure 12-7. Fast-track algorithm. The planning of a "fast-track" course is another example of a patient management plan initiated by anesthesiologists. It requires some explanation. All patients should be considered candidates except for the very high risk patients. It should be remembered that other patients are routinely extubated following large operations, and except for the "rewarming" that sometimes complicates the early postoperative course of cardiac patients, there is little reason to keep the normally convalescent cardiac patient intubated for longer than 6 hours.

QUALITY IMPROVEMENT

INFORMATION THAT SHOULD BE FOLLOWED AS QUALITY INDICATORS OF A CARDIAC CENTER

Mortality by procedure and diagnostic code (*eg*, after CABG, PTCA, and acute myocardial infarction)

Transfusion requirement by procedure and diagnostic code

Infection incidence by procedure and diagnostic code

Myocardial infarction after all procedures

Prolonged ventilation after all procedures

Renal failure by procedure and diagnostic code (*eg*, after CABG, PTCA and acute myocardial infarction)

Stroke by procedure and diagnostic code (*eg*, after CABG, PTCA and acute myocardial infarction)

Reintubation

Length of stay

Cost of hospitalization by procedure and diagnostic code (*eg*, after CABG, PTCA and acute myocardial infarction)

Figure 12-8. Information that should be followed as quality indicators of a cardiac center. This table lists information that should be followed in an ongoing quality-improvement program. A successful cardiothoracic program must have a rigorous ongoing quality-improvement program that has the full support of the medical staff and hospital administration. There is no substitute for consistent and periodic peer review of the quality of the care given in a heart center. A committee appointed by the appropriate authorities should review

on an at least a quarterly basis the morbidity and mortality of the various procedures of patients cared for in the facility. Members of the QI committee should be physicians of all the involved specialties as well as a nursing representative and a hospital administrator. For this committee to function optimally there must be an information system in place that has vital information regarding each patient, each procedure or diagnostic code, and the clinical outcome. There must be an ongoing method to track major complications, and access to the information is greatly facilitated if it is automated. An effort to "benchmark" the results with other programs should be done so that not only can the local quality be followed but it also can be contrasted with national numbers that are available from several sources. Every procedure and operation has its own set of quality indicators that are not necessarily listed in this table, *eg*, return to surgery and excessive bleeding, use of inotropes, and requirement for intra-aortic balloon pump are additional quality indicators along with length of intubation for the coronary artery bypass graft (CABG) surgical procedure. PTCA—percutaneous transluminal coronary angioplasty.

INFORMATION THAT SHOULD BE FOLLOWED AS QUALITY INDICATORS OF A CARDIOTHORACIC ANESTHESIOLOGIST

Mortality

Intraoperative hypotension and hypertension

Failed intubation

Prolonged intubation

Postoperative stroke

Postoperative myocardial infarction

Requirement for intra-aortic balloon pump

Use of inotropes

Reintubation

Cost of anesthetic drugs per case

Figure 12-9. Information that should be followed as quality indicators of a cardiothoracic anesthesiologist. There are also specific quality indicators that are germane to anesthesia. Some of these indicators are best measured with an automated anesthesia information system [4]. Any QI program should have the ability to risk adjust the patients so that practitioners who always care for the highest risk patients are not penalized. Risk adjustments for CABG[5–6] and for postoperative stroke [7] can be found in the literature. The quality assurance data when compiled should be kept confidential, but if one or more practitioners has more complications than expected, this information must be given to the individual and the chief of service.

SUGGESTED CURRICULUM FOR CLINICAL TRAINING OF THE CARDIAC ANESTHESIA FELLOW

Clinical Training	Time estimated
Orientation lectures	1 wk
ACLS training (if not already certified)	
Provide educational materials	
Primary management of adult cardiac anesthesia	4–8 mo
Patients (graded responsibility)	
Coronary and valvular surgery	
Transplantation	
Other	
Pediatric cardiac anesthesia	3 mo
Congenital heart surgery	
Catheterization laboratory	
Intensive care	
Echocardiography	
Attend combined anesthesia, cardiac surgery, and pediatric cardiology conference	
Special training	
Transesophageal echocardiography	6–8 wk
Cardiac intensive care	4 wk
Cardiac diagnostic laboratory	Elective
Cardiopulmonary bypass team, heart assist devices	Elective
Supervisory role in cardiac anesthesia cases	?

Figure 12-10. Suggested curriculum for clinical training of the cardiac anesthesia fellow. Formal education is obtained either in a subspecialty year during the residency or as a fellow in cardiothoracic anesthesiology [8]. The curriculum of a complete fellowship is listed in this table.

CLINICAL COMPETENCE OF CARDIAC ANESTHESIA RESIDENTS

Knowledge development
  Attitude and character
  Scholarship
  Continuing education
Skill Acquisition
  Disciplines of medical field
  Technical skills and correct use
  Monitoring capabilities
  Pediatric and adult care capabilities
Delivery of care
  Judgment
  Risk evaluation and assessment
  Planning and execution
  Follow-up
Extension of Basics
  Research
  Teaching and writing
  Community health objectives

Figure 12-11. Clinical competence of cardiac anesthesia residents. These are criteria used in determining clinical competence in cardiac anesthesiology. (*Adapted from* Reves and Schell [8] and Flynn and Fogdall [9].)

RECOMMENDED TRAINING COMPONENTS DESIRABLE FOR THOSE PERFORMING AND INTERPRETING TEE

Component	Duration	Number of cases
Level II background	6 months/equivalent	≈ 300
TEE examination	Variable	≈ 50
Continuing education	Annual	≈ 50–75

Figure 12-12. Recommended training components desirable for those performing and interpreting TEE. These are recommendations regarding training in transesophageal echocardiography. There is now an examination (Society of Cardiovascular Anesthesiologists Perioperative Transesophageal Echocardiography Certification Examination) that certifies cardiothoracic anesthesiologists in this special competency. (*Adapted from* Pearlman and coworkers [10] and Reves and Schell [8].)

TRAITS OF EFFECTIVE CLINICAL TEACHERS

Overall instructional effectiveness depends on
    Allocating time for teaching
    Creating a teaching/learning environment or trust
    Demonstrating clinical credibility
A complete educational experience requires
    An initial orientation
    A final evaluation
Teaching rounds are facilitated when
    Learners are able to present a case
    Teachers manage the case presentation
    Didactic sessions are used to enhance clinical case material
    Teaching takes place at the bedside, allowing students to learn physician-patient relationships
    Teachers and students discuss psychosocial issues
Maintained teaching effectiveness occurs when:
    Attention is paid to transferring the teaching responsibility

Figure 12-13. Traits of effective clinical teachers. Teaching is not always optimally accomplished in a lecturer-audience format. The operating room offers an excellent opportunity for fellows to learn instructional skills on a personal level. Residents who have been instructed by the fellow can critique that individual's effectiveness. Whether the goal of the cardiac anesthesiology fellow is to become an academician or a private practitioner, the teaching skills acquired during fellowship training enhance communication with both medical and nonmedical personnel. (*Adapted from* Reves and Schell [8] and Mattern and coworkers [11].)

POSSIBLE CRITERIA FOR HOSPITAL ACCREDITATION OF CARDIOTHORACIC ANESTHESIOLOGISTS

Formal fellowship in cardiothoracic anesthesia
Extensive clinical experience in cardiothoracic anesthesia—ongoing practice (≥ 50 cases per year)
Knowledge and experience of cardiopulmonary bypass and other mechanical assist devices
Knowledge of transesophageal echocardiography and electrocardiography
Knowledge of postoperative care
Membership in the heart center
Membership in the Society of Cardiovascular Anesthesia and evidence of attendance at the annual meeting or CME programs

Figure 12-14. Possible criteria for hospital accreditation of cardiothoracic anesthesiologists. There are certain criteria that might be considered in the credentialing of a cardiothoracic anesthesiologist. Some of these criteria are listed in this table, but this is not an inclusive list and is given only as a suggestion for the individual setting. We believe strongly in the concept that hospital credentialing should remain an individual hospital function. Nobody knows physician competency better than those who work with the individual and who share patient care responsibility with the individual physician. One belief that we do have is that cardiothoracic anesthesia is best conducted by those who do it regularly and who have had training or experience with it. This is true for other specialists as well such as cardiologists and cardiothoracic surgeons. CME—continuing medical education.

REFERENCES

1. Benumof JL: *Anesthesia for Thoracic Surgery*. Philadelphia: WB Saunders; 1987.

2. Hodgins L, Kisslo JA, Mark JB: Perioperative transesophageal echocardiography: the anesthesiologists as cardiac diagnostician. *Anesth Analg* 1995, 80:4–6.

3. Lubarsky DA, Glass PSA, Ginsberg B, *et al.*: The successful implementation of practice guidelines: analysis of associated outcomes and cost savings. *Anesthesiology* 1997, 86:1145–1160.

4. Coleman RL, Stanley TI, Gilbert WC, *et al.*: The implementation and acceptance of an intra-operative anesthesia information management system. *J Clin Monit* 1997, 13:121–128.

5. Mark DB, Nelson CL, Califf RM, *et al.*: Continuing evolution of therapy for coronary artery disease: initial results from the era of coronary angioplasty. *Circulation* 1994, 89:2015–225.

6. Parsonnet V, Dean D, Bernstein AD: A method of uniform stratification of risk for evaluating the results of surgery in acquired adult heart disease. *Circulation* 1989, 79:I-3–I-12.

7. Newman MF, Wolman R, Kanchuger M, *et al.*: Multicenter preoperative stroke risk index for patients undergoing coronary artery bypass graft surgery. *Circulation* 1996, 94(Suppl II):II-74–II-80.

8. Reves JG, Schell RM: Education of the Cardiac Anesthesiologist. In *Cardiac Anesthesia: Principles and Clinical Practice*. Edited by Fawzy G, Estafanous FG, Barash PG, Reves JG. Philadelphia: JB Lippincott; 1994, 815–828.

9. Flynn M, Fogdall R: Educational Training of the Cardiac Anesthesiologist. In *Acute Cardiovascular Management*. Edited by Ream AK, Fogdall R. Philadelphia: JB Lippincott; 1982, 877.

10. Pearlman, AS, Gardin JM, Martin RP, *et al.*: *Guideliness for Physician Training in Transesophageal Echocardiography*. Recommendations of the American Society of Echocardiography. *J Am Soc Echocardiogr* 1992, 5:187–194.

11. Mattern WD, Weinholtz D, Friedman CP: The attending physician as teacher. *N Engl J Med* 1983, 308:1129–1132.